PITUITARY CHROMOPHOBE ADENOMAS

A CLINICAL STUDY
OF THE SELLAR SYNDROME

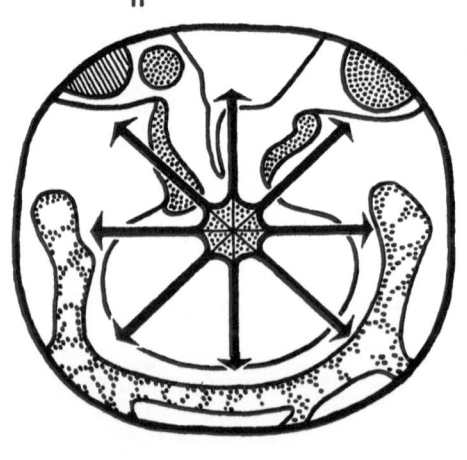

PITUITARY
CHROMOPHOBE ADENOMAS

NEUROLOGY
METABOLISM
THERAPY

By **JOHN I. NURNBERGER, M.D.**
Research Associate, The Institute of Living, and Assistant Clinical
Professor of Medicine (Neurology), Yale University School of Medicine

and **SAUL R. KOREY, M.D.**
Associate Professor of Neurology, The School of Medicine,
Western Reserve University

Springer Science+Business Media, LLC

ISBN 978-3-662-37660-7   ISBN 978-3-662-38456-5 (eBook)
DOI 10.1007/978-3-662-38456-5
Copyright Springer Science+Business Media New York 1953
Originally published by Springer Publishing Company INC in 1953.
Softcover reprint of the hardcover 1st edition 1953

Library of Congress Catalog Card Number: 53-7676

To

M. C. N.
and
D. B. K.

PREFACE

In the present study we have attempted to correlate information from several medical disciplines in order to portray the syndrome of chromophobe adenoma of the pituitary in its setting of pathologically modifield function. The book will serve a purpose if this segment of neurology is rejoined to the continuum of internal medicine and made readily available to the inquiring physician with general interests. Indeed this monograph has been written in awareness that some of the material included is beyond the range of the authors' immediate field of study. This investigation and resume is dedicated in all humility to the rapprochement of neurology to general medicine and to the reappearance of those compelling currents of medical thought which prevailed in American neurology under the influence of Cushing and Bailey.

It is idle to describe the vicissitudes involved in the publication of such a monograph: "the appeal is too limited," "the general practitioner won't be interested," etc. We are thankful to Mr. Bernhard Springer for publishing the work even in view of such opinions. We feel confident that if the material has been presented comprehensively, any physician will greet the work with interest; no more have the authors or the publisher a right to expect.

Our gratitude is extended to Dr. H. Houston Merritt whose aid and confidence in this study were sustaining factors to us. We also wish to thank Dr. Robert F. Loeb, who instructed us during the early stages of the work and gave us thoughtful guidance. Dr. Abner Wolf offered the pathologic material for review and conscientiously led us to a conservative estimate of the data obtained. Without the interest and cooperation of the Drs. Henry A. Riley and the late Irving M. Pardee, the realization of comprehensive clinical investigations of endocrine problems in patients admitted to the Neurological Institute of New York would not have been possible. Dr. Ernest Wood critically reviewed the chapter on therapy and graciously supplied typical x-rays for incorporation into the text. Dr. Paul Hoefer supplied information and comment relative to the results of electroencephalography. Both Dr. Sidney Werner and Dr. Joseph Jailer furnished observations originating in their respective laboratories. We are indebted to Dr. J. R. Nickerson of the Department of Physiology, College of Physicians and Surgeons, for the facilities of his laboratory, where we did the plasma volume studies. Dr. G. B. Mudge performed flame photometric determinations of sodium and potassium on the patients and advised us as well. The attending physicians of Presbyterian Hospital have kindly allowed us to include in this series many patients studied under their personal supervision. Mr. Ivan Summers graciously lent his talents for the illustrations. For performing the arduous task of editing the manuscript we gratefully thank Dr. L. Rowland.

We gladly acknowledge the privilege extended to us by the many publishers who have graciously allowed us to include reproductions from their texts and journals. The following publishers contributed greatly to the present monograph: C. V. Mosby Company, St. Louis; Charles C Thomas, Springfield; The Williams and Wilkins Company, Baltimore; The Wistar Institute of Anatomy and Biology, Philadelphia; Paul B. Hoeber, Inc., New York; George Banta Publishing Co., Menasha; The Macmillan Company, New York; Longmans, Green and Co., New York; Archives of Ophthalmology, Chicago; Archives of Neurology and Psychiatry, Chicago.

JOHN I. NURNBERGER
SAUL R. KOREY

CONTENTS

I

INTRODUCTION

During the years 1907 to 1912 pioneer studies of critical importance first stressed the relationship of hypopituitary states to chromophobe adenomas. It is not surprising, therefore, that descriptions of probable chromophobe adenomas prior to that period should have been devoted more to clinical abnormalities than to physiologic or pathologic mechanisms. Thus Mohr in 1840[cited in 37, 43] described a "sarcoma of the hypophysis" associated with unusual obesity, and Babinski and Onanoff in 1900[cited in 43, 296] reported an "epithelioma" of the pituitary which pressed on the tuber cinereum and was likewise associated with obesity. Fröhlich in 1901[181] published a detailed clinical study of a patient with a probable pituitary tumor associated with peculiarly disposed obesity and genital dystrophy. This case was not confirmed anatomically until 1907[296] and was then considered as a pituitary carcinoma or precancerous adenoma with cyst formation. Striking painful adiposity was a prominent finding in a patient studied both clinically and anatomically by Dercum and McCarthy in 1902.[124] Autopsy disclosed a large "eosinophilic" adenocarcinoma, ill-defined changes in the thyroid gland and fatty infiltration of the liver. The authors did not make clear the possible role played by the pituitary tumor but did suggest that the previous emphasis on thyroid disease as primary in such a disturbance might not be fully justified. In the light of present knowledge it is probable that all of these were examples of chromophobe adenomas.

1

By the end of 1912 the stage was set for an adequate presentation of chromophobe adenoma as an entity whose predominant clinical accompaniment was that of hypopituitarism. Erdheim and Stumme[145] had already published a classic article reviewing with clarity the various cytologic elements of the anterior pituitary. Dean Lewis had emphasized[304] the relative ease in differentiating lesions of the pituitary gland histologically, though interestingly enough he did not discuss chromophobe adenomas. Cushing had published his remarkable monograph[100] describing in a decisive and well documented manner not only hypo- and hyperfunctional pituitary states, but also their histopathologic correlates. He, as well as Geotsch shortly thereafter,[202] stressed the relative frequency of chromophobe adenomas in the pathogenesis of hypopituitarism. Yet the stage appears to have been set prematurely. Fully fifteen years passed during which only Cushing and those associated with him utilized this early knowledge to complete advantage.

In the interim from 1912 to 1930 chromophobe adenomas were accorded limited attention as a determinant of hypopituitary states. Despite Cushing's studies, the consistent lack of appreciation of their relative frequency made their consideration a remote and disinterested one in some clinical treatises of the period as, for example those of Gilford,[197] Engelbach,[141] and later those of Rowe and Lawrence[397] and Hartoch.[138] In some instances[154, 192, 339] chromophobe adenomas were considered worth mentioning only because they appeared to be unassociated with acromegaly or gigantism. An even greater number of workers was concerned with the possible role of such tumors in the production of pathologic obesity, with or without disturbance of genital structure and function.[45, 46, 216, 296, 356, 533] Careful endocrine and metabolic studies were exceptional.[46, 533] These clinical investigations nevertheless gave a necessary stimulus to the resultant intensive experimental study of the hypothalamus and its functions. In the late 1920s the possible relationship of such tumors to pituitary cachexia was discussed[390, 470] albeit general treatises of the period[43, 533] mention this problem summarily. Endocrine and metabolic investigations often lacked clearly defined clinical or pathologic criteria[2] though exceptions can be found.[182] Histopathologic differentiation of tumor type received little attention,[247, 356] in studies of juxta-hypophyseal pressure disturbances.

During the period just mentioned, which finds a faithful echo even in recent years,[441] a small group labored to categorize chromophobe adenomas, not only as a histopathologic entity but also as a unique determinant of metabolic dysfunctions. This labor has continued to the present. Cushing, as previously mentioned, laid the foundations for this work in 1912. Von Monakow,[348] Illig,[266] and Bailey and Cushing[24, 103] have advanced this approach; the latter authors have defined an entire subgroup of transitional or transitory hyperfunctional states as distinct from the condition of hypopituitarism characteristic of chromophobe tumors. More recently Schnitker and his co-workers,[416] Henderson,[239] Foley and co-workers,[167] Foster and McCarter,[170] Starr and Davis,[456] German,[193] Globus and his associates[200] and workers from the Lahey Clinic[294a, 531a] have considered the myriad problems associated with chromophobe adenomas. An increasingly mature and sophisticated interest in the dynamic metabolic disturbances associated with this tumor is manifest in these studies.

No attempt has been made to assign precedence to any worker or group in this introduction. Our purpose has been rather to stress the dominant trend in clinical studies of each period. Undoubtedly the struggles, distinctions and polemics of the so-called "syndrome" period served to direct attention to neurohypophyseal mechanisms later confirmed by controlled animal experimentation. It is hoped that the clinical analysis which comprises the bulk of the present study may serve, in some small measure, as a stimulus to continued experimental study. We have attempted to interpret signs and symptoms from the standpoint of the disturbed neurophysiology and metabolism concerned in their elaboration. Through this broader analysis an evaluation of the resources available to the patient with a chromophobe adenoma for enduring environmental exigencies can be made. The core of this report is the data obtained from patient records but the explanation of the observations involves discussion of neural and endocrine mechanisms of general significance.

II

ANATOMY OF THE PITUITARY

The pituitary gland arises from epithelial and neural elements in the usual tortuous manner of developing organs. The anlagen juxtapose but their constitutent cells do not intermingle. In the adult the main glandular mass occupies a secure position within a bony pit in the middle cranial fossa and by means of a dural investment is separated from the subarachnoid space. The vicinal neural organs are somewhat removed from the body of the pituitary but its relations to these structures become brutally apparent when neoplastic expansions of the gland disorganize their sensitive nervous tissue.[179] Blood reaches the pituitary through a portal system of vessels and directly from the internal carotids. Venous drainage is to the cavernous sinus and perisellar plexuses. The pituitary is innervated by autonomic nerves and by a definite bundle of fibers arising in the hypothalamus and ending in the neural lobe. The secretions of the gland probably enter the blood stream and to a lesser degree ascend toward the third ventricle of the brain.

EMBRYOLOGY

In the head end of the embryo there exists an area of adherence, (the neuro-ectodermal plate) between the inferior surface of the neural tube and the roof of the stomodeum.[196] In the course of the general

5

development of the head, mesenchymal tissue invades this region of contact and restricts the extent of the area of adherence to a median position, circumscribed by mesodermal elements (fig. 1). From the torsions produced on this region by the developmental flexions of the

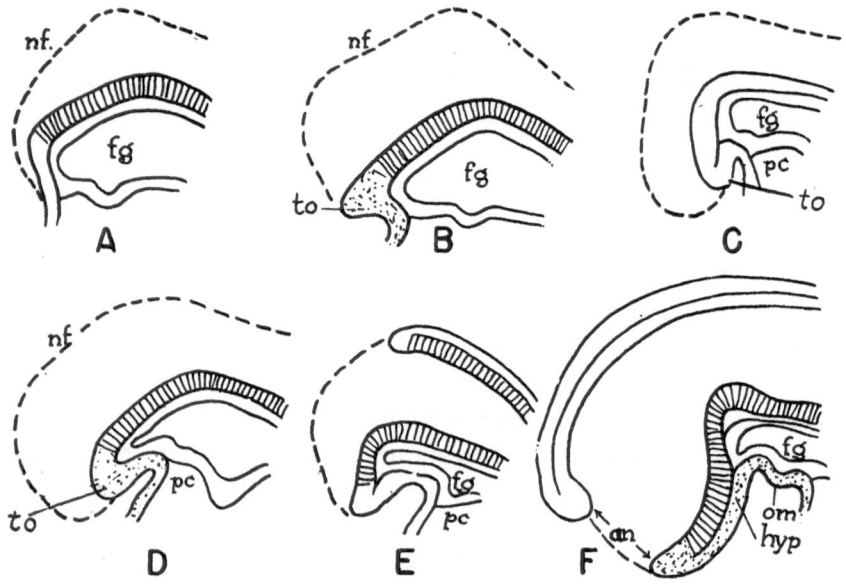

Fig. 1—Median sagittal sections of the anterior end of young human embryos: (A) 2 somite; (B) 7 somite; (C) 8 somite; (D) 10 somite; (E) 13 somite; (F) 16 somite.

These diagrams illustrate the fusion of the neural folds and surface ectoderm (thatched area) in the region of the torus opticus without the intervention of mesodermal elements. It it within this and the proximately caudal area, the region of neuroectodermal adherence, that the hypophysis develops.

Key: an, anterior neuropore; fg, foregut; hyp, hypophyseal area; om, oral membrane; pc, pericardial cavity; to, torus opticus.

From original of figure 2, Gilbert, M. S.: Some factors influencing the early development of the mammalian hypophysis. Anat. Rec. 1935, 62: 347.

cephalon and by active local growth an outpouching of the roof of the stomodeum results. This is Rathke's pouch, which develops into the anterior lobe of the hypophysis. According to Gilbert,[196] in the early stages Rathke's pouch remains adherent to the neural tissue, which will later become the infundibulum of the diencephalon. The cells of the infundibular region do not appear to be increasing in proportion to the configurational changes occurring at this time. This has led to the supposition that the outpocketing of the infundibulum is induced initially by the mechanical effects of rotation of the neuro-ectodermal plate from a dorso-ventral to a cephalo-caudal plane.

The concept expressed above states that the neural and stomodeal parts of adenohypophysis are in immediate connection with each other; the rearrangements of one element are reflected by its partner in development. Moreover, the development of both depends upon spatial changes occurring in the course of the general organization of the differentiating head.

The more usually accepted hypothesis of the dual origin of the adenohypophysis asserts that local evaginations proceed from the stomodeum and neural tube. Under the influence of "biotaxis," perhaps a synonym for a local organizer,[494] these outpouchings become associated with each other. Their interdependent orientation and configurations are the responsibility of local processes supposedly acting at each evagination. The later development of pituitary does not present similar controversy.[17, 481, 482]

The anterior lobe of the hypophysis is differentiated from Rathke's pouch (figs. 2, 3, 4). The tubular connection of this latter structure with the stomodeum elongates as the stomodeum becomes increasingly separated from the neural tube by ingrowing mesenchyme. The juxtaneural extremity of the tube expands into three evaginations. The central outpouching enlarges and becomes the pars distalis, the main component of the anterior lobe. The lateral projections elongate and fuse across the midline and, as the pars tuberalis, apply themselves to the median eminence. A thickening of the dorsal lip of the main midline evagination develops into another pair of pouches which also coalesce and envelope all but the dorsal aspect of the infundibular process and represent the pars infundibularis in the adult state. These latter protrusions contain the cavity of Rathke's pouch which is narrowed to an insignificant slit in the adult. A downward extension of the pars infundibularis separates the anterior lobe from the diencephalic posterior lobe. In the adult this downward extension is called the pars intermedia. The cleft-like residuum of the stomodeal cavity lies between the pars distalis and the pars intermedia.

During the early stages of pituitary development the tubular neck of Rathke's pouch disappears, terminating the connection of the mouth with the pituitary anlage. It is believed that embryologic rests from the dental ridges which have been incorporated into the walls of the oropituitary canal may persist and occasionally develop into cranio-pharyngiomas in the region adjacent to the stalk of the infundibulum.

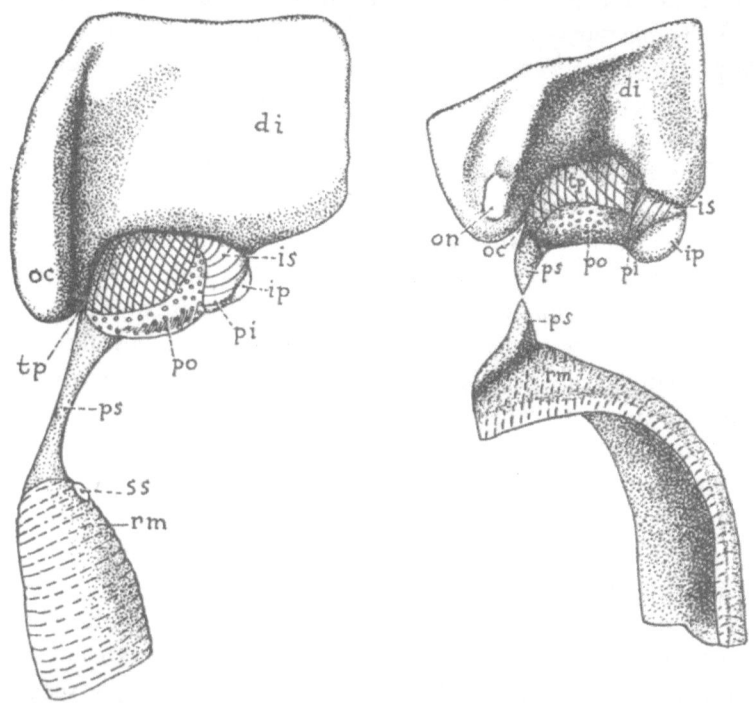

Fig. 2—(A) Left lateral view of reconstruction of pituitary region in 16 mm. human embryo. (B) Left lateral view of pituitary region in 24 mm. embryo.

The expansion of the juxta-neural end of the oropituitary tube comes into intimate relationship with the diencephalic region, enfolding the infundibular stem. The oropituitary canal becomes pinched off and the connection between the stomodeum and the future adenohypophysis is lost.

Key: di, diencephalon; ip, infundibular process; is, infundibular stem; oc, optic chiasm; on, optic nerve; pi, pars infundibularis; po, pituitary pouch; ps, pituitary stalk; rm, roof of mouth; ss, Sessel's pocket; tp, tuberal process.

From original of figures by Tilney, F.: The development and constituents of the human hypophysis. Bull. Neurol. Inst. New York 1936, 5: 387.

In common with the type of developmental abnormalities seen in other organs ectopic tissue derived from stomodeal outpouching may exist along the course of the oropituitary canal and pouch, e.g., in the roof of the mouth or in the bridge of the sphenoid bone (which differentiates from the mesoderm surrounding the oropituitary canal).

The neural division of the pituitary originates from the hypo-

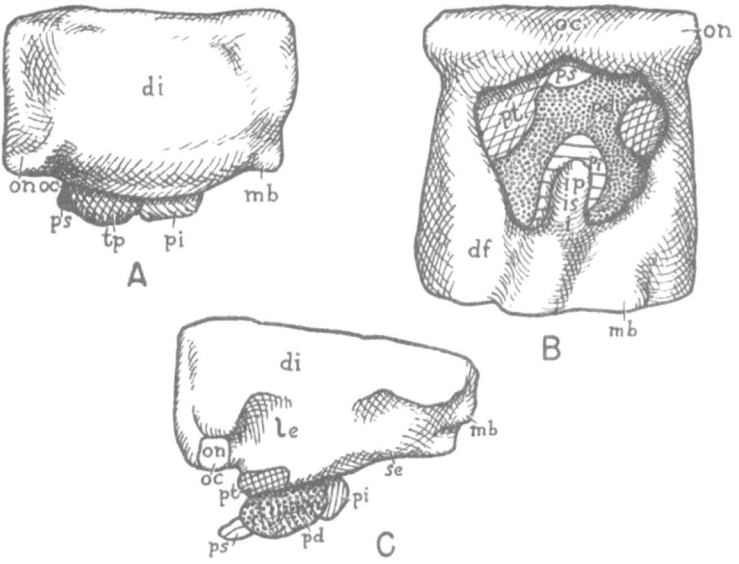

Fig. 3—Left lateral and basal views (A, B) of reconstruction of hypophyseal region in a 30 mm. human embryo. (C) Lateral view of reconstruction in a 55 mm. embryo.

In (A) and (B) the pars tuberalis is seen to be formed by the fusion of the tuberal processes across the midline, eventually completely investing the median eminence. The basal view indicates the glandular collar about the infundibular stem and process. In (C) the pars tuberalis is applied to the increasingly prominent median eminence of the tuber cinereum. The infundibular stem and process are enclosed by the infundibular component of the adenohypophysis.

Key: df, diencephalic floor; di, diencephalon; i, infundibulum; ip, infundibular process; is, infundibular stem; le, lateral eminence; mb, mammillary body; oc, optic chiasm; on, optic nerve; pd, pars distalis; pi, pars infundibularis; ps, pituitary stalk remnant; pt, pars tuberalis; tp, tuberal process; se, saccular eminence.

From original of figures by Tilney, F.: The development and constituents of the human hypophysis. Bull. Neurol. Inst. New York 1936, 5: 387.

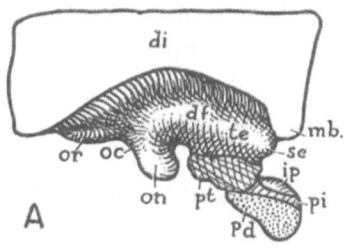 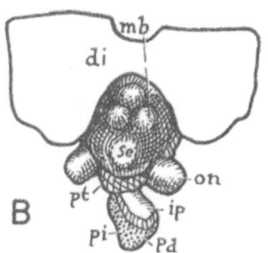

Fig. 4—Lateral and caudal aspects (A, B) of reconstruction of hypophyseal region in a 5 month human fetus.

As the infundibular stem lengthens the pars tuberalis becomes visible at the region where it envelopes the median eminence. The change in the axis of the infundibular stem permits the settling of the glandular mass into the sella turcica. The appearance of both lateral and caudal views approaches that of the adult.

Key: df, diencephalic floor; di, diencephalon; ip, infundibular process; le, lateral eminence; mb, mammillary body; oc, optic chiasm; on, optic nerve; pd, pars distalis; pi, pars infundibularis; pr, preoptic recess; pt, pars tuberalis; se, saccular eminence.

From original of figures by Tilney, F.: The development and constituents of the human hypophysis. Bull. Neurol. Inst. New York 1936, 5: 387.

thalamus between the optic chiasm and mammillary bodies (fig. 5). In this region a ventral bulging, the median eminence, is notable in man. Just posterior to it the infundibular evagination arises. The median eminence, the infundibulum, and its expanded process comprise the major part of the posterior lobe (fig. 6). On cytologic grounds, Bucy[501] believes that only the posterior part of the median eminence is concerned in the development of the neural component. The tensions impressed upon this area, the median eminence and infundibular region, by the rotation of the neuro-ectodermal plate and growth pressures from the surrounding hypothalamus are thought to be responsible for the evagination of the infundibular anlage of the neurohypophysis. Gilbert's work[196] in regard to the number of mitoses found in contiguous areas of the infundibular region and hypothalamus indicates relative inactivity of the infundibular cells. Nevertheless, the presently popular view suggests an active outpouching of the infundibulum which extends to its buccal counterpart, both finally constituting the pituitary gland.

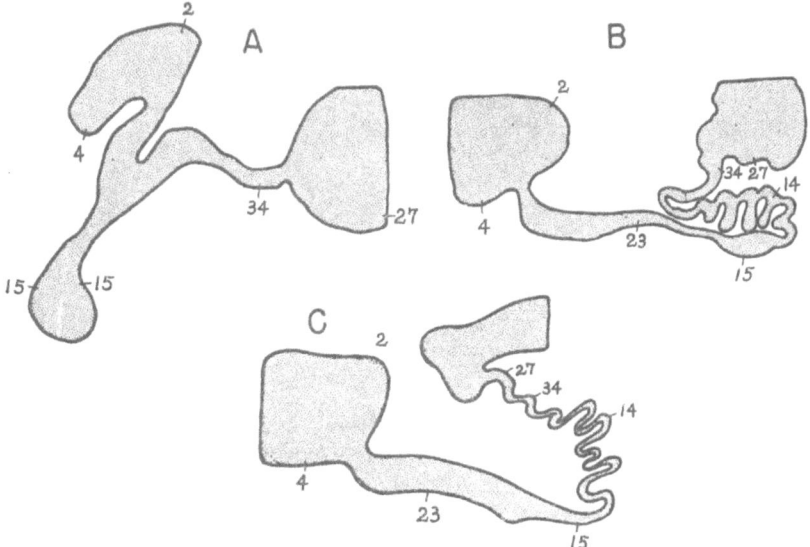

Fig. 5—Comparative series of infundibular region. (A) man; (B) fowl; (C) dog-fish. The saccus vasculosus may be represented in man by part of the infundibular wall but there is no direct evidence for this.

Key: 2, chiasmatic process; 4, chiasm; 14, infundibular process on saccular surface (saccus vasculosus); 15, infundibular process on pituitary surface; 23, median post chiasmatic groove; 27, mammillary body (posterior lobe); 34, postinfundibular eminence.

From original of figure 1, Tilney, F.: The morphology of the diencephalic floor—a contribution to the study of craniate homology. J. Comp. Neurol. 1915, 25: 216.

The infundibular protrusion lengthens and becomes expanded at its extremity into the main component of the neural lobe. From comparative data part of the infundibular wall has been related to the saccus vasculosus of lower orders (fig. 5). The latter is a floor gland of the brain of unknown function. Were it to persist in man it might support the belief that the hypothalamus is in part a secretory organ. However, it does not appear to be represented in the development of the neural division of the hypophysis in man.[482] As the infundibulum extends downward the third ventricle follows, but becomes obliterated in this area in the adult. The infundibular stem and process are then a solid structure. They are intimately invested by the upward ex-

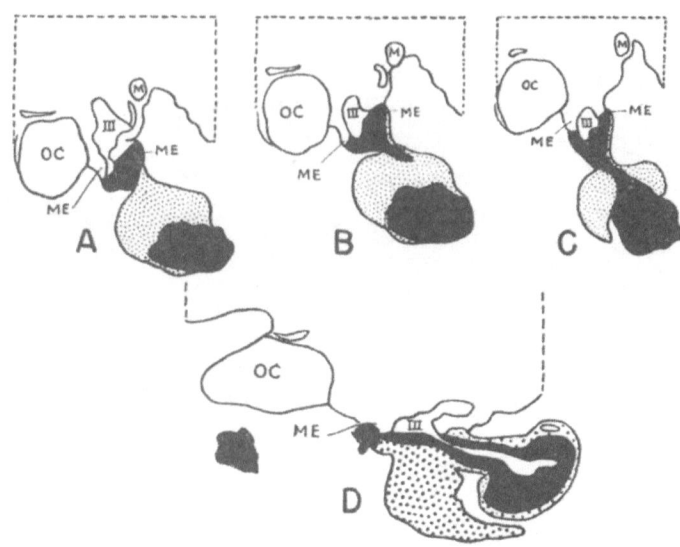

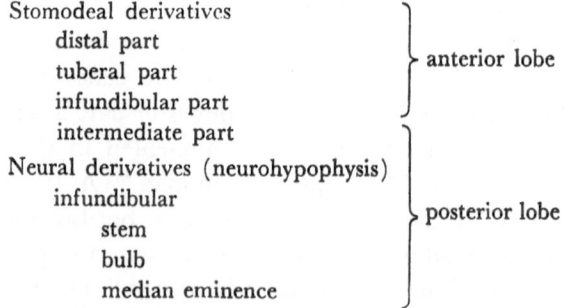

Fig. 6—The components of the neurohypophysis. The hypothalamus is white, the neurohypophysis black and the adenohypophysis stippled. (A) Parasagittal section just lateral to hypophyseal stem. (B) Sagittal section medial to A. (C) Sagittal section through the stem (A, B, C—monkey). (D) Sagittal section through the infundibular stem (cat).

Key: ME, median eminence; OC, optic chiasm; M, medial mammillary nucleus; III, third ventricle.

From original of figures by Weaver, T. A. and Bucy, P. C.: The anatomical relationships of the hypophyseal stem and the median eminence. Endocrinology 1940, 27: 227.

tensions of the stomodeal evagination. The final orientation is represented in figure 7.

The divisions of the pituitary gland are[373]:

Stomodeal derivatives
    distal part
    tuberal part   } anterior lobe
    infundibular part
    intermediate part
Neural derivatives (neurohypophysis)
    infundibular
        stem   } posterior lobe
        bulb
        median eminence

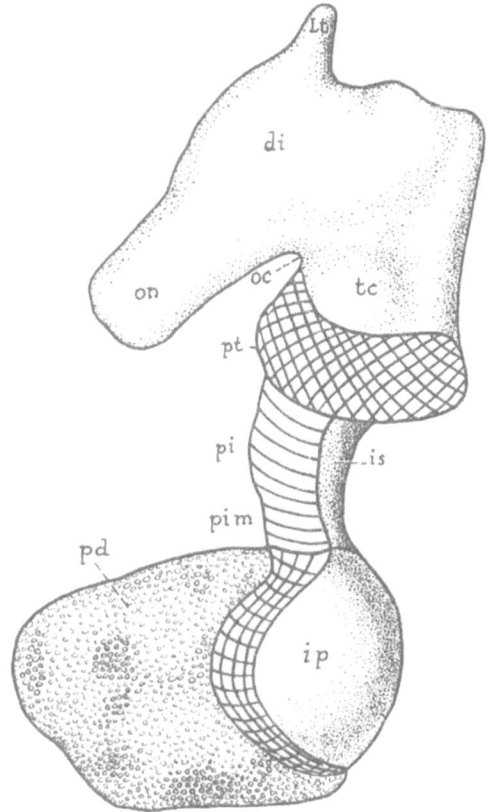

Fig. 7—Reconstruction of hypophysis and related portion of diencephalic floor of adult female.

Key: di, diencephalon; ip, infundibular process; is, infundibular stem; le, lateral eminence of tuber cinereum; lt, lamina terminalis; oc, optic chiasm; on, optic nerve; pd, pars distalis; pi, pars infundibularis; pim, pars intermedia; pt, pars tuberalis.

From original of figures by Tilney, F.: The development and constituents of the human hypophysis. Bull. Neurol. Inst. of New York, 1936, 5: 387. Figure modified by Rasmussen.

CYTOGENESIS

The cytogenesis of the hypophysis appears to be a complicated and unsettled problem. In the human stomodeal derivative indeterminately stained cells are present exclusively until the stage of the nine month fetus. At first they are arranged in irregular cords and masses. By the twentieth week many of the convoluted cell cords form acini. There are apparently two representative types of cells, either faintly or deeply staining; their mature destiny remains unclear. The deeply staining juxtaneural cells show some tendency to invade the infundibular process and stalk. The gland is vascularized about the fourteenth week. The blood vessels appear rather indiscriminate, the major vascularization being lacunae which are bordered by deeply tinted cells. Connective tissue appears in the adenohypophysis about this time and a fine reticulum is woven through the gland. It is only in the nine month fetus that a mass of acidophiles appears within the extensively vascular central area of the adenohypophysis. During the period of infancy the acidophiles increase in number but remain more or less confined to the central parts of the gland though variably present in other areas. Basophiles are also differentiated and become grouped into acini. The basophiles are distributed in the central areas, the periphery and the juxtaneural region as the sole cells. Both the basophiles and acidophiles vary in the intensity with which they stain. Less granulated and indefinitely stained cells represent chromophobic elements.[480]

The histogenesis of the neurohypophysis has not been defined satisfactorily. Within this division glia-like cells, the pituicytes, mast and wandering cells have been recognized, but their origin and development are not clearly apprehended. Presumably the pituicytes are derived from supporting ectodermal spongioblasts and resemble astrocytes. Bucy considers the pituicytes the characteristic cell type of the neurohypophysis. They are found in the neural lobe, infundibular stalk and median eminence. These cells have long processes which branch profusely, their extremities being lost in the dense network of the infundibular process. The soma and nuclei are morphologically variable. It is likely that wandering and mast cells are associated with the stromal connective tissue and blood vessels.[64]

Anatomy of pituitary gland and sella turcica

The hypophysis is ovoid in shape and measures about 12 mm. in its transverse and 8 mm. in its anterior-posterior diameters. It lies within the sella turcica in a median position in the middle cranial fossa. The hypophysis is joined superiorly to the hypothalamus by means of the infundibular stalk, which passes upwards and backwards from the gland, through the dural roof of the sella turcica, to become continuous with the floor of the third ventricle. The infundibular stalk is related most frequently to the posterior edge, rarely to the anterior aspect, of the optic chiasm.

The pituitary is related superiorly to the optic chiasm and tracts, the hypothalamic floor of the third ventricle, and in front, to the inferior surface of the frontal lobes. The lateral relations are: the cavernous sinus and its constituents, the third, fourth, sixth and the first and second divisions of the fifth cranial nerves. The internal carotid artery and the perivascular sympathetic nerves are included in the cavernous sinus. More remotely, the optic tracts and medial aspect of the temporal lobe face the gland. The crura pedunculi and the free edge of the tentorium cerebelli are posterior to the pituitary (fig. 8).

The sella turcica is formed by the union of the various components of the sphenoid bone with the basilar process of the occipital bone. This protective fossa lodges the pituitary body (fig. 9). The landmarks of the sella turcica are important for interpretation of the x-ray picture found with expanding lesions of the pituitary. The body of the sphenoid constitutes the floor and part of the anterior wall of the pituitary fossa. The remainder of the anterior wall results from fusion of various elements of the anterior aspect, body and lesser wing of the sphenoid bone. In the midline the anterior superior lip of the sella turcica presents an eminence, the tuberculum sellae, which is roentgenographically recognizable (figs. 10, 11). Some intracranial tumors, e.g., meningiomata, arise in this region and thicken the tuberculum sellae. Chromophobe adenomas, when they press forward, have a tendency to undermine the tuberculum sellae. The anterolateral angles of the sella turcica are formed by the anterior clinoid processes which are projections of the free edges of the lesser wings of the sphenoid. They, as well as the posterior clinoids, serve as attachments for the tentorum cerebelli. The posterior boundary of the sella turcica is formed by a vertical flat plate of cancellous bone, the dorsum sellae. The upper and lateral

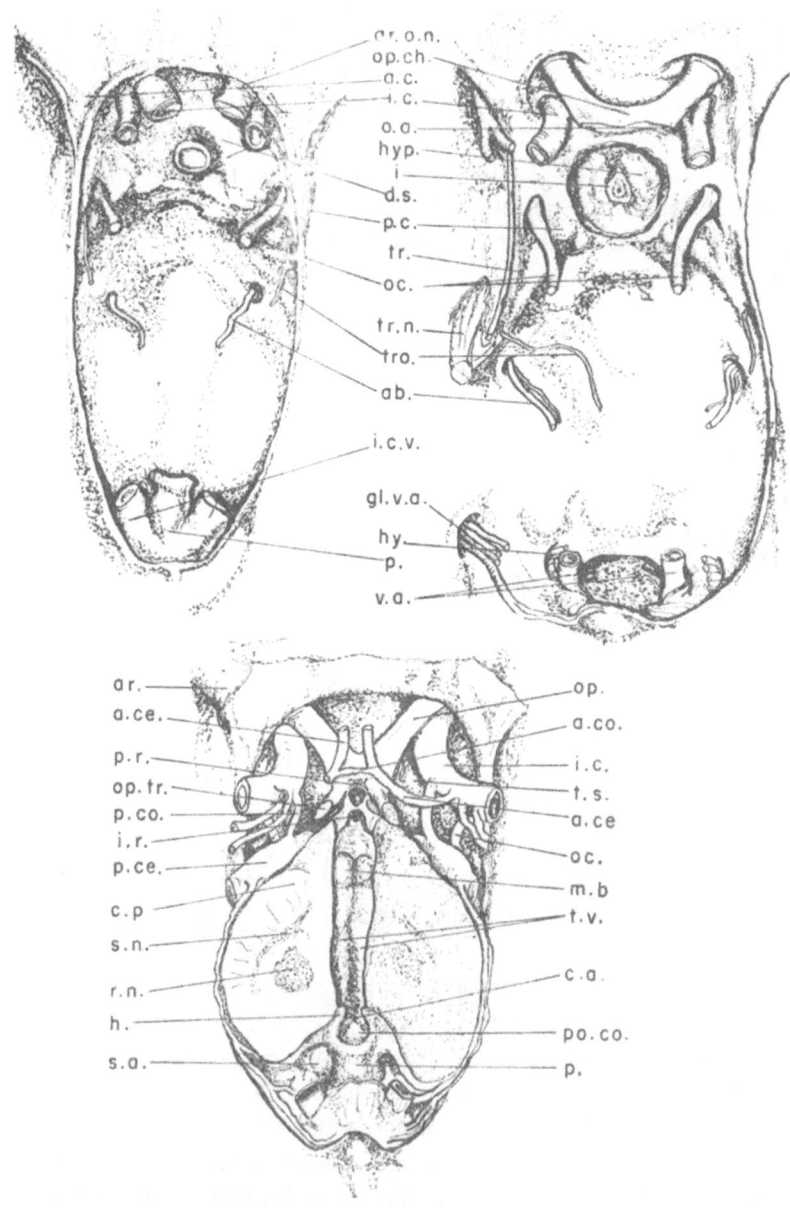

Fig. 8—The tentorial notch and its relations. See legend, facing page.

angles of the dorsum sellae are extended to form the posterior clinoid processes. The dorsum sellae may extend directly up, slope backward or curve forward. It may be well pneumatized, extremely vascularized or dense. Erosion of this part of the sella turcica is a common accompaniment of pituitary tumors. Its displacement and changes in density exhibited in the x-ray are especially significant. The clinoids attached to the dorsum likewise reflect changes in locally as well as generally increased intracranial pressure in a manner similar to the dorsum sellae.[135]

Fig. 8—The tentorial notch and its relations. Three stages of dissection in three different heads: *Lower middle,* from a mesocephalic head, showing the structures which occupy the notch itself and the arachnoid in place about the notch; *Upper left,* from a dolichocephalic head, the central neural structures and arachnoid having been removed, the diaphragma sellae being still in place. *Upper right,* from a brachycephalic head, the diaphragma having been removed, exposing the hypophysis. The left side of the tentorium has been cut away.

Redrawn from original of figure by Mettler, F.: Neuroanatomy, ed. 2. St. Louis, C. V. Mosby, 1948 p. 53.

KEY

ab.—abducens
a.c.—anterior clinoid pcs.
a.ce.—anterior cerebral artery
a.co.—anterior communicat. artery
ar.—arachnoid (cut edge)
ar.o.n.—arachnoid sheath of optic nerve
c.a.—cerebral aqueduct
c.p.—base of cerebral peduncle
d.s.—diaphragma sellae
gl.v.a.—glossopharyngeal, vagus and accessory nn.
h.—habenula
hy.—hypoglossal
hyp.—hypophysis
i.—infundibulum
i.c.—internal carotid artery
i.c.v.—internal cerebral vein
i.r.—infundibular recess
m.b.—mammillary body
o.a.—ophthalmic artery

oc.—oculomotor nerve
op.—optic nerve
op.ch.—optic chiasm
op.tr.—optic tract
p.—pineal
p.c.—posterior clinoid process
p.ce.—posterior cerebral artery
p.co.—posterior communicat. artery
p.r.—preoptic recess
po.co.—posterior commissure
r.n.—red nucleus
s.a.—subtentorial arachnoid covering cisterna ambiens
s.n.—substantia nigra
tr.—triangular field
tr.n.—trigeminal nerve
tro.—trochlear nerve
t.s.—tuberculum sellae
t.v.—third ventricle
v.a.—vertebral artery

An additional set of clinoid processes may arise from the anterior wall of the sella turcica. The clinoids can be joined together by ligaments which ossify (fig. 11). Perhaps such restraint as is mechanically exerted by the existing ligaments influences the direction of the expansions of a pituitary tumor.

The sphenoid bone is irregularly pneumatized, the various types of which are illustrated in figure 12. The degree of pneumatization may

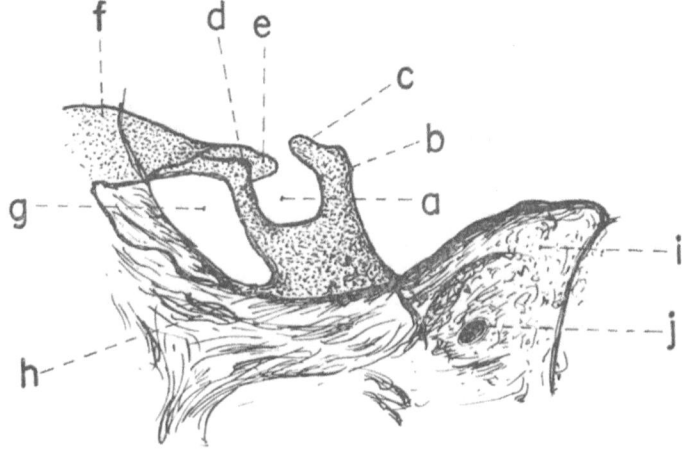

Fig. 9—Semi-diagrammatic view of the sella turcica.

Key: a, pituitary fossa; b, dorsum sellae; c, posterior clinoid process; d, tuberculum sellae; e, anterior clinoid process; f, floor of the middle cranial fossa; i, superimposed mastoid and petrous portions of the temporal bone; j, external auditory meatus.

From original of figure 2 in Kornblum, Karl: Alterations in the structure of the sella turcica as revealed by the roentgen ray. Arch. Neurol. & Psychiat. 1932, 27: 307.

affect the rate of development of neurologic symptoms from chromophobe adenomas. A highly pneumatized sphenoid body and dorsum sellae may offer less resistance to downward and backward extension and osseous invasion than would solid bone or ligamentous structures. A virtual decompression with retardation of symptom formation may result from intrusion of a pituitary tumor into a capacious sphenoidal sinus. However, one may anticipate bacterial infection of the meninges in some instances of such natural decompression.

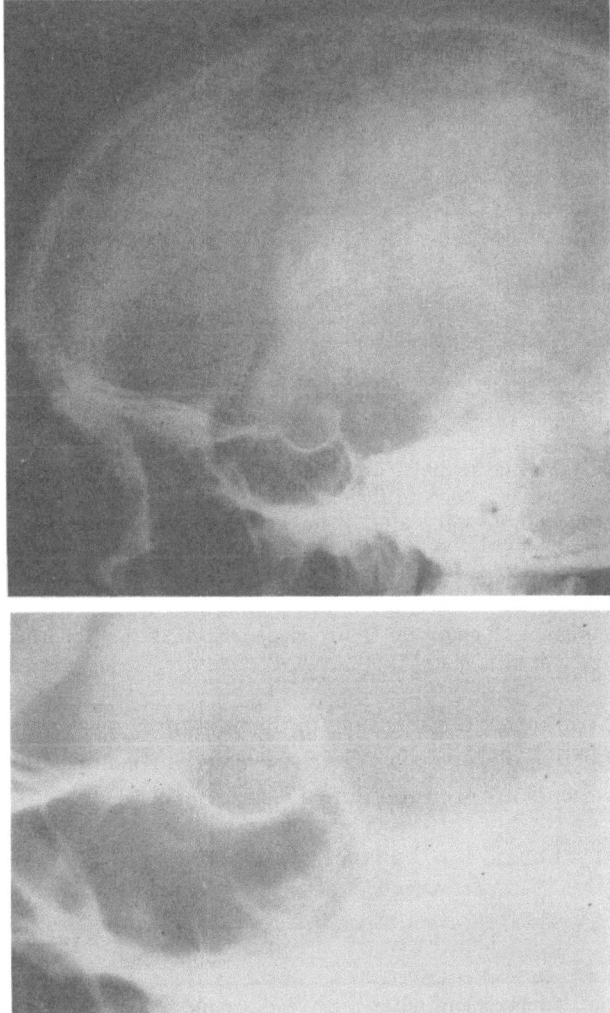

Fig. 10—Normal adult skull. Lateral view (*top*) and detail (*bottom*) of the pituitary fossa. The landmarks of the sella turcica are well defined. Anteriorly the fusion of the lesser wings with the body of the sphenoid forms the forward wall of the fossa. The medial extension of the lesser wing, the anterior clinoid process, and the tuberculum sellae constitute the other anterior limits of the sella turcica. The floor of the pituitary fossa is distinct and overlies a well pneumatized sphenoid sinus. Posteriorly the dorsum sellae extends upward with its projections the posterior clinoid processes. In this instance it is not significantly pneumatized. The caudal root of the dorsum sellae terminates at the occipitosphenoidal suture.

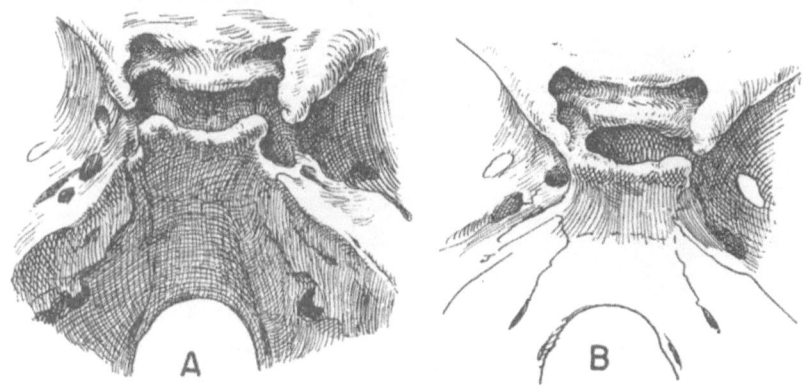

Fig. 11—The intracranial aspect of the sella turcica. The anterior clinoid processes are attached solely at their bases in A, whereas in B there is a junction of the anterior, middle and posterior clinoid processes on the left and the anterior and middle clinoids on the right. In the latter instance, the bony restraints afforded to an expanding lesion of the pituitary obviously may alter the direction of its growth.

From original of figure by Howe, H. S.: Normal and abnormal variations in the pituitary fossa. Neurol. Bull. 1919, 2: 235, figs. 2, 3.

The contour and dimensions of the sella turcica are quite variable. The silhouettes of the sella turcica revealed in examination of forty normal patients are seen in figure 13.[259]

TABLE 1—*Diameters of Hypophyseal Fossa*

Diameter	Landmarks	Method of Examination	Dimensions (mm.)
A – P	tuberculum sellae to post-clinoid process	radiographic and direct	7–15
Transverse	medial borders of carotid grooves	direct	8.5–17.5
Depth	at greatest diameter from the floor to a horizontal line joining the post-clinoids to tuberculum sellae	radiographic and direct	6–14

The dimensions of the hypophyseal fossa are related to the cranial circumference.[374, 379] The figures in table 1 are derived from several sources[259, 360, 379] and represent the extremes recorded.

The range of the size of the sella turcica is wide, but dimensions exceeding 12 mm. anterior-posterior by 10 mm. transverse may be tentatively considered abnormal. Changes in contour are of a significance equal to increase in size. Shape and size are, in fact, complementary aspects of the picture produced by expanding lesions of the pituitary.[360]

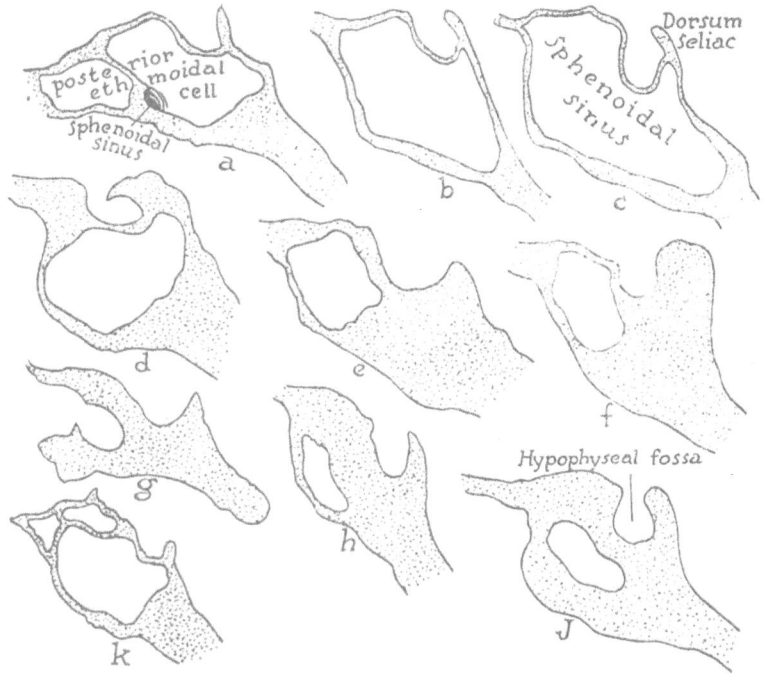

Fig. 12—Line figures indicating the several degrees of pneumatization of the sphenoid bone as well as the various sizes and shapes of the hypophyseal fossa.

From original of figure 7 in Schaeffer, J. P.: Some points in the regional anatomy of the optic pathway, with especial reference to tumors of the hypophysis cerebri and resulting ocular changes. Anat. Rec. 1924, 28: 264. Figure modified by Pancoast, H. K., Pendergrass, E. P. and Schaeffer, J. P.: Head and Neck in Roentgen Diagnosis. Springfield, Charles C Thomas, 1942.

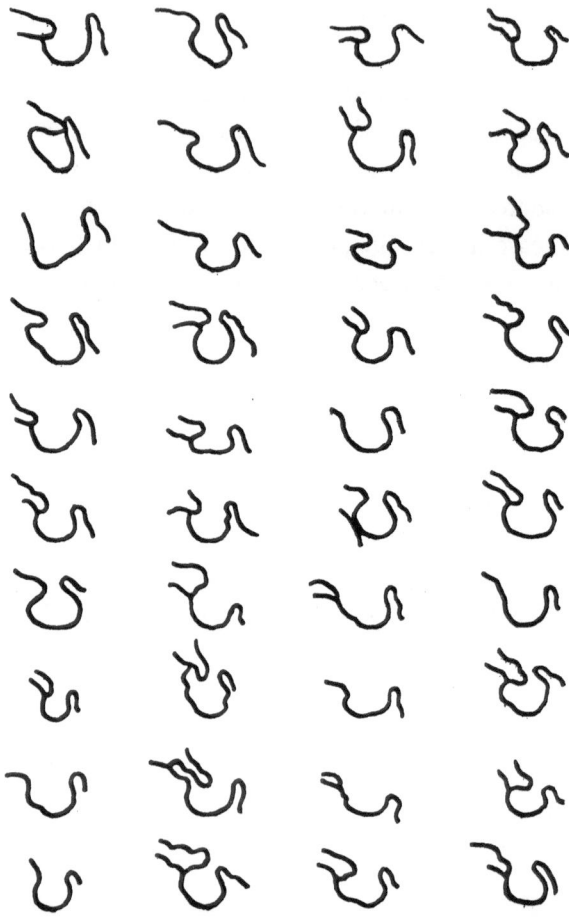

Fig. 13—Traced outlines of 40 normal pituitary fossae showing the marked variation in size and shape.

From original of figure by Howe, H. S.: Normal and abnormal variations in the pituitary fossa. Neurol. Bull. of New York, 1919, 2: 234.

Meningeal relations

The dura mater bridges the superior surface of the sella turcica and is attached to the clinoid processes and the anterior lip of the fossa. The dura passes down into the hypophyseal fossa in apposition with both the periosteum and the periglandular investment. There is no intervening intra- or subdural space present about the pituitary body.

The diaphragma sellae, the dural roof of the sella turcica, is perforated by an opening of variable diameter through which the infundibular stalk is continued to the hypophysis. The size of this orifice may determine to some extent the direction of tumor extension. The dura itself has considerable resistance to pressure but the diaphragmatic opening may offer an adequate avenue for the upward escape of an adenoma.

The pia-arachnoid encapsulates the pituitary stalk, but usually does not pass into the sella to any considerable extent.[521] When the diaphragmatic orifice is large it is possible that extensions of leptomeninges, with their enclosed spaces, may protrude into the upper part of the sella in contact with the superior aspects of the anterior and posterior lobes of the gland.[461] Since the subarachnoid space usually terminates above the sella it is unlikely that hormones of the hypophysis will follow this route for passage away from the gland.

The pia mater is applied closely to the brain but the arachnoid often bridges the space between adjacent neural structures. The space thus formed between the pia and arachnoid expands along the base of the brain to form the basal cisterns. Invasions of the neighboring subarachnoid cisterns by pituitary tumors may be revealed by pneumoencephalography. Figures 14 and 15 illustrate the position of the perisellar cisterns in diagrammatic and roentgenographic form.

Blood supply

The significant aspects of circulation in the hypophysis are: (1) its independent vascularization relatively distinct from nearby neural structures such as the hypothalamus; (2) the presence of portal veins; (3) the paths of venous drainage; (4) the effect of adenomas and surgery on the blood supply of the gland.

The hypophyseal arteries consist of the superior hypophyseal groups supplying the infundibular stalk, the median eminence and the adenohypophysis, and the inferior hypophyseal arteries destined for the infundibular process. The pars intermedia is supplied by both divisions which anastomose with each other in this region.

The superior hypophyseal arteries arise from the internal carotid and posterior communicating arteries of the circle of Willis in the subarachnoid space and pass to both anterior and posterior aspects of

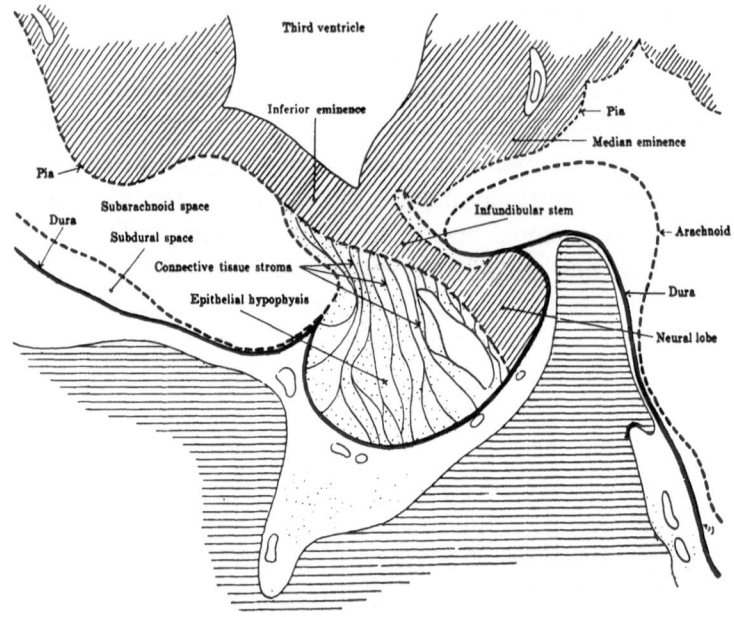

Fig. 14—Diagram of the meninges of the hypophyseal region of a 160 mm. human fetus, copied from Wislock (original drawing by E. Piotti).
From figure by Mettler, F.: Neuroanatomy, ed. 2. St. Louis, C. V. Mosby, 1948, p. 56.

the infundibular stalk at the junction of the stalk and the pars distalis. Those vessels that pass to the stalk penetrate the pars tuberalis and then branch on the surface of the stalk under cover of the pars tuberalis. The vessels either remain superficial and end as capillaries or invade the stalk and form arborizing tufts of capillaries within its substance.[522, 523] The blood of the surface capillaries eventually is re-collected in sinusoidal channels of the pars distalis. Both the superficial and the deep capillaries become continuous with venules which coalesce to form the portal system of the hypophysis.[375, 522, 523] A posterior group of superior hypophyseal arteries is applied to the posterior aspect of the stalk in a manner similar to that of the anterior group. The capillaries here are formed into skeins, rather than into terminal tufts, which likewise lead into venules and a portal system of vessels.[206] There are other posterior hypophyseal arteries which do not participate in the above arrangement. At the junction of the stalk and pars distalis they

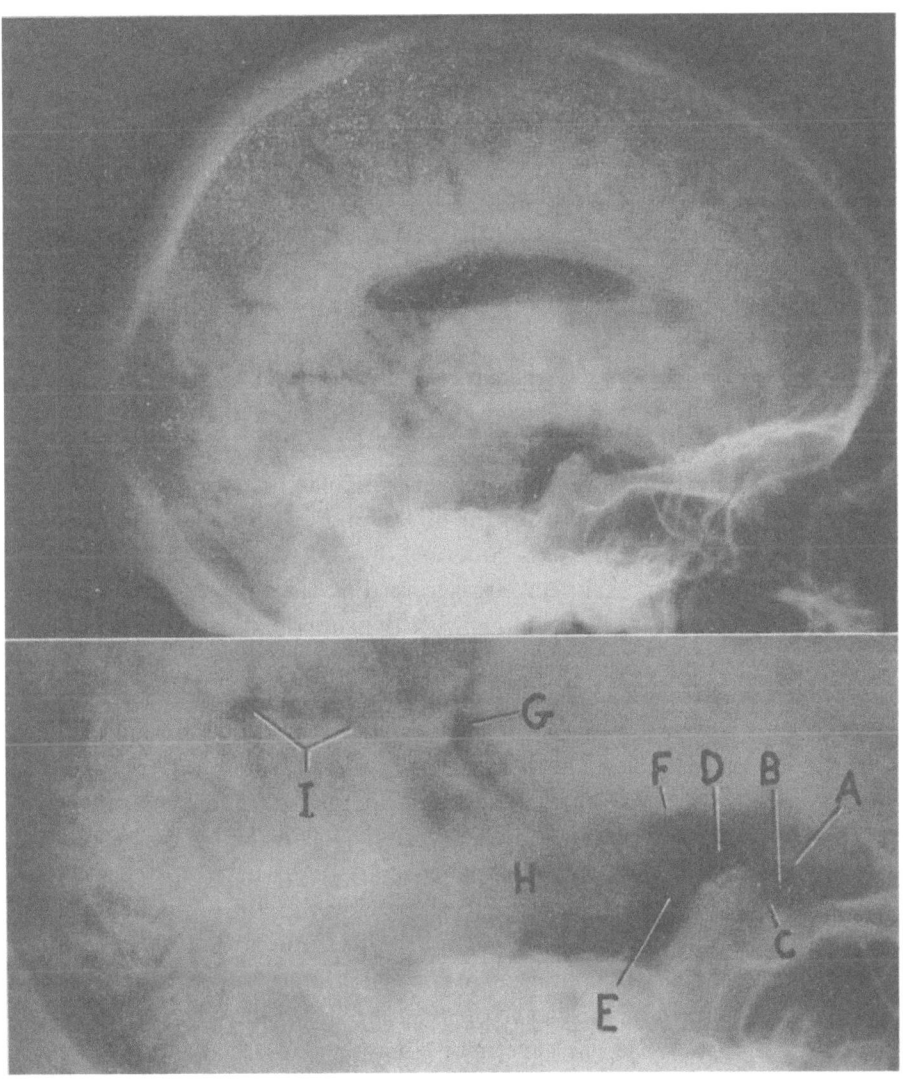

Fig. 15—Pneumoencephalograms. Lateral view (*top*) and inset (*bottom*) of perisellar cisterns.

Key: A, optic chiasm and nerves; B, chiasmatic cistern; C, sellar diaphragm; D, interpeduncular cistern; E, pontine cistern; F, region of the mammillary bodies; G, region of the ambiens cistern and internal subarachnoid pathways; H, cerebral peduncles; I, air over the cerebellar foliae.

enter the latter structure and divide into smaller vessels which drain into the sinusoids of the pars distalis. According to Green[206] the pars tuberalis is deficient at the point of entry of this posterior group, near the origin of the infundibular stalk. In place of the pars tuberalis a specialized neurovascular zone is found. The area contains a few islands of glandular cells, many blood vessels and nerve fibers which end mainly in apposition with the perivascular connective tissue. The source of the nerve fibers is not yet defined but they are assumed to be vasomotor in function. The physiology of the neurovascular zone is as yet uninvestigated.

The capillary net of the superior hypophyseal arteries, which do not go directly to the pars distalis, supplies the area of the median eminence as well as the substance of the infundibular stalk. No other important hypothalamico-hypophyseal vascular interconnections have been proved to exist. Evidently the direction of blood flow is downward from the stalk to the pars anterior through the portal system of veins.[522, 523] The portal veins arise from the coalescence of the venous capillaries which are continuous with the superior hypophyseal capillaries. As a result of the conjunction of the venules larger channels are formed on the surface of and within the stalk. These pass downward and once again splay out in the pars distalis to form the sinusoids of the pars distalis. The blood of these sinusoids is a mixture of arterial blood direct from branches of the superior hypophyseal, and venous blood from that filtered through the infundibular stalk and median eminence.[375, 523] The sinusoids of the pars distalis are bordered by the secreting cells of this part of the gland. It is probable that the hormones of the pars distalis are secreted directly into the sinusoids. The sinusoids become organized into emissary veins which unite to form the lateral hypophyseal veins. These leave the lateral poles of the pars distalis and empty into the adjacent cavernous sinuses.

The inferior hypophyseal arteries arise from the internal carotids while the latter are still in the cavernous sinus. As the hypophyseal arteries approach the free pole of the neural lobe, they branch and anastomose with each other before entering the infundibular process. Within the process a capillary system is found which eventually is formed into veins that pass out of the neural lobe through the investiture of the pars intermedia to reach the cavernous sinus. The cavernous sinus is the chief outlet of venous drainage of the entire hypophysis.

The arteries of the stalk, median eminence and adenohypophysis are pial in origin, whereas the arteries of the infundibular process are from the dural circulation. The communication between the pial and dural vascular beds is scanty. Wislocki believes that development of the portal system stems from pial veins which after passing with their membranes into the hypophyseal stalk lose external connections with their parent vessels. Thus the superior hypophyseal arteries are not accompanied by veins.[523]

Apparently chromophobe adenomas do not seriously compromise the circulation of the pituitary. Some of these tumors are extremely vascular but their circulatory demands are usually fulfilled. However, pressure of the tumor on the surrounding vascular bed and larger vessels conceivably may become great enough to diminish the blood flow in other parts of the pituitary. Some hemorrhages arise as a result of stasis due to obstruction of circulation by the tumor. Hemorrhages of all types exist in less than 3.0 per cent. More significantly, surgery in this area meets with the hazard of an extremely vascular organ. Postoperative hemorrhage is more common than preoperative hemorrhage. Edema, subsequent to hemorrhage of whatever source, may decrease the functioning of the anterior lobe and lead to acute pituitary insufficiency. Similar signs may occur in the case of acute hypothalamic failure, and the distinction between acute pituitary insufficiency and hypothalamic disturbances often is an uncertain one. Blood that escapes from the confines of the pituitary may cause reaction in the juxtahypophyseal neural structures. In this manner hypothalamic symptomatology may arise from pituitary hemorrhage.

There is no lymphatic system evident in the hypophysis.[80]

Nervous innervation

If nervous control of the pituitary could be experimentally established, the central nervous system could be viewed as the prime integrator and regulator of many psychologic mechanisms both by virtue of its own activity and through the mediation of the pituitary. The latter holds such a compelling position with regard to the other endocrine glands that its regulation by the nervous system would effectively subordinate the peripheral glands to neural control. Because of the attractiveness of such a physiologic principle and because of interest in the control of the pituitary as a problem in itself, considerable investigative work has been concerned with neurohypophyseal relationships. At present sufficient experimental evidence has been adduced to conclude that the neural lobe is under control of the hypothalamus but the neuroadenohypophyseal relation has not been similarly defined. It may be affected by nervous mechanisms but probably operates in the main independent of nervous regulation.

Consideration of the innervation of the pituitary body evokes two queries: (1) what nerves pass to the gland? (2) what are their functions? Although we discuss these questions separately, modern research no longer isolates the study of anatomy from the physiology of the structure examined.

The cells of origin of the sympathetic supply to the hypophysis are not definitely known. Presumably they arise in spinal segments C8 and T1. They pass as sparsely myelinated fibers from the corresponding superior cervical ganglion to the pericarotid plexus. They accompany the internal carotid intracranially and intermingle with the parasympathetic system on the surface of this vessel. Sympathetic nerve fibers leave the pericarotid plexus while the artery lies within the cavernous sinus and pass to the capsule of the hypophysis and into the anterior lobe. The fibers appear to be related chiefly to the vessels of the gland. However, a relatively limited number of fine fibrils do intertwine with the cell cords of the pars distalis. They are most prominent in the periphery but are also noted in restricted areas deep in the anterior lobe. Some sympathetic fibers enter the infundibular process and are lost in this division. Other fibers ascend and on the surface of the infundibular stalk join branches from the sympathetic plexus of the anterior and posterior communicating arteries. The latter pass with the superior hypophyseal arteries to the stalk. The nerves about the stalk are associated with the vessels of this region, a few being directed downward into the anterior lobe.[110, 387]

There has been no definite demonstration of the participation of parasympathetic nerves in the innervation of the pituitary. Evidence has accumulated that the sensory component of the seventh cranial nerve contains vasodilator fibers which may be distributed to pituitary vessels. The cells of origin of these fibers are in the geniculate ganglion. Their proximal extensions end in the tractus solitarius. Distally these fibers are continued in the greater superficial petrosal branch of the facial nerve and after commingling with sympathetic fibers finally end in the sphenopalatine ganglion. It is surmised that recurrent branches from the sphenopalatine ganglion, or from the junction of the autonomic nerves are conducted to the pituitary along with the superior sympathetic supply.[79, 532]

There is no significant evidence that the autonomic supply of the pituitary gland is concerned with control of its secretion.

Although the presence of unmyelinated nerve fibers passing from the hypothalamus through the infundibular stalk was noted by Cajal[66] and others, their detailed course and functional attributes were studied most carefully by Fisher, Ingram and Ranson.[162]

In the rostral part of the hypothalamus a condensation of neurons forms the supraoptic nucleus. Fibers which arise from this nucleus constitute the main component of the hypothalamico-hypophyseal tract. A smaller contribution is made by the paraventricular nucleus which is located in the anterior part of the hypothalamus adjacent to the third ventricle. This nucleus is similar in origin and histology to the supraoptic nucleus.[50] From a more general area, the tuber cinereum, fibers whose sources are not specifically assigned to any nuclear collection descend to the neurohypophysis in association with the supraoptic and paraventricular hypophyseal fibers, the total comprising the hypothalamico-hypophyseal tract.

The fibers of the supraoptic and paraventricular nucleus descend to the infundibular area and through the anterior part of the stalk. The tubero-hypophyseal component of the hypothalamico-hypophyseal tract lies more posteriorly in the stalk in its course to the neural lobe. The hypothalamico-hypophyseal tract disposes fibers to the median eminence and the infundibular stalk and process—the neurohypophysis. Occasional fibers are found in the partes tuberalis, infundibularis and intermedia, but their presence in these areas would appear fortuitous.[387] The termination of the nerve fibers has not been related to any particular structures within the infundibular lobe. In part this has been due to the complex histomorphology of the neurohypophysis. One should like to know whether the fibers innervate the pituicytes, but definite statements to this effect have not been forthcoming.

This hypothalamic-posterior pituitary axis has been shown to be related to the regulation of the renal output of water[162, 283, 284, 372, 492] and will be discussed in the following chapters.

Pathways of secretion

The pendulum of opinion has come a full period since Cushing declared that neurohypophyseal secretions pass into the third ventricle and are there reabsorbed into the vascular system. On the basis of experimental work, Rioch[393] has suggested that the natural outlet for secretions of all parts of the hypophysis are the venous channels which drain the gland. He does not deny that some of the products of the median eminence may diffuse into the third ventricle but believes this is an unimportant route for both neuro- and adenohypophyseal secretions. However, in Borell's work [51] the course of thyrotrophic hormone is traced from the adenohypophysis to the choroid plexus of the third ventricle. Extracts of pituitary and parapituitary areas were injected into guinea pigs and changes in their thyroidal cell heights were noted in subsequent sectioning. Increase in thyroidal cell heights was taken to indicate the presence of thyroid-stimulating hormone (TSH). By this means TSH was believed to be followed from the adenohypophysis to the stalk, tuber cinereum and choroid plexus of the third ventricle. Other confirmatory experiments were done as well. Borell does not exclude the vascular route as the chief one for the exit of TSH from the pituitary but emphasizes the possibility of an alternate pathway through the stalk to tuber cinereum, third ventricle and finally reabsorption by the choroid plexus into the systemic circulation.

The trend of experimental investigations would appear to be directed to the venous pathway as the main and immediate route by which hormonal secretions leave the pituitary.

III

FUNCTIONAL ANATOMY OF
THE PERISELLAR REGION

In terms of clinical comprehensiveness it seems unwise to distinguish too strictly between the morphology of the structures of the region into which chromophobe adenomas may extend and the physiology of its constituents. This chapter describes the functional anatomy of the perisellar structures which may become compressed or stretched by an expanding pituitary tumor. Often we shift the descriptive focus from an anatomic to a functional one, following what seems most relevant to the explanation of the development of symptoms.

SUPERIOR RELATIONS

The optic nerves, chiasm and tract, the hypothalamus and somewhat more remotely the inferior aspect of the frontal lobes are situated above the pituitary and are vulnerable to the effects of its expansion.

Optic nerves

The optic nerves converge from the optic foramina to form a chiasm lying one-half to one cm. above the diaphragma sellae.[413] The chiasm, in which rearrangement of the nerve fibers occurs, is related to the underlying sella turcica in the fashion illustrated in figure 16. Between the edge of the chiasm and the tuberculum sellae the anterior

31

aspect of the pituitary body is visible and accessible in all but the pre-fixed type of chiasm. The infundibular stalk passes superiorly and somewhat posteriorly in contact with the inferoposterior aspect of the optic chiasm. The posterolateral angles of the optic chiasm are drawn out as the optic tracts, embracing their respective cerebral peduncles en route to the lateral geniculate bodies.

The chiasm lies within an expansion of the subarachnoid space,

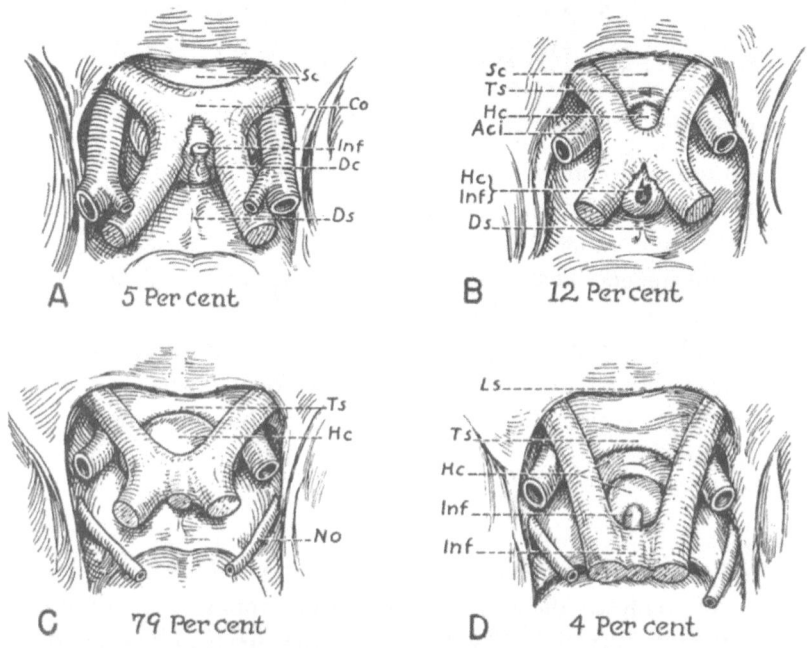

Fig. 16—The positions of the optic chiasm.

A. Optic chiasm lying partially in chiasmatic sulcus and on the diaphragma sellae (prefixed chiasm). Found in 5 per cent.

B. Chiasm located above diaphragma sellae. Found in 12 per cent.

C. Chiasm lying on the diaphragma sellae and projecting onto the dorsum sellae. Found in 79 per cent.

D. Chiasm located on and behind dorsum sellae. Postfixed chiasm. Found in 4 per cent.

From originals of figures 1 to 4 in Schaeffer, J. P.: Some points in the regional anatomy of the optic pathway, with especial reference to the tumors of the hypophysis cerebri and resulting ocular changes. Anat. Rec. 1924, *28*: 253.

which forms the basal cisterns, intimately related to the third ventricle and in effect forming part of its floor.

The internal carotid arteries lie inferolateral to the chiasm. The anterior cerebral branches pass up and over the optic nerves as these enter the chiasm. The anterior communicating vessel connects the two anterior cerebrals above the optic nerves. The posterior communicating arteries arise from the internal carotids and course alongside the chiasm and beneath the optic tracts to join the basilar artery. Thus the chiasm and its immediate extensions are cradled by the circle of Willis. An aneurysmal dilatation of any of these vessels may compress the visual paths of this region and simulate the effects of a pituitary tumor. When such visual defects as result are associated with partial destruction of adenohypophyseal tissue by the expanding aneurysm and with the development of hypopituitarism, it is difficult to differentiate between intracranial aneurysm and pituitary adenoma without resorting to arteriography. A point of importance stressed by Jefferson[273] is the relation of the anterior cerebral arteries to the optic nerves. As a chromophobe adenoma extends it may push before it the overlying chiasm and entering nerves. Further upward deflection of these structures presses them against the relatively fixed anterior cerebral arteries. Thus the nerves and anterior part of the chiasm are compressed between the firm pulsating vessels and the underlying tumor. Visual impairment may be the consequence of this mechanical derangement.

To understand the nature of defects produced by pressure on or stretching of the visual tracts or their blood supply, the correspondence of the visual field to the topography of the nerve fibers within the juxtachiasmal intracranial portion of the optic nerve, the chiasm and the beginning of the optic tracts must be appreciated.

The retina is arbitrarily divided into two halves, the vertical line of bisection passing through the macula. The temporal or lateral half contributes fibers which are uncrossed and terminate in the homolateral occipital cortex. The nasal or medial half of the retina gives origin to fibers which cross within the optic chiasm and reach the contralateral cortex. The fibers of central vision are believed to be bilaterally represented in the cerebral cortex; on this basis one infers that they consist of crossed and uncrossed elements. The presumed areas which the optic fibers of each retinal division occupy within the optic nerve, chiasm and beginning optic tract are shown in figure 17.

Essentially the fibers occupy positions in their course through the optic nerves which correlate with their retinal origins. Within the chiasm the scheme of Wilbrand and Saenger[516] is tentatively followed (fig. 18). The crossing fibers occupy much of the body of the chiasm before concentrating in the inferomedial aspect of the optic tract. Of these fibers the inferonasal retinal quadrantic group crosses ventrally in the anterior part of the chiasm. Some of these fibers form a genu in the heterolateral optic nerve before turning back to pass along the side of the chiasm. In the beginning of the optic tract they are in the ventromesial quadrant. The superonasal retinal quadrant fibers cross in the middle and posterior parts of the chiasm, also ventrally situated, and occupy the dorsomesial quadrant of the opposite tract. This retinal division also contributes some groups which reach the inception of the homolateral optic tract, bend within its origin and then join their associates by crossing the posterior part of the optic chiasm to enter the heterolateral tract. Fibers from the temporal quadrants pass directly back, those of the superior temporal quadrant lying mesial to the fibers of the inferior temporal quadrant. The temporal group enters the homolateral optic tract, adopting a dorsolateral position therein.

The macular fibers are placed within the core of the optic nerve, the uncrossed temporal group lying lateral to the crossed nasal group. Within the chiasm the crossing macular fibers decussate in the dorsal and intermediate layers of the chiasm in its middle and posterior parts, whereas the uncrossed macular fibers pass directly back deeply situated within the lateral half of the chiasm. The macular fibers are reassembled within the central part of the optic tract. The crossed fibers remain mesial to the uncrossed (fig 18).

The correspondence of the retinal quadrants to the visual field is well known, in that the retinal image in any quadrant is derived from the diagonally opposite field quadrant, e.g., the superior temporal visual field is projected onto the inferonasal retinal quadrant.

The relation of the optic chiasm to the underlying sella turcica and the direction and rapidity of tumor growth are determinants in

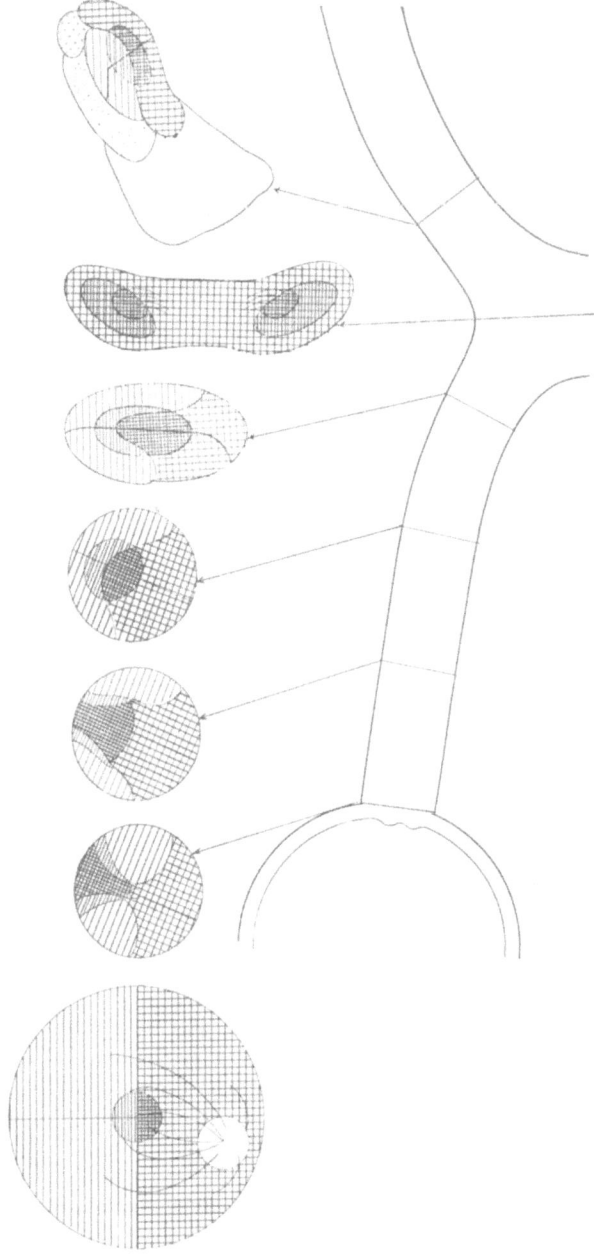

Fig. 17—The distribution and course of the nerve fibers in the retina, optic chiasm, and tract of the right side (Henschen's scheme, modified. The chiasmal section is slightly modified from Wilbrand and Saenger).

After Traquair, H.: An Introduction to Clinical Perimetry, ed. 4, St. Louis, C. V. Mosby, 1944, fig. 31, p. 76.

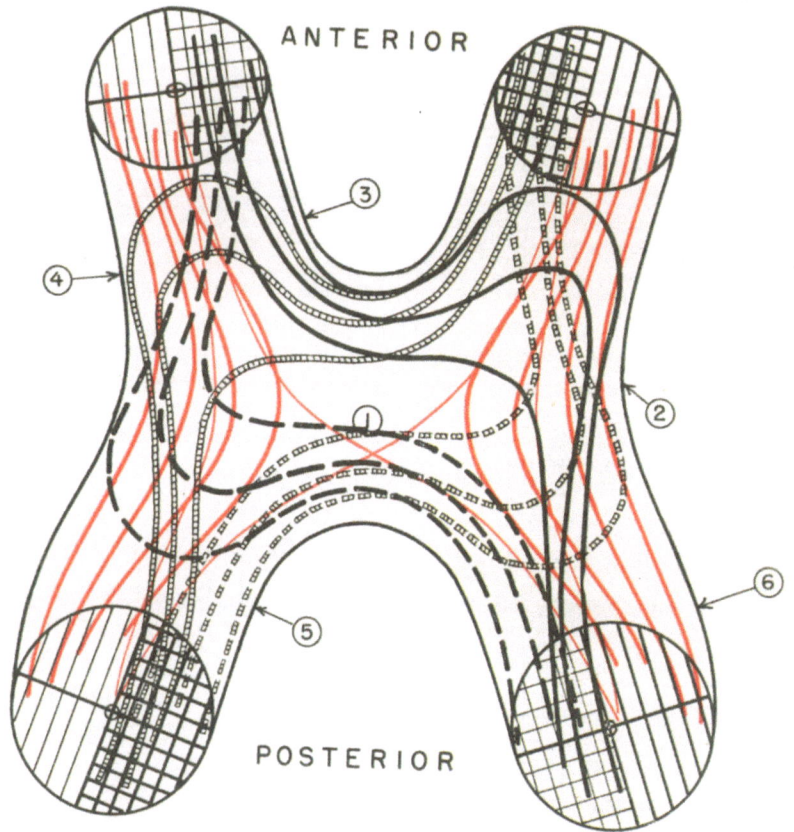

Fig. 18—The chiasmal crossing.

┅┅┅┅┅┅ Fibers from inferior quadrant of right optic nerve cross in the anterior part of the chiasm, form a genu at the termination of the contralateral optic nerve and pass to the lower quadrant of the left optic tract.

━━━━━ Corresponding fibers from inferior quadrant of left optic nerve.

▭▭▭▭▭▭▭ Fibers from superior quadrant of right optic nerve descend along the same side of the chiasm to its posterior angle and then cross in the posterior part of the chiasm to enter the upper inner quadrant of the left optic tract.

━━ ━━ ━━ Corresponding fibers from superior quadrant of right optic nerve.

the typical visual interference observed in cases of chromophobe adenoma. The median and upward surge of a pituitary tumor interferes with nervous function of the optic pathways by direct pressure on the

───────────

━━━━━━━━━ Direct fibers of the optic nerves pass back along the homolateral side of the chiasm and into the corresponding optic tract. The superior quadrant fibers extend more dorsally than those of the inferior quadrant. Both enter the corresponding quadrants of the optic tract.

─────────── Macular fibers cross within the chiasm and pass back directly. They lie in a posteroventral position in the optic tract.

Possible sites of lesions of the chiasm, as indicated by the numbers on the diagram, are as follows.

1. In the presence of midline involvement, bitemporal hemianopia may occur. Central scotomas are associated with effects on the posterior part of the chiasm.

2. Here a complex defect results. The direct uncrossed fibers are implicated and a defect appears in the nasal field of the homolateral eye. Both the crossing fibers of the same side from the superior nasal retinal quadrant and those of the opposite side from the inferior nasal retinal quadrant may suffer. The inferior temporal field of the homolateral and the superior temporal field of the contralateral eye are diminished. This type of defect is rare in cases of chromophobe adenoma.

3. Pressure at this region may cause temporal hemianopia or blindness of the eye on the same side and a defect in the superior temporal quadrant of the opposite eye. However, if the effect of pressure is directed equally to both optic nerves a bitemporal hemianopia may develop.

4. Here the direct uncrossed fibers of the temporal quadrants and the crossing fibers of the inferior nasal quadrant are affected producing an ipsilateral nasal and contralateral superior temporal defect, a fragmentary homonymous hemianopia.

5. Involvement of crossing fibers from the opposite nasal quadrants and uncrossed fibers from the homolateral temporal quadrants produces a homonymous hemianopia that is complicated by an inferior temporal quadrant defect of the eye homolateral to the site of lesion. It is apparent that with lesions of the optic tract the presence of the consequent homonymous hemianopia is opposite to side of the lesion.

6. Lateral lesions of the posterior part of the chiasm produce defects in the homolateral nasal field and in the heterolateral temporal field as a result of involvement of direct uncrossed temporal and crossed nasal fibers respectively. Persistence of the inwardly directed pressure may cause destruction of the entire field on the side of the compression.

After Traquair, H.: Introduction to Clinical Perimetry, ed. 4, St. Louis, C. V. Mosby, 1944, Plate III, p. 229.

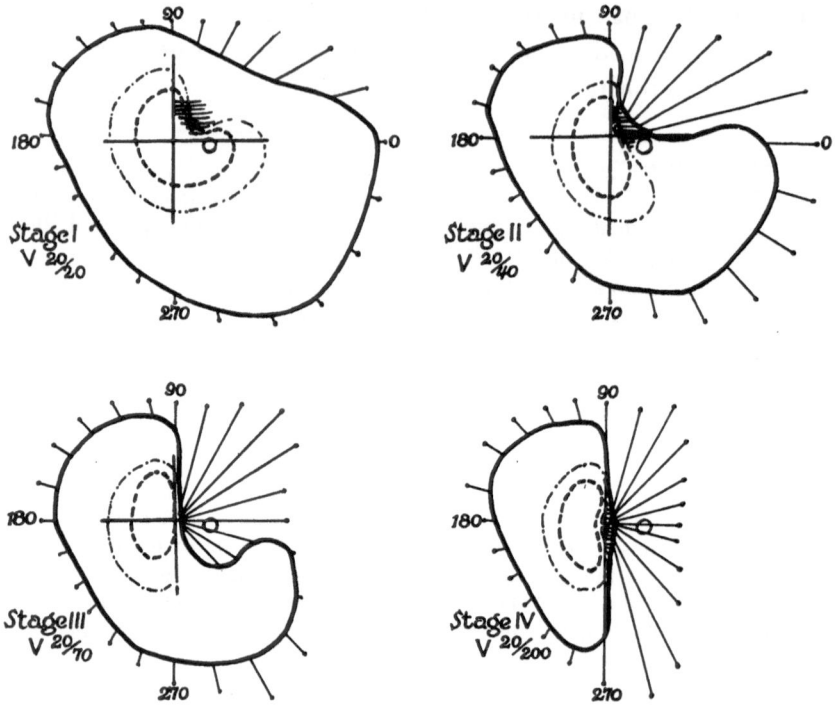

Fig. 19—The progression of a right temporal deficit. *See facing page for continuation of figure and complete legend.*

neural fascicles or on their venous drainage, less probably on their arterial supply. Based on the summary of the anatomic details described above a satisfactory interpretation of the changes noted in the visual fields can be given. Cushing and Walker[106] and Traquair[484] have clarified the development of field changes seen with expanding lesions of the pituitary body. Typically the encroachment of a pituitary tumor on the optic chiasm occurs from below, in the midline and within the middle one-third to anterior half of the chiasm. Thus those fibers which are in the ventral layers of the optic chiasm, in the midline and in the anterior half are involved initially. These are the crossing fibers of the inferonasal retinal quadrants arising from both the paracentral and peripheral regions of these quadrants. The field defect (fig. 19) is noted, therefore, in the upper temporal quadrants of both eyes, frequently

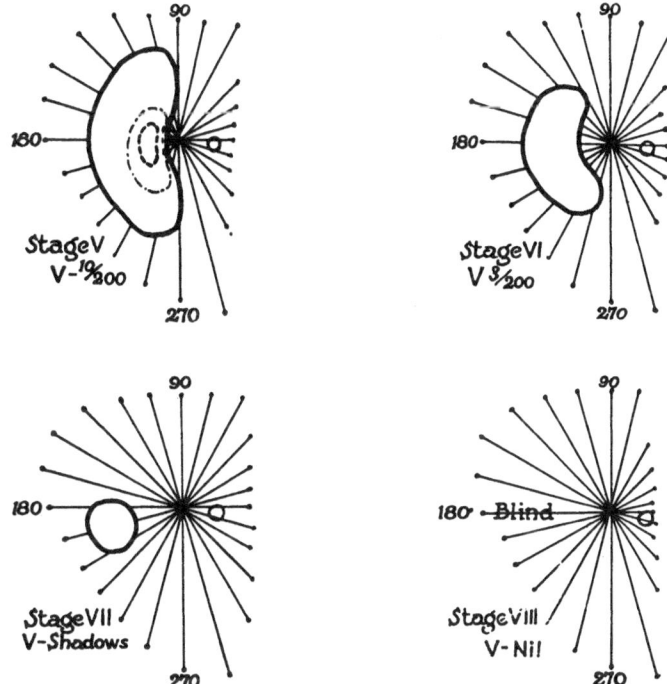

Fig. 19 (*above and facing page*)—The progression of a right temporal deficit. The hook-like extension of the advancing defect is seen particularly well as it passes from the upper into the lower temporal field.

From original figures by Cushing, H. and Walker, C. B.: Distortion of the visual fields in cases of brain tumor. Chiasmal lesions with special reference to bitemporal hemianopsia. Brain 1915, *37*: 341.

more marked in one than the other. Because of anatomic or spatial particularities, it is possible that there is a preponderant effect either on the fibers from the central or from the more peripheral areas, the former being more common. It is usual then to see failing vision in the region of the inner isopters of the upper temporal field. A pericentral or central scotoma develops, distinctly bounded by the diameter vertically bisecting the visual field, but diminishing less abruptly in intensity at the equatorial plane. A gradual retreat of the peripheral field develops. The extending central scotoma coalesces with the peripheral visual defect to produce an upper temporal quadrantopsia. In a hook-like configuration the visual defect descends into the lower temporal quadrant. The failure of vision in this quadrant indicates the progression of the pathologic effects of pressure on the chiasm to the more posteriorly located crossing fibers of both central and peripheral origin.

Within the temporal half of the visual field there may be relative sparing of a part of the peripheral field so that larger test objects at lesser distances are perceived in a remnant of the temporal field, while the internal isopters are significantly drawn inward. This formation is supposedly characteristic of the effect produced by midline expansions of pituitary tumors and is called the temporal island. It is separate from the central scotoma and lies within the temporal field externally circumscribed by areas of diminished visual acuity. The persistence of a functional temporal field is explained hypothetically by supposing that the course of the crossing fibers concerned is more lateral and dorsal than the bulk of the other nasal retinal fibers. By virtue of their situation, removed from the immediate neighborhood of maximal pressure, these fibers are partially spared.

At this stage there is bitemporal hemianopia with involvement of the central and peripheral regions of the visual field. Progression of the field changes is not inevitable. However spontaneous regression is unusual. For the moment we shall continue as if the adenoma persists in its aggressive expansion to damage further the optic pathways.

The visual defect turns clockwise in the right field and counter clockwise in the left. The route of its invasion is from superior to inferior temporal quadrant, followed by entry into the inferornasal and then superonasal areas. As one would expect, the involvement of the nasal fields is the result of upward lateral pressure on the chiasm affecting the direct uncrossed fibers arising in the temporal retinal quadrant. Since the fibers of the superotemporal retinal quadrant arch mesially, en route to the ipsilateral optic tract, they are compressed by a midline tumor before those of the inferotemporal retinal quadrant. The depression of the nasal half of the visual field passes from periphery centrad. Once again there may be a combination of central scotoma and diminution of peripheral field. The visual fields are thus extinguished.

There are variations in the manner and the degree of involvement. A frequently found progressive field change is one in which the central scotoma is not a major defect. Rather the loss is limited to the peripheral fields, the visual impairment pursuing a course similar in sequence to the above.

If the optic chiasm is prefixed the fibers in the posterior part of the chiasm, mainly the crossing macular fibers, may be significantly altered while the peripheral crossing fibers are relatively spared. This leads to bitemporal central scotomata and only later to peripheral changes. With a postfixed chiasm all but the anterior crossing fibers of the lower nasal retinal quadrant may escape damage. Their involvement results in superior temporal quadrantopsia, which may remain stationary as the adenoma enlarges without further compressive effects. With a postfixed chiasm, lateral expansion of an adenoma without median involvement may produce total blindness in one eye and a superior temporal quadrantic defect of the visual field of its mate. Those inferonasal retinal fibers which cross anteriorly suffer the pressure effects at their genu in the hilt of the contralateral optic nerve prior to its entry into the chiasm.

A homonymous hemianopia is not infrequently found in cases of chromophobe adenoma. It is possible that here the chiasm is prefixed, the tumor pressing laterally against one optic tract to cause this visual deficit. Occasionally one may see further compromise of the fields with homonymous hemianopia. An inferior temporal quadrantic defect may be added to this field homolateral to the compressed optic tract. This latter condition is the result of interference with the genu of the crossing fibers of the superonasal retinal quadrant in the homolateral optic tract.

The degree to which the central and fixation regions are affected is also variable. It is possible to see central scotomata of different intensities and extent in any of the above lesions. Moreover central scotomata with intact peripheral fields may occur. In the presence of depressed visual acuity which cannot be accounted for by intraocular pathology there is presumptive damage to the retro-ocular visual pathways. A case of surgical bisection of the optic chiasm studied by Evans and Browder[152] revealed the expected central scotoma only under very careful examination. These authors accept the usual explanation for the difficulty in determining such scotomata, that is, eccentric fixation by the retina adjacent to the macula which then assumes the physiologic center of the visual field. It is technically difficult to detect eccentric fixation because of the nystagmoid movements of the eyes occurring in normals and, to a greater extent, in those with decreased visual acuity. Strict immobility of the eyeball is a virtual impossibility. In the course of routine examinations for central vision the methods we and others have employed are not exact enough to determine the extent of central impairment. We assume that a central scotoma exists when visual acuity is diminished to 20/200.

In addition to the depression in visual field and acuity there are hallucinatory episodes reported due to tumor on the optic pathways. Classically visual hallucinations have been thought to arise from disturbances of the temporal or occipital visual fibers.[496] It is difficult to imagine that the ungraded and unorganized effects due to pressure should afford appropriate stimuli for a complex psychologic formation. However, cases of chromophobe adenoma exhibiting visual hallucinatory episodes have been recorded, in which the pressure was directed to the chiasmal and perichiasmal area.[505]

Hypothalamus

The elucidation of symptoms due to pituitary tumors involves the differentiation of hypothalamic from hypophyseal functions. At the present time there is a tendency to attribute an increasingly significant role to the hypothalamus in the control of the secretory activity of the pituitary, making distinctions between these two more difficult. But apart from this aspect of hypothalamic physiology there are independent neural mechanisms in which the hypothalamus participates; its disturbance induces neurologic symptomatology in cases of chromophobe adenoma. They are presented here briefly to provide an interpretative background for our study. Although clinical material has produced the impetus for investigation, well founded concepts of hypothalamic physiology have evolved mainly from experimental data.

The hypothalamus extends from the optic chiasm to the caudal border of the mammillary bodies. It is removed from the superior surface of the hypophysis by a scant 15 mm. Within its substance there are nuclear groups that are concerned with: (1) thermoregulation, (2) the state of wakefulness, (3) appetites and emotional behavior, (4) conservation and distribution of body water, (5) the autonomic systems, (6) cortical facilitatory mechanisms and (7) sexual functions.

The diagrammatic outlines of figure 20 along with the following breakdown of the nuclear groups of the hypothalamic area may serve to acquaint the reader with the anatomic orientation of the region.[265]

The five regions of the hypothalamus, each listed with their nuclear groups, are:

1. *Anterior:* supraoptic nucleus, paraventricular nucleus, suprachiasmatic nucleus, diffuse suprachiasmatic nucleus, anterior hypothalamic area, preoptic region. (Although the preoptic region is not an anatomic part of the hypothalamus, it is considered with it functionally.)

2. *Middle:* ventromedial nucleus, dorsomedial nucleus, dorsal hypothalamic area, posterior hypothalamic area.

3. *Lateral:* lateral hypothalamic area, lateral tuberal nucleus.

4. *Posterior:* pre- and supramammillary area, mammillary intercalate nucleus.

5. *Periventricular:* preoptic and arcuate nuclei.

The thermostatic action of the hypothalamus is subserved by nuclei of its anterior and posterior areas. Division between the thermoregulatory functions of these areas is not distinct. However, a hypothalamic center associated mainly with the dissipation of body heat resides in the preoptic and supraoptic areas.[30, 382] Although vasodilatation and sweating are reflex acts which can be performed in the absence of hypothalamic control, they have been observed to appear upon direct stimulation of the anterior hypothalamic area.[331] In experimental animals lesions of the preoptic and supraoptic areas, or of the pathways leading from them through the lateral hypothalamus, result in hyperthermia, without accompanying panting and increased respiratory rate. These moderating reflexes appear to have been impaired and hyperthermia ensues. The effect of lesions of the anterior hypothalamus on sweating in primates has not been fully described, but it is probable that an integrative center for sweating and vasodilatation is likewise present in this area.

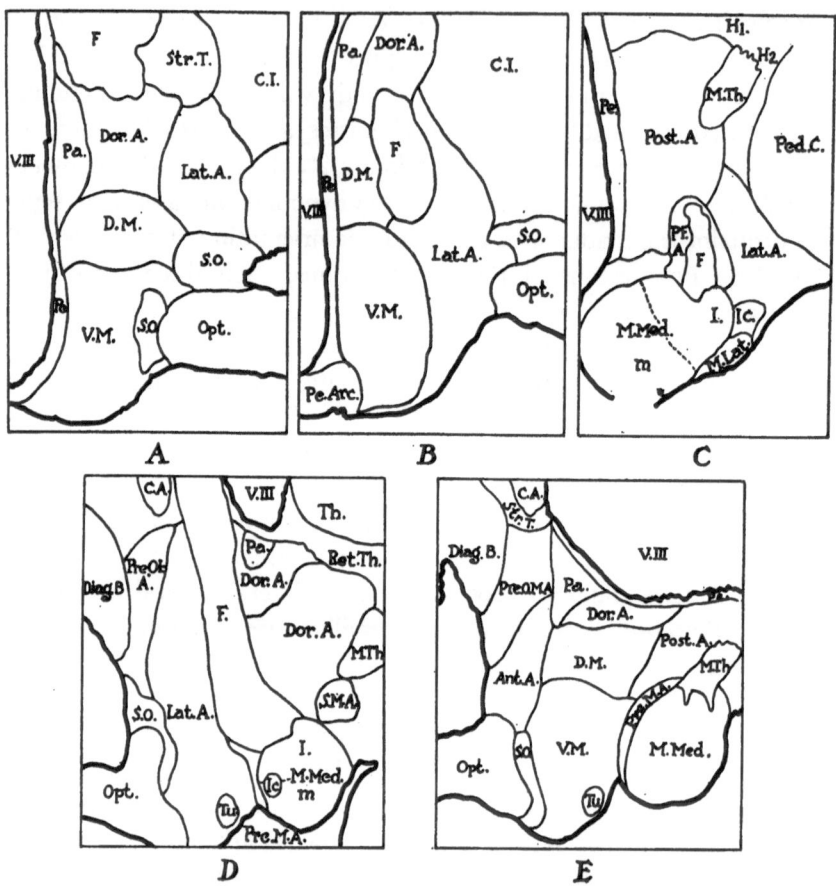

Fig. 20—Diagrammatic representation of several regions of the hypothalamus. Three coronal sections A, B, C through the human hypothalamus. A is just caudal to the infundibulum; B lies between infundibulum and mammillary bodies; C is through the rostral pole of the mammillary bodies. Two sagittally directed sections D, E through the human hypophysis. D is a parasagittal section through the lateral hypothalamic area and E is between the fornix and third ventricle.

Key: Ant. A., anterior hypothalamic area; C.A., anterior commisure; C.I., capsula interna; Diag. B., diagonal band; Dor. A., dorsal hypothalamic area; D. M., dorsomedial nucleus; F, fornix; H_1, H_2, fields of Forel; Ic, nucleus intercalatus; Lat. A., lateral hypothalamic area; M. Lat., lateral mammillary nucleus; M. Med., medial mammillary nucleus (N. Med. 1, lateral division and N. Med. m, medial division); M. Th., mammillothalamic tract; Opt., optic chiasm and tract; Pa, paraventricular nucleus; Pe, periventricular system; Pe Arc, periven-

Damage to the posterior hypothalamus or to the caudal part of the lateral hypothalamus containing descending pathways interferes with the protective reflexes of vasoconstriction and piloerection. Animals with lesions of this region maintain normal body temperature under ordinary circumstances but become more readily hypothermic in extreme cold. These experimental results seem to indicate that even though other mechanisms are associated with the function of heat conservation, the hypothalamus is an important central neural thermoregulator.

The anterior hypothalamus also responds to the stimulus of cold by mediating, through an unknown circuit, a shift in water from the blood to interstitial and intracellular locations.[30] Due to consequent diminution in peripheral volume flow, less heat is lost from the organism by conductance. Primarily the liver and then the spleen and muscles are reservoirs for the displaced water. Systemic ergotization and denervation of the liver are said to eliminate this water shift induced by cold, whereas adrenalectomy prevents the loss of electrolytes from the circulation. It has been noted also that injury to the posterior hypothalamus alters the usual water shifting responses provoked by cold. The changes in electrolytes, osmotic pressure and specific gravity of the blood associated with redistribution of water, although supportive to the events described, have not been fully investigated. There would appear to be a dynamic balance between anterior and posterior centers with regard to shifts of water caused by changes in temperature. Experimental extensions and further corroboration of the existence of a water shifting mechanism have not been noted in recent reports. In man, the nature of hypothalamic responses to cold has not been so clearly defined.

Fig. 20—*Continued*
tricular arcuate nucleus; Ped C, cerebral peduncle; Pf. A., perifornical area; Post. A., posterior hypothalamic area; Pre. M.A., premammillary area; Pre. OLA, lateral preoptic area; Pre. OMA, medial preoptic area; Ret. Th., thalamic reticular nucleus; S M A, supramammillary area; S O, supraoptic area; Str. T, bed nuclei of stria terminalis; Th., thalamus; Tu, lateral tuberal nucleus; VIII, third ventricle; V.N., ventromedial nucleus.

After Rioch, D., Wislocki, G. and O'Leary, P.: The Hypothalamus. Research Publ. A. Nerve & Ment. Dis., Baltimore, Williams & Wilkins, 1940, vol. 20, p. 3.

Evidence derived from the clinic confirms the importance of the hypothalamus in the regulation of body temperature.[115] In human cases damage to the hypothalamus usually is not discrete, but there is general agreement with the data presented above. The cases usually are complicated by terminal systemic disease which obscures the issue.

Although previous studies indicated that stimulation of the posterior hypothalamus would induce somnolence, Ranson and his collaborators,[381] demonstrated a coordinative center, present within the mammillary bodies, responsible for maintaining a state of wakefulness. The center is bilateral and lesions of the mammillary bodies on both sides are associated with production of sleep. Ranström[385] believes that within the cells of the nucleus tuberomammillaris and the nucleus of the raphe of the mesencephalon there are colloidal droplets representative of secretions that under appropriate conditions diffuse into the environs and cause local changes predisposing to sleep. Aside from this conditional finding Ranström confirms the work of Ranson with regard to a waking center situated in the region of the mammillary bodies. Stimulation and injury in several regions of the hypothalamus are known to affect normal cortical electroencephalographic patterns.[309] Whether the "waking" center is associated with the appearance of cortical alpha rhythm has, however, not been investigated directly.

Davison[116] has reviewed the clinical literature and presented additional observations concerning the location of a waking center. Although the data are not equivalent to those gained through animal experimentation, it appears that the hypothalamus is related to the preservation of wakefulness in humans as well.

The hypothalamus has been regarded as the neural center which impells the organism to act upon its instinctual needs. The appetites for water, food, sleep and perhaps sex are governed in part through the agency of the hypothalamus. The origins and mechanisms of the forces that drive the hypothalamus are only incompletely identified. No doubt these are dependent on the functioning of the entire organism and influence the hypothalamus through neural and perhaps humoral means.

Many workers have agreed that abnormal obesity may be referred to hypothalamic lesions.[23, 69] The observation of Hetherington and Ranson[244] that adiposity induced by hypothalamic lesions is not affected by total hypophysectomy supports the independent influence of the hypothalamus. In a more recent series of animal experiments it was found that lesions of the ventromedial nuclear area are associated with changes of food intake and body weight.[57, 243] The animals so affected exhibit an unusual voracity associated with the wolfing of food offered. They spontaneously select a diet similar to that of the controls but consume it promptly, rather than abiding with their usual habits of eating. On an unlimited diet there is a rather marked gain in weight with the consequent accumulation of great depots of fat. However the utilization of the stored fat appears to be normal. Carbohydrate consumed is converted to fat at an accelerated rate and is metabolized as such. The extent of the obesity attained by the rats cannot be accounted for by reduction in heat formation or voluntary activity.[58, 473] It is to be reemphasized that removal of the hypophysis does not effectively prevent the development of the obesity.[242] The necessarily bilateral lesions associated with the state described are in the ventromedial nuclei, ventromedial portion of the lateral hypothalamic area and the ventrolateral region of the central gray. Brobeck[55] states that in the rat, "the neurons involved . . . are in the region of the ventromedial nuclei; that their axons run from the inferior and lateral borders of these nuclei into the regions above and lateral to the mammillary bodies, and from there into the mesencephalic tegmentum."

The clinical corollary of these investigations is found in the obesity of some postencephalitic patients in whom damage to the hypothalamus is known to occur.[519] The voracity exhibited by some of these patients is striking. In contrast, Aschner, as early as 1912,[14] considered fatal cachexias to be the result of tuberal and infundibular lesions. Bailey and Bremer[cited in 189] concluded, from experimental data of greater precision, that widespread tuberal lesions were incompatible with life, even in the presence of an intact pituitary gland. Heinbecker and White[232] have recently advanced the opinion that loss of anterior lobe tissue, without concomitant hypothalamic depression, does not lead to cachexia, but that the combination of both most probably does.

This problem awaits further study, the trend being, nonetheless, clearly away from the anterior pituitary gland alone.

In connection with their studies on obese rats Brobeck, Tepperman and Long[473] observed proteinuria and cylindruria, reporting fatty droplets within the renal tubular epithelium and hyaline casts intraluminally. In a functional study of these renal changes Stevenson[460] observed a subnormal glomerular filtration rate and renal plasma flow. He confirmed the presence of diminished urinary output in comparison with the water load and the low water to food ratio described by Leyendecker.[cited in 460] Although these observations were noted originally in obese rats, the examination of other rats with similar lesions yielded parallel results before development of obesity. These data, however, do not have a recognized clinical application as yet.

Investigators from the time of Bailey and Bremer[cited in 23] and Camus and Roussy[69] have suggested that permanent diabetes insipidus appears to be associated with lesions of the hypothalamus. This topic has been discussed elsewhere in the text. Whether tissues in the floor of the third ventricle are capable of secreting an antidiuretic substance is not established.[23] The work of Heinbecker and his associates,[232, 234] in great measure extending the studies of the Ranson group, strongly indicates that the origin of such a substance is actually not from the hypothalamus but rather from the neurohypophysis, specifically the median eminence. Such a distinction is of far more than academic importance because Heinbecker and his associates have thus given experimental confirmation to the concept that anterior lobe tissue is, in fact, quite unnecessary for maintaining any except maximal diabetes insipidus. They have found the disturbance equally persistent with or without anterior lobe tissue present, provided that the entire neurohypophysis (including the median eminence) is totally denervated or destroyed.

Within the area that includes the hypothalamic nuclei related to appetite for food there is a center whose destruction releases rage patterns.[511] Bilateral lesions of the nucleus ventromedialis of the middle region produce a hyperirritable inconsolable animal. Presumably the presence of this nuclear mass is necessary to appropriate emotional expression. Bard and Mountcastle[32] apparently have shown in experiments on cats that the removal of amygdala and the rhinencephalic and transitional cortex produces marked rage after a latency of several weeks. After de-neocortication, on the other hand, a placid animal emerges. In accord with these findings it is possible that the rhinencephalic and transitional cortex act via the amygdala on the ventromedial nucleus to inhibit excessive and inappropriate expressions of rage. The neocortex may act as a suppressor on the remainder of the fore brain through the amygdala or by-pass this median complex and act as an excitant of the rage reaction. However, Bucy's[65] work on monkeys is apparently in direct conflict with the data presented by the Hopkins group. The system of checks and balances of Bard may be overextended.

Whether the apparent rage corresponds to the feelings one experiences under appropriate stimulation has been debated for some time. It has been impossible to condition animals to rage reactions by following the condition stimulus with local hypothalamic stimulation. When the rage reaction produced by hypothalamic stimulation interrupts goal directed and highly motivated behavior, experimental neuroses do not develop. There is an on-off quality to the rage, present with stimulation and absent on its cessation. This lack of emotional after-discharge does not resemble closely what is observed in the true affect.[341, 528] Without participating in this type of research one's opinion must be prudently restricted. However, the animals that Bard[32] recently described give the appearance of being quite nasty, in a bad mood much of the time. They convincingly mimic beasts experiencing anger.

It may be stressed at this time that complex interrelationships exist between the various parts of the nervous system and the hypothalamus. There are no independent centers in the nervous system which are projected exteriorly as a function. Neural areas probably serve as regions of organization and final common pathways. Because a colligation of fibers and concentration of neurons occur in these areas their destruction results in major functional deficits. To reverse the argument and imply that these areas are generators of events is, however, not equally true. In this respect it might serve current neurophysiology·well to declare a retreat from concepts of organization by levels and to seek operational definitions in keeping with biochemical and electrical data. Attempts to correlate emotional attitudes of human cases suffering from hypothalamic pathology with the functional attributes of the hypothalamus are certainly worthy.[10] However, they beg such issues as the qualitative aspects of emotions, their central origins, the neural circuits and areas concerned. In short the complexity of the problem is sacrificed for the statement that the hypothalamus is involved, which frequently it is, in clinical cases with pronounced changes in mood.

Although the general extent of hypothalamic mechanisms is but approximated, its role in relation to autonomic functions has been extensively examined.[383, 384] Generally the anterior and posterior regions of the hypothalamus are believed to be related to the parasympathetic and sympathetic systems respectively, but such a division is not rigidly maintained. Many of the older experiments depended on the direct observation of the viscera as affected by stimulation or localized injury of the hypothalamus. Perhaps in this manner disagreement in the description of hypothalamico-autonomic relationships arose. A method such as employed by Pitts et al.[59] lends itself to more definable results. These investigators stimulated the posterior and lateral hypothalamic regions and recorded the action potentials set up in single or multi-fibered postganglionic sympathetic cardiac axons. In keeping with the results of previous work, the hypothalamus was found to be unnecessary for the maintenance of blood pressure or cardiac rate or for the homeostatic reflexes concerned with them. Medullary centers appeared to suffice for these mechanisms, the hypothalamus being adjunctive to their functioning. These investigators further observed a ratio greater than one between the number of stimuli applied to the hypothalamus and the action potentials recorded in the isolated autonomic axons, as well as a delay in the appearance of the action potentials in the peripheral fibers. The assumption was made that there are nuclei within the hypothalamus which dispose their discharges through neural nets that are linked to other centers intervening between the hypothalamus and the autonomic outflows.

It is of interest to note that the rate and intensity of stimulation applied to a particular hypothalamic area may result in peripheral inhibitory or facilitory effects, as revealed in the frequency of action potentials recorded in the sympathetic axon. It is not always certain, therefore, that so-called parasympathetic or sympathetic effects obtained with a less rigorous technic can be accepted as such. They may rather represent varying effects of the same system.

The role of hypothalamic centers in the excitation or inhibition of gastro-intestinal motility and secretion is not clear. In a review of this problem Sheehan[431] reports that stimulation of the supraoptic, preoptic and tuberal areas increased the motility of the stomach and caused an outflow of watery secretions, whereas posteriorly directed stimuli resulted in decreased gastric movement. This is in accord with the parasympathetic and sympathetic representation within the interbrain. Of significance are the reports that large hypothalamic lesions may cause bleeding, erosions and ulceration of the stomach and occasionally of the duodenal wall.[277, 278, 500] Sympathectomy prevents the hemorrhage but not the ulceration. In a case of a cytologically undefined extra-axial tumor of the tuber cinereum, without disruption of the tuberal cytoarchitecture, duodenal ulceration was found postmortem.[351] In this regard the therapeutically encouraging work of Dragstedt[475] who vagotomized patients with peptic ulceration, represents the effective application of the theories of many workers in neurophysiology. Investigation of the hypothalamus and its role in the movements and secretions of the remainder of the gastro-intestinal tract and bladder has not yielded results which can be summarized fruitfully. It is probable that diencephalic discharges affect the physiology of the gut and the urinary bladder but the details are not clear.[294]

The recent work of Gellhorn,[353] who has demonstrated a facilitory effect on the corticospinal system induced by activation of the hypothalamus and enhanced by elimination of sympathetic influences, serves as a bridge between visceral and somatic functions. This author believes the hypothalamic region discharges through mammillothalamic and periventricular tracts to the dorsomedial nucleus of the thalamus. From there impulses pass to the frontal cortex. The details have not been elaborated but the idea that the hypothalamus is associated with the corticospinal system and thus perhaps with somatic functions is given experimental support.

In cases of chromophobe adenoma with hypothalamic compression or with operative injury to the diencephalon, many signs of disordered autonomic physiology may become apparent: e.g., tachycardia, cardiac arrhythmia, gastro-intestinal immobility and ulceration. The difficulty lies in defining the causes of such symptoms. However, the knowledge that disturbed hypothalamic mechanisms may produce functional and even structural pathology is of assistance in the management of the patient.

There has been a resurgent interest in the relation between hypothalamus and sexual functions, stimulated by the finding that extra-axial neoplasms in the region of the tuber cinereum may be associated with marked sexual precocity in infants and children. These patients may exhibit large genitalia, marked secondary sexual characteristics and accelerated general growth patterns.[392a, 506] However, emotionally and behaviorly the children do not appear otherwise advanced. In most instances hormonal assays in the urine have been incomplete, but wherever tested high or normal androgenic and normal gonadotrophic and estrogenic urinary levels have been found. Active spermatogenesis has been demonstrated in some cases.[60, 215, 485] Hypothyroidism and perhaps other endocrine abnormalities may occur. The hypothalamic tumor usually is confined to the posterior part of the floor of the third ventricle in the region of the tuber cinereum or median eminence, may be mainly extra-axial and does not compress the pituitary body. Histologically the tumor varies in type, being glial, sparsely cellular, or as cellular as and similar to the tuber cinereum.[50] It does not appear to contain secretory cells.

Whether the hypothalamic tumor and tuberal disruption are part of a general syndrome and not its author, cannot be apprehended from the literature. Bronstein's[506] case of a 22 month old female revealed on autopsy, in addition to the tuberal tumor and advanced sexual changes, hyaline and fatty aortic placques and myocardial hypoplasia. Scholz has discussed a similar case of an 8 year old girl with generalized arteriosclerosis.[392a] In the absence of ovarian and adrenal tumors precocious sexual changes may arise from hypothalamic dysfunction.

The results of animal experimentation designed to determine the part played by the hypothalamus in sexual physiology do not fall into a clear pattern. In contrast to Evans and others,[14, 40, 69] many have turned to the hypothalamus for an explanation not only of sexual dysfunction but even of gonadal atrophy. Evidence summarized by Brookhart and Dey[61] indicates that bilateral hypothalamic lesions placed latero-centrally in the vicinity of pituitary stalk and optic chiasm produce conspicuous disturbances in rhythmic, cyclic sexual activity and in reflex copulatory motor patterns, irrespective of sex. These disturbances are observed in the presence of quite normally maintained gonadal structure. This concept would seem more readily reconcilable with the majority of experimental observations.

However, the more recent studies of Hillarp[245] demonstrate that in the guinea pig anterior hypothalamic injury reduces the secretion of luteinizing hormone, whereas damage to the median eminence diminishes the output of both this hormone and the follicle stimulating hormone. Genital atrophy ensues. In rats, large anterior lesions, extending to but not including the paraventricular nuclei and lying lateral to the medial forebrain bundle, do not interfere with oestrus. Although large follicles are present, corpora lutea do not develop in the ovary. Other data indicate that injury to the tuber cinereum of rats may cause obesity and sexual dystrophy. Stimulation of this area in rabbits induces ovulation.[219, 243] The sum of experimental findings tends to the conclusion that there are areas within the hypothalamus concerned with the control of adenohypophyseal secretion of gonadotropins.[121, 126, 229, 336]

When the stalk is sectioned experimentally there is no apparent uniformity in the results. In the rabbit, where coitus is followed by ovulation in a short time, interruption of the direct connection between hypothalamus and pituitary well within this time prevents post coital ovulation.[62, 156] However, in various other species, section of the stalk appears to yield variable disturbance in sexual rhythms and gonadal atrophy depending on the experimentor.[121, 130, 279, 510] In Dandy's[111] case, stalk section in a young woman did not interfere with menstruation or pregnancy. The general objection that a regrowth of vascular communications between hypothalamus and pituitary may occur unless specifically guarded against applies to most of the investigations, with few exceptions.[510]

The sexual behavior of animals with hypothalamic lesions is not remarkable if the neural axis from a region just anterior to the mammillary bodies caudad is preserved.[31] The mesencephalic reticulum appears to be the more important area in coordinating primitive sexual patterns.

The paucity of neural connections between the hypothalamus and the adenohypophysis suggests that the influence of the hypothalamus is mediated by a vascular route. It does not appear necessary to assume that the only vascular channels available are in the portal system, since access to the general circulation is not denied to the hypothalamus in the event of stalk transection. However, it is evident that the currents are running strong for subordinating many hypophyseal functions to neural direction.[184] For example, in addition to influencing hypophyseal gonadal relations the hypothalamus is thought to affect the regulation of other adenohypophyseal secretions through nervous pathways.

It is clear, nevertheless, that after experimentally transplanting the hypophysis to places remote from its origin most of the essential functions ascribed to this gland are preserved to a degree. The belief that the pituitary can function sufficiently to maintain metabolic balance in the absence of neural stimulation is well grounded, though it may still be true that the hypothalamus secretes hormones which reach the hypophysis via the blood stream.

After producing electrolytic lesions in the anterior hypothalamus of dogs, Hume and Wittenstein[261] demonstrated that eosinopenic response to stress is diminished. Since the release of ACTH may be associated with the depression of eosinophils in the peripheral blood, they deduce that the hypothalamus is concerned with stimulating the adenohypophysis to produce ACTH. Destruction of small areas 1 to 2 mm. within the ventral periventricular hypothalamus deprived the adenohypophysis of its indirect neural stimulation. These authors further state that section of the infundibular stalk and interruption of nervous and vascular pathways from the hypothalamus to the pituitary does not diminish the eosinopenic response to stress or that induced by remote control stimulation of the hypothalamus. It would also appear that neither epinephrine nor the sympathetic fibers to the pituitary are essential to the process of secretion of ACTH. The conclusion is that on demand a hormone is elaborated within the hypothalamus which passes into the general circulation and returns to the pituitary causing it to secrete ACTH. The direct evidence for this is not yet evolved nor have further confirmations come from other laboratories.

Hume and Wittenstein place weight on the findings of Scharrer and Scharrer[414] who have reviewed the comparative basis for hypothalamic secretion. The latter workers have found that in many animal species including man there are morphologic characteristics of the neurons suggestive of secretory activity within the areas related to the supraoptic and paraventricular nuclei. Injection of extracts of the hypothalamus has yielded negative results in the hands of the Scharrers, but Hume and Wittenstein indicate that their work in this regard is promising. Although the study just described would appear convincing, the theory of glandular activity within the central nervous system does not sit agreeably with many neurophysiologists. On the other hand the scarcity of nerve fibers within the adenohypophysis is difficult to reconcile with the expected safeguarding and extensive control of such an important function as regulating secretions of the adenohypophysis.

Aside from the indication that the hypothalamico-hypophyseal connections are important in preserving the hypertrophic response of the thyroid cells to cold, the adenohypophysis seems to operate independently of the hypothalamus in its production of TSH.[487,488] Recently Greep[208a] has demonstrated that thyroidal cell height and total thyroid size are dependent on the presence of an intact hypothalamus. Lesions in the anterior hypothalamus of the rat interfere with the thyroidal cellular hyperplasia in response to the administration of thiouracil. In other experiments this investigator has removed the adenohypophysis to an intraocular location and shown that under these circumstances total thyroid mass is reduced below that of the controls. However, in both types of experiments—when hypothalamic lesions are made or when the adenohypophysis is transplanted—the thyroid still remains capable of fulfilling its metabolic functions.

In man, hypothalamic tumors without involvement of pituitary tissue, notably in the case reported by Collins,[85] produce marked depressions of basal metabolic rate (BMR). A fair statement might be that the thyroid can be influenced by the hypothalamico-hypophyseal unit, but that the basal secretory activity induced by the adenohypophysis is relatively independent of the hypothalamus.[487]

The relation of neural control of the hypophysis to secretion of the "diabetogenic" hormone and indirectly to the action of insulin is confused. The reader is referred to discussions of these questions in pertinent articles.[56, 219, 319, 333]

It would seem that if such a relationship exists it is yet to be defined.

Frontal lobes

The further removed and superiorly located structures which occasionally suffer distortion and compression due to the expansion of pituitary tumors are the frontal lobes, mainly the rhinencephalic and orbital regions and parts of the ventricular system. Although a full discussion of the frontal lobes cannot be undertaken here, it may be of interest to mention that animal studies[311] indicate that the orbital gyri may be concerned with autonomic activities, e.g., blood pressure, vasomotor phenomena, and neural mechanisms related to the renal vascular shunt described by Trueta.[486] The shunt mechanism is believed to be absent in man. Ablation of the orbital region causes hyperactivity of experimental animals and vasodilatation of their extremities. There is no detectable clinical correspondence to these experimental findings. More significantly, persistent expansion of a tumor into the anterior perforated substance may interfere with venous drainage of the anterior capsular area. Circulatory insufficiency and subsequent signs of an upper motor neuron lesion may appear. Pressure directed more anteriorly can affect the function of the olfactory tract and produce hyposmia. The extension of a chromophobe adenoma into the main mass of the frontal lobes is unusual. However a small percentage of tumors do involve the central white matter of the frontal lobes. Personality abnormalities attributed to the effects of such frontal lobe invasion are presumed to be located in the sphere of behavioral adaptation to novel situations. Patients with unilateral frontal lobe lesions or lobotomies are said to be unable to adapt readily to new environmental conditions, especially when abstraction capacity is required.[216a] Their affective reactions are determined in part by previous personality structure although their intellectual deficits are quite similar.

Ventricular system

The ventricular system is of particular interest to us. Its deformation affords a means of determining the presence and origin of intracranial tumors. The ventricles are contained within the cerebral hemispheres, the interthalamic and hypothalamic area, the tegmentum of the mesencephalon and the rhombencephalon. In figure 21 the ventric-

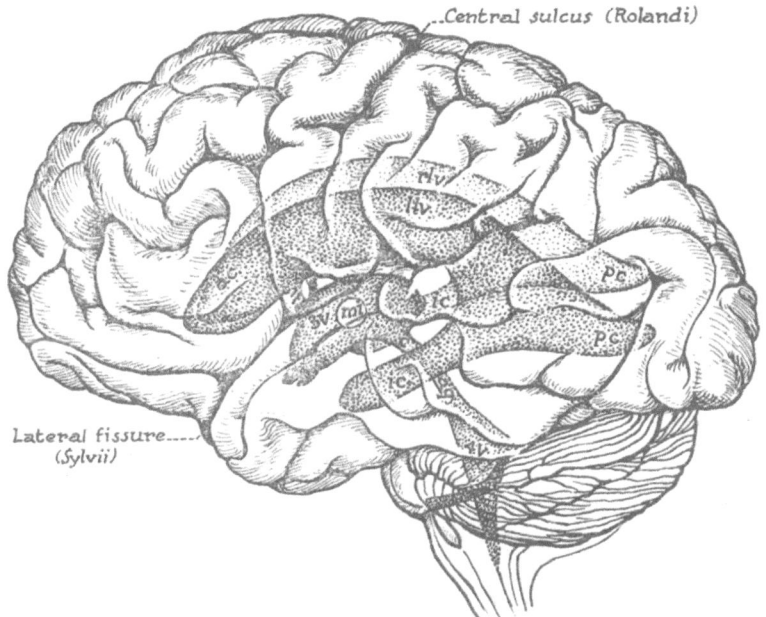

Fig. 21—Lateral view of the ventricular system within the brain.

Key: rlv, llv (right and left lateral ventricles); ac (anterior horn of lateral ventricle); pc (posterior horn of lateral ventricle); ic (inferior or temporal horn of lateral ventricle); if (interventricular foramen of Monro); 3V (third ventricle); mi (massa intermedia); eaq (aqueduct of Sylvius); 4V (fourth ventricle).

From original of figure by Pancoast, H. K., Pendergrass, E. P. and Schaeffer, J. P.: Head and Neck in Roentgen Diagnosis. Springfield, Charles C Thomas, 1942, p. 905.

ular system is projected within the contours of the brain. The third
ventricle is most proximate to the hypophysis; its floor, in fact, consists
of the optic chiasm, infundibulum, tuber cinereum, the mammillary
bodies and the posterior perforated space. Irregularities of its outline
induced by chromophobe adenoma are frequently of diagnostic import.

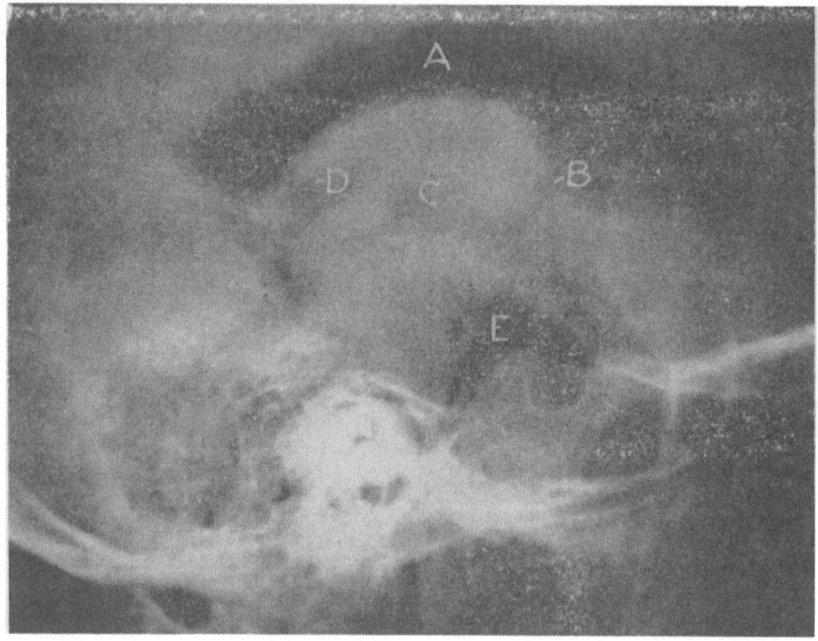

Fig. 22—Lateral view of normal pneumoencephalogram revealing the ventricular system and subarachnoid cisterns; (A) lateral ventricles; (B) foramen
of Monro; (C) third ventricle; (D) suprapineal recess; (E) subarachnoid
cisterns.

Figures 22 and 23 indicate the radiographic representation of the
ventricular system partially filled with air. The sensitive points of the
ventricular system are the foramina of Monro and the aqueduct of
Sylvius. The larger cavities of the lateral, third and fourth ventricles
allow for considerable encroachment without impairment of the circulation of cerebrospinal fluid. However, compression and blockage of
the narrow necks of the foramina and aqueduct produce internal
hydrocephalus. Tumors of the pituitary may invaginate the walls of

the third ventricle or elevate the lateral ventricles. It is the exceptional tumor, however, which extends to involve the aqueduct of Sylvius or the foramen of Monro. In these instances, the cerebrospinal fluid secreted by the choroid plexuses of the lateral and third ventricle accumulates ahead of the obstructed passageway. There is distension of the ventricular system and a rise in intracranial pressure. As a consequence

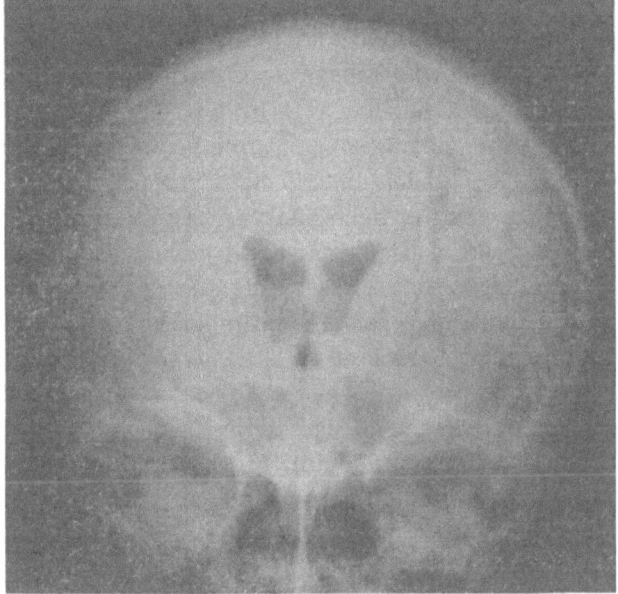

Fig. 23—Anteroposterior projection of normal pneumoencephalogram. Lateral ventricles are clearly defined as butterfly shaped shadows. The tear drop contour lying in the midline is the third ventricle.

any of the classical signs of intracranial hypertension may occur, e.g., headache, vomiting which is occasionally projectile, choked disc, bradycardia, an increased systolic blood pressure and a clouded sensorium.

LATERAL RELATIONS

The structures situated lateral to the hypophysis are the cavernous sinus, its contents and somewhat more remotely the medial surface of the temporal lobes.

Cavernous sinus and its contents

The cavernous sinus is a spongy trabeculated venous channel which passes from the superior orbital fissure to the level of the tip of the petrous bone. It drains the periocular, ocular and retinal areas through the superior and inferior ophthalmic veins and the central vein to the retina. It has connections with the superficial, middle and inferior cerebral veins. The sinus communicates with its mate, forming a circumsellar net, with the pterygoid plexus and with the pericarotid venous plexus. The flow of venous blood continues into the transverse sinus and the internal jugular vein by way of the petrosal sinuses. Partial obstruction by compression or thrombosis of the cavernous sinus frequently causes congestion and edema of the periocular, ocular and retinal regions. Swelling of the orbital tissues with proptosis, venostasis of the retina with local hemorrhage and papilloedema may develop.

The neural findings associated with the syndrome of the cavernous sinus[504] arise from impairment of the function of the third, fourth, sixth and ophthalmic branch of the fifth nerves (fig. 24). The corresponding symptoms consist in palsy of the extraocular muscles, supraorbital and ocular pain and changes in the sensibility of the area innervated by the first branch of the fifth. The lateral extension of pituitary tumors rarely causes the entire syndrome of the cavernous sinus to develop. The clinical picture is usually fragmentary. The relationships of the various structures within the cavernous sinus are demonstrated in the accompanying diagrams (fig. 24 a to f). Following is a complete description of the diagram, as it originally appeared in F. B. Walsh's article (Bilateral ophthalmoplegia with adenoma of the pituitary gland; report of 2 cases; anatomic study. Arch. Ophth. 1949, *42*: 653):

A wide variation exists in the size and arrangement of the sinuses and the ophthalmic veins in normal persons. The superior petrosal sinus is inconstant. The intercavernous sinuses are variable in size. The transverse (basilar) sinus, which connects the inferior petrosal sinuses, is shown in A but is not identified in the drawing. It is always a large sinus.

Nerves in the cavernous sinus: The sixth nerve is shown at the base of the skull in A. It passes within the inferior petrosal sinus under the petrosphenoid ligament to enter the body of the sinus, where it lies lateral and inferior to the carotid artery. In C it can be seen that the sixth nerve enters the sinus before the third and fourth nerves. In the posterior part of the cavernous sinus only the sixth nerve and the first and second division of the fifth nerve are present. Farther forward in the sinus the sixth nerve becomes lateral and inferior (E, D). It enters the superior orbital (sphenoid) fissure inferiorly and laterally (B, A).

The third nerve enters the cavernous sinus at the junction of the posterior and middle third (F, E). Its position anteriorly and directly lateral to the carotid artery is seen (E, D). It passes through the superior orbital fissure medial to and above the sixth nerve (C, B). This nerve divides into its superior and inferior branches within the cavernous sinus (Gifford, H., Jr.: Arch. Ophth. 41: 5, Jan. 1949); this is not shown in the drawing.

The fourth nerve enters the sinus just posterior to and below the entrance of the third nerve. Its course through the sinus is shown in A. Its position in the lateral wall of the sinus is seen in A and D. It goes through the upper part of the superior orbital fissure after passing medial to the third nerve (B).

The gasserian ganglion is seen to lie in Meckel's cavity (C, B). The sensory root and the three divisions are seen in B. The ophthalmic and maxillary nerves are seen to lie in the posterior part of the sinus (B, F). The position of the nerve in the lateral wall of the sinus is seen in E and D. The branches of the ophthalmic division are shown in A and B.

In the absence of secondary thrombosis, lesions of the nerves in their intracavernous course are due to direct pressure, to stretching of their fibers or of nutrient vessels, by the enlarging pituitary tumor. The sequence of appearance and extent of the symptoms depend on the variable anatomy of the contents of the cavernous sinus and the pathway impressed upon the expanding adenoma. The first branch of the fifth nerve is protected by distance. Its early involvement is not usual. One may also attribute the infrequent impairment of the first branch of the fifth nerve to the lesser susceptibility of sensory than of motor nerves to pathologic changes induced by pressure.[123]

The damage produced by pressure and stretching consists in injury to peripheral nerves. To some extent this simplifies the explanation of the disabilities of extraocular movement seen in cases of chromophobe adenoma with extension into the cavernous sinus. A brief description of the extra-axial courses of the third, fourth and sixth nerves may indicate the regions of their vulnerability.

The third nerve, the oculomotor, containing fibers for all the extraocular muscles except the superior oblique and the lateral rectus, as well as autonomic

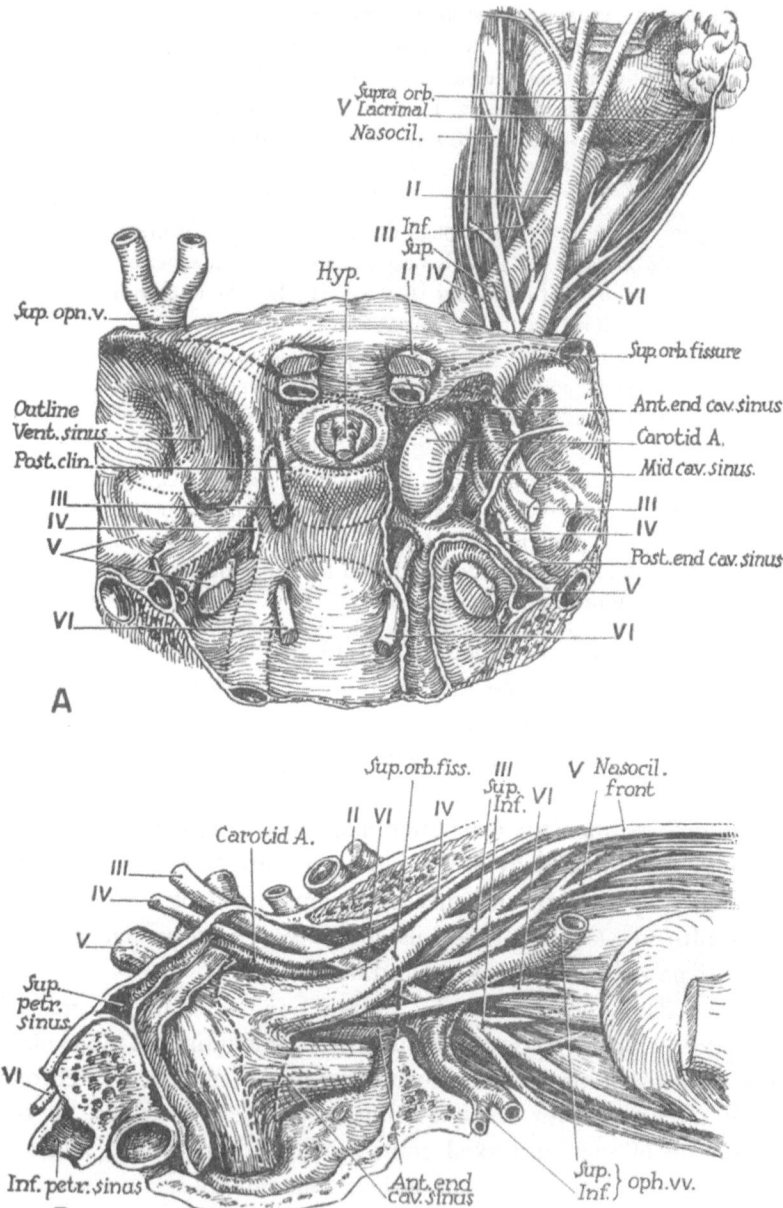

Fig. 24—The cavernous sinus. See facing page and text pages 60, 61.

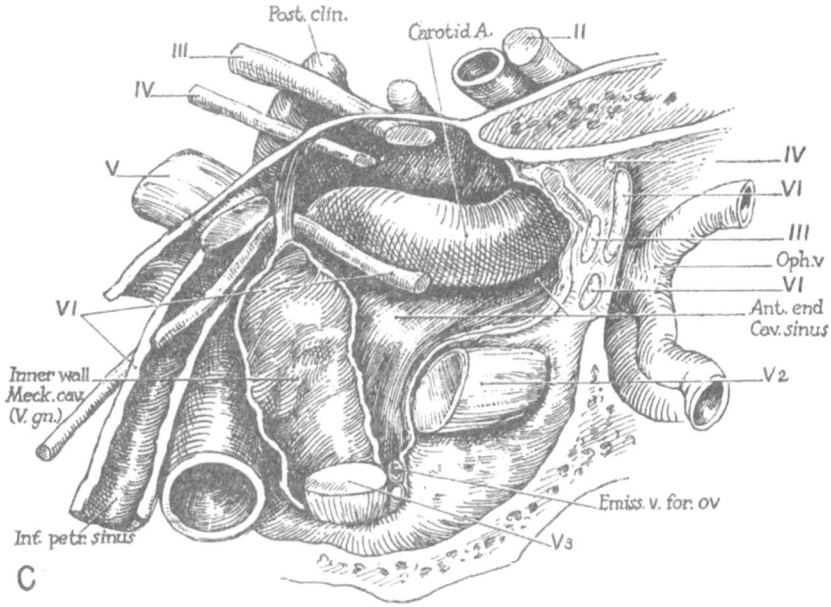

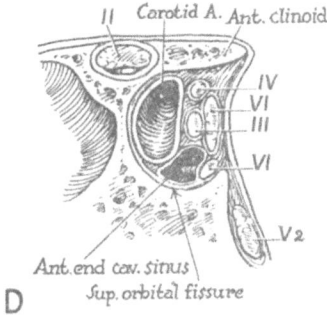

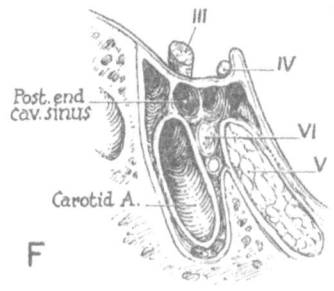

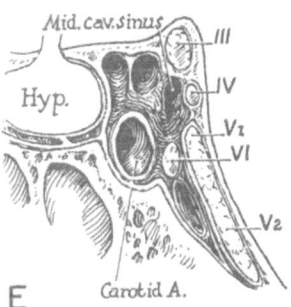

Fig. 24—The cavernous sinus. (A) Top view: dotted lines indicate position of sinuses; right side is dissected. (B) Right lateral view: wall of sinus is dissected away and position of nerves is shown. (C) Deeper dissection than that shown in B; tip of petrous bone is removed. (D, E, F) Vertical sections through posterior, middle and anterior parts of cavernous sinus, respectively. See pages 60, 61 for further description.

innervation for the pupil, emerges on the medial surface of the cerebral peduncles anterior to the basilar sulcus of the pons. This is the first fixed point of attachment. It is closely related to the vessels of the circle of Willis and as such is subject to the effects of aneurysmal dilatation or perivascular inflammation. The nerve passes forward from the interpeduncular fossa lateral to the posterior communicating vessel to enter a triangular area between the free and attached borders of the tentorium cerebelli. It courses through the subarachnoid space and perforates the dura mater at the level of the posterior clinoid and in this interval is relatively immobile. After passing through the cavernous sinus along its lateral wall the nerve enters the orbit through the superior orbital fissure and breaks up into an upper and lower branch (fig. 24a to f). The walls of the superior orbital fissure are bony ridges against which the nerve may press. From this description it becomes apparent that dislocation of the nerve from its usual pathway by an expanding mass along its course may induce angulation at its origin, where it penetrates the dura to enter the cavernous sinus, or at the rim of the superior orbital fissure.

The fourth nerve, the trochlear, is equally exposed to the effects of an expanding sellar or parasellar lesion but the detection of paresis of the superior oblique, the only muscle it innervates, is difficult. Except for the rare instance of an isolated and advanced superior oblique palsy, partial disability of this nerve is usually overlooked. This is especially true when paresis of other extraocular muscles is present. This nerve winds about the brain stem to pass forward lateral to the third nerve. It likewise enters the triangular area formed by the tentorial extremities. The trochlear proceeds through the subarachnoid space and dura mater below the free edge of the tentorium cerebelli at the level of the posterior clinoid to arrive within the cavernous sinus. The fourth nerve passes along the lateral wall of the cavernous sinus below the third to enter the orbit through the superior orbital fissure. Essentially, the regions of fixation are similar to those of the third nerve but by virtue of its early lateral position it is somewhat removed from the vessels composing the circle of Willis and is therefore less affected by pulsatile pressures or aneurysmal dilatation.

The sixth nerve, the abducens, which supplies the lateral rectus, is regarded as the most vulnerable extraocular nerve because of its long and angulated course. Emerging at the ventral surface of the pons the abducens is directed forward in the cisterna pontis. It leaves the subarachnoid space opposite the dorsum sellae and penetrates the dura mater. Then bending sharply forward it crosses the superior surface of the petrous part of the temporal bone close to its apex and below the petrosphenoidal ligament and enters the cavernous sinus. Coursing along the lateral wall of the sinus the sixth enters the orbit through the superior orbital fissure. The length, the several fixation points, the angularity at the level of the petrous bone and the exposure to ligamentous and osseous edges predispose this nerve to injury.

The extraocular muscles innervated by these nerves are six in number. They act in pairs or in more complex combinations. The mate of an actively contracting muscle reciprocally relaxes in a gradual fashion. The yoke muscles, the lateral and medial recti, horizontally abduct or adduct the globe respectively. The other major actions of the extraocular muscles are outlined as follows: the superior rectus elevates the eyeball and inferior rectus depresses it when the eyeball is in the abducted position; the obliques act dominantly as vertical movers

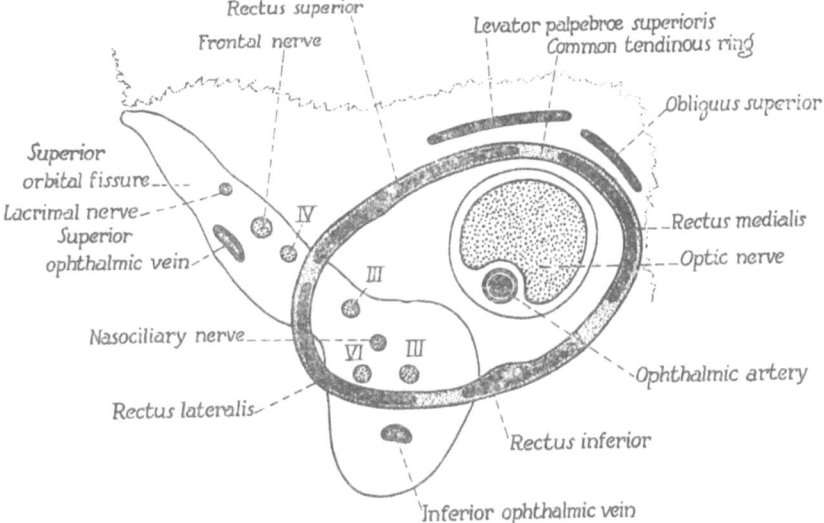

Fig. 25—The superior orbital fissure (left). Occasionally an adenoma may extend forward to compress the structures entering the orbital cavity through the fissure. The fissure may be demonstrably enlarged. More frequently the structures are distorted by the tumor and forced against the bony ridges of the fissure.

Original figure by T. B. Johnston, in Gray, H.: Anatomy Descriptive and Applied, ed. 26, edited by Johnston, T. B., London, Longmans Green & Co., fig. 1038, p. 1164.

when the eye is adducted fifty degrees. The inferior oblique is then an elevator and the superior oblique a depressor.

As a consequence of their fixed attachments, the action of the external ocular muscles depends on the relation of the axis of the globe to the longitudinal axis of the muscle at work. The influence of a muscle is not dominant for a particular movement until the axes of the globe and the muscle are aligned appropriately.

The eye at rest may reflect the presence of a paretic muscle by deviation from the normal position. As the eye is directed into the field of movement of a paretic muscle or complex, the effects of muscular weakness become more apparent. The directed movement is not accomplished, or only inadequately, and diplopia may be noted subjectively. To facilitate the examination of the patient for perception of double image, a colored glass is used to cover one eye and light is shown at various points of the visual field. When diplopia appears the patient is able to designate the position of the separate images by their color. Diplopia appears in that part of the field which engages the paretic muscle and by bringing the object further into this region of the field there is an increase in the diplopia. When false and true image correspond in laterality to the paretic and normal eye, the diplopia is uncrossed. This occurs in the presence of paresis of muscles with an abducting action. The obverse, crossed diplopia, appears with palsies of the adducting group.[47]

After examination of the extraocular muscles the palsies detected can be expressed in terms of the nerves involved. This is true in cases of chromophobe adenoma where the nerve injury is at the level of the peripheral nerve and the neuromuscular defect is apparent in all reflex and voluntary ocular movements. This pervasive type of impairment usually is not seen with lesions of the cortico-regulatory tracts to the extraocular muscle nuclei. In the latter case bulbar reflex eye movements may be retained.[281]

As a consequence of weakness of the external ocular muscles nystagmoid movements of the eye may occur. When, in addition to muscular paresis, visual acuity is diminished, fixation nystagmus combines with paretic nystagmus to produce fairly obvious and easily elicited oscillatory movements of the eyes.[47, 281, 454]

Medial surface of temporal lobe

There are established cases of chromophobe adenoma which, in their lateral drift, press upon the medial surface of the temporal lobe. Further extension may result in their investment by a mantle of temporal lobe tissue (fig. 26). The signs of temporal lobe invasion are usually few, but occasionally characteristic. When the rhinencephalic area in the region of the uncus is effected, a psychic equivalent state may appear. It is associated with changes in the state of consciousness, feelings of strangeness or familiarity and olfactory and visual hallucinations. There are evidently several varieties of this sort of seizure. The nervous mechanisms are as yet unknown.

Allen[9] has demonstrated that the corresponding area in animals is concerned with the retention of conditioned olfactory reflexes. In man, the physiology of the rhinencephalon is virtually unexplored. Recently Glusman[201] has shown that the region of the uncus has parameters of stimulation which are similar to those of the motor cortex.

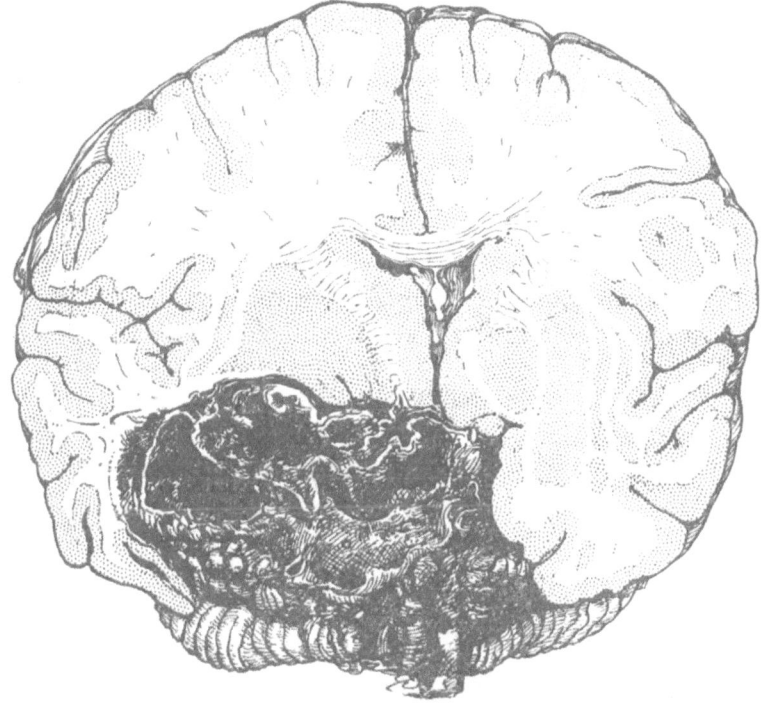

Fig. 26—The expansion of a large adenoma into the right temporal lobe. The patient exhibited visual impairment but apparently did not have extensive neurologic changes.

From original of figure by Cushing, H.: Intracranial Tumors. Springfield, Charles C Thomas, 1932, p. 76.

Moreover, on stimulation of the uncus definite changes in respiration and blood pressure appear. Because this work was done on patients under general anesthesia, the effect of uncal stimulation on the consciousness of the patient could not be investigated. Invasive pathology of the temporal lobe is associated with convulsive disorders of other than uncinate type.[195] Psychomotor[26] and generalized motor seizures have been ascribed to this cerebral division. Convulsions are not a frequent complication of chromophobe adenoma and their temporal origin appears to be rare.

Extension of the tumor towards and into the temporal lobe may affect the optic radiations and produce an homonymous hemianopia involving the macular field. Compression of the subcortical region of the dominant temporal lobe, through which communication is maintained between the frontal and posterior parts of the cerebrum, may cause aphasic disturbances. More extensive temporal lobe involvement may result in personality changes which are believed to be manifested by emotional and intellectual disorganization and regression.

The understanding of cerebral synthesis of language and of personality structure is a major aim of neurology. It is not evasion but caution and ignorance that proscribes further discussion of their disturbances due to the effects of pituitary tumors on the temporal lobes.

THE INFERIOR RELATIONS

Less usual routes of extension of chromophobe adenoma are into the sphenoid sinus and into the interpeduncular space and posterior fossa.

Sphenoid sinus

Variations in the dimensions of the sphenoid sinus have been described by Onodi.[358] When the sinus is reduced in size and the perisinusoidal walls compactly thickened, it is probably a less available avenue of escape from the pituitary fossa. Other factors may play a role as well. The restrictive effects of the diaphragma sellae may favor a downward growth into the sinus rather than intracranial extension. In addition, the origin of the tumor toward the superior or inferior surfaces of the pituitary may have an influence in the direction of its spread. Once the floor of the sella turcica has been eroded and the sphenoid sinus invaded, further extensions into the nasopharyngeal and superior nasal cavities are possible. It has been claimed that such a course of events is not too unusual.[513] The general experience of several clinics including our own indicates that this complication is rare.[114, 239] With the advent of intrusion into the cavities of the sinuses and nose, blood streaked nasal discharge, occassionally cerebrospinal fluid rhinorrhca and obstruction to breathing may appear. Infection of the meninges may develop spontaneously or from local surgical manipulation. The occurrence of meningitis was a major reason for the abandonment of the transphenoidal approach to chromophobe adenomas.

Interpeduncular fossa

The adenomas that reach the interpeduncular fossa in their wayward course have a rich opportunity to produce neurologic symptoms by pressure directly against the cerebral peduncles, the vessels supplying them or by displacement of these structures against the free edge of the tentorium cerebelli. The cerebral peduncles, which form the lateral boundaries of this region, contain a variety of nervous tracts but mainly the corticospinal, cortico-bulbo-reticular, corticobulbar and corticopontine tracts. In addition, an extrapyramidal nucleus and the substantia nigra are situated in the interval between the mesencephalic tegmentum and the peduncle. It is possible that these structures are accessible to the effects of pressure by an enlarged pituitary tumor.

Increasing expansion of the tumor within the interpeduncular fossa is accompanied by the appearance of paresis and spasticity in the affected extremities, due to disturbances in the contralateral cerebral peduncle. The third and, by extension, the fourth and sixth nerves may be compromised as well. Disorders of the extraocular muscles ensue. Occasionally, spontaneous and involuntary movements of the limbs may occur. These dyskinesias have no established mechanism but are related to disturbances of the extrapyramidal system, of which several interpeduncular tracts, the subthalamic nucleus and the substantia nigra are neighborhood representatives. Finally, interference with the great corticopontocerebellar system can induce ataxia and other cerebellar motor discoordinations. Of this group of symptoms, paresis, with or without spasticity, is the most frequent. The mechanisms of spasticity are among the most hotly debated subjects in clinical neurophysiology,[132a, 332] and the interested reader is referred to recent discussion of this.

The spread of chromophobe adenomas is not confined to the regions discussed. Rather these are most closely related to the pituitary. Extension beyond their limits is possible although unusual. An attempt has been made to give an additional dimension to the structural anatomy of the region by relating it to the physiology of its components. The neurologic symptomatology to be described will be set into this pattern.

IV

METABOLISM

PERTINENT PHYSIOLOGIC DATA

Clinical studies and correlated laboratory investigations have proceeded hand in hand (the latter actually leading the way only on rare occasions) in the clarification of disturbances associated with chromophobe adenomas. It may be desirable first to follow the trends established by clinical and pathologic studies before considering the data of controlled laboratory procedure.

Reference of the dominant endocrine and metabolic disturbances of chromophobe adenomas to hypopituitarism rather than to hyperpituitarism was clearly stated and documented by Cushing in 1912.[100] The conspicuous differences between these two fundamental states of glandular activity were further confirmed by subsequent studies of both a metabolic[105] and clinico-pathologic [24, 25] nature and the hypopituitary characteristics of chromophobe adenomas reemphasized in studies of increasing scope.[103, 193, 239] Only Berblinger[43] has suggested a partial hyperpituitarism in pure "chief-cell adenomas," manifested in what he terms a hyperhormonal amenorrhea.

Simmonds' first descriptions of anterior hypophyseal cachexia[438, 439] and the appreciation of clear-cut similarities between this and some cases of chromophobe adenomas[175] added early evidence that Cushing's thesis was sound. Subsequent studies of Simmonds' disease[310, 432, 434] indicate that the predominant trends differ only quantitatively from those in chromophobe adenomas. Likewise Erdheim's studies of craniopharyngiomata[145] indirectly verify the association of pituitary deficiency with chromophobe tumors since the metabolic symptoms produced by these two types of tumors are frequently indistinguishable. Moreover, recent studies of so-called pituitary myxedema[71, 302] associated with fibrosis of the anterior pituitary gland further supplement the evidence in favor of an associated insufficiency state in destructive diseases of the hypophysis.

Falta[154] and Berblinger,[43] summarizing available evidence of clinico-pathologic nature more than fifteen years ago, emphasized that all was not to be attributed to pituitary hypofunction alone. They referred the occasional associated diabetes insipidus to hypothalamic compression or destruction, rather than to hypopituitarism. Globus and his associates[200] recently suggested that either hypothalamic or pituitary lesions may be associated with pathologic obesity, sexual dystrophy, diuresis and "vegetative dysfunction."

Through all of the literature there is almost general agreement that the deficiency state in an individual with a chromophobe adenoma is predominantly one of pituitary hypofunction with a variable hypothalamic component; further that such a state is ultimately a reflection of peripheral endocrine gland deficits in gonadal, thyroidal and adrenal spheres. The parathyroid glands, bone marrow, liver and lymphoid structures have been more obscurely implicated.

These clinical observations and conclusions lead us to seek information concerning the dysfunctions resulting from chromophobe adenomas first from studies in experimental animals, where the consequences of partial and complete hypophysectomy as well as of hypothalamic lesions have been delineated.

Total hypophysectomies

In older studies, the so-called total hypophysectomies implied removal of the adenohypophysis, more or less complete removal of the pars tuberalis and removal of neural lobe with a variable portion of the infundibulum. Concepts of pituitary functions were few and fragmentary up to 1910.[352, 411] Even E. A. Schäfer, in 1909, while conceding a growth regulating function to the anterior lobe, dwelt much more extensively on the posterior lobe with its extracts of remarkable properties. Studies of this early period[202, 335] were occupied with the question of the pituitary gland's possible role as a vital organ. Crowe, Cushing and Homans[99] made the first comprehensive statement about hypopituitary states. In partially hypophysectomized animals these experimenters noted the appearance of obesity, secondary hypoplasia of genitalia in adult animals (persistent infantilism in preadolescents), polyuria, glycosuria, significant alterations in skin structures, decrease in body temperature and lowered resistance to infection and disease. They carried such animals successfully through temporary crises with pituitary gland transplants. Here, indeed, were findings justifying further study since so many of them mirrored observations even then coming to be appreciated as associated with clinical pituitary disease. Aschner in 1912[14] reported complete and careful studies of essentially similar nature, concluding, inter alia, that obesity was much less common than his predecessors had thought. He was inclined to ascribe its occurrence to lesions of the base of the brain. Aschner noted decreased body temperature and adrenalin glycosuria and decreased resistance to trauma in hypophysectomized animals. He considered persistent hypogonadism conspicuous only in animals deprived of their pituitary glands early in life. He described minimal and unimpressive gonadal changes in adult animals. In hypophysectomized frog larvae P. E. Smith in 1916[442] observed decrease in skin pigmentation, decreased or arrested growth and striking atrophy or failure of development of the thyroid gland.

This knowledge was actually not expanded on the basis of total hypophysectomy experiments[154] until 1930, when P. E. Smith[443] reviewed his crucial studies in hypophysectomized rats with intact stalk, pars tuberalis and hypothalamus. In rats operated upon before maturity he observed inhibition of skeletal growth and persistent infantile characteristics. His adult animals usually became cachectic, only rarely slightly obese. Histologic studies revealed regressive atrophy of adrenal cortex, thyroid and genitalia. Follicular growth ceased while corpus lutea persisted for relatively long periods. Spermatogenesis was markedly diminished in male animals; liver, spleen and kidneys appeared smaller than normal. Daily anterior pituitary homotransplants effected total or almost total restoration. These and similar studies led Smith to conclude that obesity was probably a result of hypothalamic injury. He tested this thesis by injecting chromic acid into the hypothalamic area. The resulting observations confirmed Aschner's previous beliefs as well as Smith's similar concepts and lent support to many careful histopathologic studies in related structural disturbances in humans. In hypophysectomized rats, shortly thereafter, hormonal studies[148] revealed the possibility of correcting such pituitary deficiencies in a more specific way. Preparations of crude growth substance free of gonadotrophin restored normal growth and reversed changes previously noted in the adrenal glands and thyroid. No changes were observed in the gonadal defects already described. However, these same animals, treated with gonadotrophin free of growth promoting substance, actually developed genital hyperplasia but showed all other deficiencies relatively unchanged. A year later it was reported[108] that some deficiency manifestations in partially hypophysectomized animals, particularly insulin sensitivity, were crudely correlated in inverse relation to the amount of residual anterior lobe tissue.

Removal of anterior or glandular lobe

Because of technical difficulties relatively few attempts have been made to remove only the anterior or glandular lobe of the pituitary (with variable portions of pars tuberalis and pars intermedia). Paulesco in 1908[202] and Crowe, Cushing, and Homans two years later[99] concluded that such ablations were equivalent to total hypophysectomy. However, long term metabolic studies were prevented by early death of their animals as a result of rapidly developing "cachexia hypophysiopriva." On the basis of the summarized evidence, Geiling, in his review of such procedures in 1926[189] verified the fundamental role of the anterior pituitary gland in the maintenance of metabolic equilibria, referring decreased or arrested growth and atrophy of the adrenal, parathyroid and thyroid glands to its loss.

Removal of neural lobe

Although the striking physiologic properties of neural lobe extracts were recognized early,[412] its antidiuretic property was not readily accepted by some.[101] Crowe and his associates[99] and Paulesco[cited in 202]

considered complete neural lobe removal (along with variable portions
of the infundibulum) to be accompanied by no gross disturbances in
function. These early workers did not appreciate the significance of
the great mass of nerve fibers traveling by way of the stalk to the
neural lobe,[110] nor did they recognize the easily overlooked structures
within the stalk itself. Houssay in 1936[251] referred only cutaneous
pallor to neural lobe ablation in the toad. He emphasized again the
striking lack of correlation between potency of extracts and removal
of extract source. That a structure of such rich nerve supply[388] apparently little of which is bound for the active anterior lobe (or, for
that matter, not even clearly terminating in or on any structure of
note in the neural lobe itself) should have such obscure functions has
been an enigma to many. The complete story still remains to be written
although comprehensive experiments[234] based on a precise recognition
of neural lobe components, have amply confirmed the fundamental
role of the total neural lobe in production of antidiuretic hormone, so
clearly indicated in the work of Ranson and his collaborators.[184]

The operation of pertinent neurovegetative reflex integrations
mediated[63, 399] through the neurohypophysis will be discussed later in
this section. It is evident that the animal organism is able to function
far more efficiently deprived of these integrations[99] than deprived of
the anterior lobe hormonal trophisms upon which this integrating
action plays.

General metabolic studies

Extensive reviews of endocrine and metabolic dysfunctions associated with hypo- and apituitary states, have stressed the regularity
with which such states are associated not only with evident disturbances
in growth, in thyroid, adrenal and gonadal functions, but also with
idiosyncrasies of sugar metabolism, nitrogen balance and dermal structural characteristics.[101, 193, 202, 251] That these are the manifestations of
deficient pituitary function normally capable of reasonably selective
and independent[122] trophic influences rather than of what were once
thought to be nonspecific autonomic discharges[107] now requires no
further proof. Only Mosonyi and associates[350] have advanced evidence
to suggest that some metabolic disturbances subsequent to total hypophysectomy (primarily alterations of serum protein, calcium, BMR

and fasting decrease in nitrogen excretion) tend to decrease or disappear within three to six months after operation. Their supposition is that neurovegetative regulatory devices may eventually substitute for the absent humoral mechanisms.

Rarely performed human chromophobe adenoma assay studies[77, 170, 425] supply indirect and questionable evidence that disturbances such as those mentioned above should probably not be attributed to any demonstrable secretory activity of the tumor tissue itself.

The functions of the neurohypophysis, aside from the control of water diuresis, are of an uncertain nature and extent. Recently Stehle[456a] has reviewed this subject with considerable thoroughness. It would seem that the main deterrent to elucidation of the problem of the endocrine activities of the neurohypophysis is the impurity of the preparations employed in the various experimental investigations. In fact it has not been determined whether the range of actions of the neurohypophysis is dependent on a single protein with multiple activities or upon several individual protein hormones. The work of Van Dyke[489] suggests that a single protein may possess antidiuretic, oxytocic and pressor characteristics. Criticism leveled at the work on which this opinion is based has not effectively controverted it.[269] In short the chemical individuality or identity of the several active principles of the posterior pituitary remains uncertain.

An action of an oxytocic principle of neurohypophyseal origin on the uterus has been described by Dale.[109] Fisher[127, 163] and Pencharz and Long[363] have contributed data which suggest that there is a disturbance in the myophysiology of labor in animals deficient in pituitrin due to hypothalamic lesions, complete ablation of the hypophysis or posterior hypophysectomy. Smith[445] noted no changes in parturition under the latter circumstances. As in all work of this type, species differences and the hormonal cycle of the animal are important factors in comparing the results of the several workers. It is believed possible that in some forms the low luteal and high estrin content of the blood at term may sensitize the uterine body to the contractile effects of the oxytocic principle and so facilitate labor.

Changes in blood pressure and intestinal motility have been described with lesions of the hypothalamus, the infundibular stalk or the neural lobe. Stimulation of the hypothalamus and infundibular stalk[158, 219] has been shown to elevate the blood pressure and increase intestinal motility, but the path of outflow and the nature of the effector organ have not been clearly demonstrated.

Because extracts of the posterior pituitary may cause contraction of involuntary muscles, the effect of hypothalamic lesions or stimulation in modifying blood pressure, gastro-intestinal and uterine motility has been ascribed to the release or retention of posterior pituitary hormones under the influence of the hypothalamus. Since the functions of the active pituitary fractions themselves have not been clarified it is difficult to categorize the experimental situation briefly. However, the hypothalamus is believed to be capable of inducing the secretion of whatever components exist within the posterior pituitary.

Summary

The data derived from clinical observations and from ablative and destructive procedures on the pituitary gland and hypothalamus justify the conclusion that the physiologic phenomena pertinent to the study of chromophobe adenomas are to be derived only in part from an analysis of pituitary and hypothalamic mechanisms per se. Perhaps even more direct and important data must be sought in an analysis of peripheral endocrine deficits appearing either singly or in combination. Finally certain clues are to be expected from a study of specific metabolic processes, for example, utilization of carbohydrate, protein, fat and the metabolism of minerals and from an analysis of mechanisms of water balance and renal function. The preceding discussion thus calls for a more detailed analysis of data relating to specific metabolic processes.

THE THYROID GLAND

In hypopituitary states there is consistent hypothyroidism[105, 146, 193, 416, 456] sometimes distinguished with difficulty from frank primary myxedema.[71, 302, 343] In acidophilic hyperpituitarism[105] a clear-cut tendency toward hyperthyroid states with occasional enlargement of the thyroid gland is seen. While the occurrence of fatty livers in hypopituitary states[100, 124] is not so clearly related to alterations in thyroid function, the concomitant disturbances in lipid metabolism suggested by many[263, 264] justify discussion under the heading of thyroid function. Likewise alterations in cardiac output observed in both primary and secondary hypothyroidism by Lequime[301] and others extend the compass of thyroid functional relationships.

Observations of a general nature

The failure of development of the thyroid gland in hypophysectomized tadpoles,[444] its functional as well as anatomic involution in hypophysectomized adult animals[252, 444] and the reversal of these observed changes following anterior pituitary transplantation (apparently not through mediation of growth promoting substance),[444] establish a close and perhaps specific pituitary-thyroid interdependency. How precisely the resultant hypothyroid state influences the integrity of the animal organism is matter for closer scrutiny.

Thyrotrophin

Although pituitary thyrotrophin (TSH) has not been isolated in chemically or physiologically pure form, the evidence is conclusive that it is a distinctive secretion of the pars distalis and probably a glycoprotein. Some have suggested that an antithyroid hormone, which would inhibit activity may also be secreted by the anterior pituitary.[418] At present there is not sufficient support of this thesis to consider it in such a summary discussion of the pituitary-thyroidal system. A single thyroid trophin may act both upon the thyroid and the extraocular tissues concerned with the production of exophthalmos in hyperthyroidism. Distinct fractions of this hormone may, on the other hand, be responsible for these two effects.[417] In this regard it has been shown that TSH may be inactivated by tissue of the thyroid, thymus, or lymph nodes.[389] TSH which ordinarily is not found in the urine may appear there when administered to thyroidectomized animals.[419] On the basis of these and similar experiments, Salter[403] and others believe that the TSH which is not inactivated by thyroid or extrathyroid lymphatic or thymic tissue may exert its main action on the extraocular and other periorbital regions related to production of exophthalmos.

The modes of action or sequence of events induced in the thyroid itself by TSH are being gradually revealed. Administration of TSH will cause thyroidal cell hypertrophy and hyperplasia, an increase in rate of release of thyroxin, enhancement in the ability of the thyroid to concentrate iodine, and acceleration of the conversion of diiodotyrosine to thyroxin.[76, 389] A balance between the output of TSH and the level of circulating thyroxin may be attained by the inhibiting action of thyroxin on the further release of TSH from the anterior pituitary.[404] The intimate mechanism by which TSH produces changes in the thyroid is unknown. It has been suggested that intracellular proteolytic enzymes are activated by TSH. These enzymes may cause a cleavage of thyroglobulin, which then can diffuse out of the thyroid itself.[125] Others have stated that TSH contributes a chemical component to the formation of thyroxin and that its own inactivation by thyroid is suggestive of this.[389] The reactivation of TSH may be effected by reducing agents including antithyroid drugs.[389]

Basal metabolic rate

The depression of "total metabolism" in hypophysectomized dogs observed many years ago by Benedict and Homans[cited in 178, 189] was later evaluated by Houssay and his associates.[252] This latter group noted that the depression of basal metabolic rate observed in a majority of hypophysectomized dogs and rats was increased by subsequent thyroidectomy, the total depression equalling that observed after thyroidectomy alone. These observations have been recently confirmed in part by White, Heinbecker and Rolf.[cited in 33] The importance of the metabolic mixture offered to such an animal deserves emphasis, since it has been observed that hypophysectomized rats which consumed a high carbohydrate diet, in contrast to high fat, showed basal metabolic rates approximately 18 per cent below all others.[405]

The signs of thyroid hyperfunction induced in both normal and hypophysectomized dogs by injections of anterior pituitary extracts are not observed if such animals are thyroidectomized previously.[252] The paradoxical depression of basal metabolic rate in both normal and hypophysectomized animals after prolonged administration of anterior pituitary extract[252] has been interpreted as a probable manifestation of antihormone production, an action traced to the protein component of relatively pure thyrotrophin.[507] Although other endocrines interplay with the thyroid, thyrotrophin is the only hormone which induces changes in the thyroid characteristic of activity and subsequently elevates the BMR. The administration of ACTH, for example, is ineffectual in augmenting the BMR in myxedematous patients.[285]

Iodine metabolism

Following hypophysectomy the concentration of total plasma iodine falls within two days. After four days about one-half of both total and protein bound iodine remains.[76] This level apparently is maintained. Thyroidectomy likewise produces a definite and persistent diminution in total blood iodine.[252] Interestingly, the total content of iodine and thyroxin of the thyroid in hypophysectomized animals is maintained. Chaikoff concludes that a lowered concentration of circulating thyroxin is not a stimulus to the thyroid to release this hormone.

The administration of iodine to a normal animal may cause diminution of TSH in the hypophysis. This may be a direct effect of iodine or of pituitary inhibition by the increased concentration of circulating thyroxin resulting from the action of iodine on the thyroid. There have been other experimental indications that the peripheral action of iodine may partially inhibit the effect of TSH on the thyroid gland.[433] However, Astwood[15] tentatively suggests, on the basis of work by Chapman,[77] that the effect of iodine is not due to its antagonism to TSH or suppression of thyroidal cellular activity. He presents the view that low concentrations of thyroidal intracellular iodine may serve as the stimulus for the thyroid parenchyma. The administration of iodine may remove this stimulus and in a sense inhibit glandular activity. The action of TSH on iodine distribution has been mentioned. Essentially the equilibrium is shifted from the inorganic state of iodine to organic combinations through the formation of diiodotyrosine and then thyroxin. The rate of formation of protein-bound iodine in the gland and plasma also is increased by administration of TSH.

Lipid constituents of blood and tissues

There are no consistent nor characteristic changes in the lipid constituents of the blood or liver following hypophysectomy alone as is evident from a comparison of the following data. Houssay's group[252] have reported slight variations in blood lipid constituents with a tendency toward decreased values in total fats, fatty acids and cholesterol. Chaikoff and his co-workers[75] noted that all lipid constituents of the blood were within the maximum normal range though cholesterol esters, in particular, tended toward the upper extreme. They found liver lipids to be normal in types and distribution. In contrast, others have reported less fat than normal in the liver of hypophysectomized animals and more in peripheral fat depots during short term experiments.[405] This was especially notable after high carbohydrate feedings.

The data concerning lipid metabolism and distribution in directly thyroidectomized animals must be interpreted in the light of two variables: (1) an apparent nonuniformity within the vertebrate scale and (2) a marked dependence upon caloric intake. Variable though consistent elevation of all lipid constituents of the blood of thyroidectomized dogs has been reported. The intensity of this elevation is directly proportional to caloric intake.[73, 74, 143, 144] Hypophysectomy alone appears to contribute very little to this response and plays a less prominent part here than in the chronic deposition of fat in the liver of such animals. The close dependence of blood lipid levels upon caloric intake offers one possible reconciliation of these facts with the contradictory observations of Thompson and Long[474] that the hypercholesterolemia of thyroidectomized dogs (diminished by subsequent adrenalectomy) is abolished by hypophysectomy.

In the monkey the response is somewhat different. Jailer, Sperry and co-workers [271, 453] have observed elevation of serum cholesterol in only 1 of 7 thyroidectomized monkeys. Their studies suggest that in this species cholesterol metabolism itself is not conspicuously altered either by thyroidectomy, bilateral ovariectomy or both. They did note, however, a significant decrease in serum cholesterol values following thyroxin therapy in normal and thyroidectomized monkeys, and a less conspicuous decrease following therapy with thyrotrophic hormone. These workers invite interpretation of the interesting observation that serum cholesterol levels rose well above normal values and remained so elevated for one month following cessation of thyrotrophin therapy in 2 otherwise intact animals. However the work has not been elaborated by the investigators.

Summary

The anterior pituitary gland exerts a powerful trophic influence over the thyroid gland. It is quite probable that the thyroid gland is capable of minimal function in the absence of any anterior pituitary influence. As regards the specific nature of the trophism of the pituitary for the thyroid, thyrotrophic hormone is known to induce thyroidal cell hypertrophy and hyperplasia, to release thyroxin, to cause incorporation of iodine in the thyroid; in brief, to shift the equilibrium, inorganic iodine $\rightleftharpoons$ organic iodine, to the right. Plasma iodine is decreased after hypophysectomy and thyroidectomy though the concentration of iodine in the thyroid of the hypophysectomized animal is in itself not decreased. Iodine itself may act either by inhibiting directly or indirectly the TSH output of the pituitary or by inhibiting the action of TSH on the thyroid gland.

Though complete absence of thyroid gland substance is associated with maximal depression of basal metabolic rate it is not at all clear that the submaximal depression following hypophysectomy is a reflection of hypothyroidism alone. In fact the contrary is probably true. Moreover, metabolic depression of whatever origin, is closely related to the nature of the ingested metabolic mixture.

Concerning lipid metabolism we are justified in assuming only that any observed blood lipid elevations in hypopituitary states are more closely related to hypothyroidism than to any other glandular hypofunction; moreover, that such elevations are an indication not so much of disturbed metabolic processes as of increased or adequate caloric intake. Likewise the evidence warrants the interpretation of total blood iodine levels and iodine uptake by the thyroid gland as measures of intrinsic thyroid function.

The relationship of the thyroid gland to carbohydrate metabolism is discussed under separate heading; that concerning cardiac output and circulation time incorporated in the section on renal function.

ADRENAL FUNCTION

In 1933, Harrop and his co-workers[223] outlined concisely the signs and symptoms of primary adrenal insufficiency as then recognized by workers in the field. In their study pigmentation of the skin and mucous membranes, hypoglycemia, increased tolerance for glucose, insulin sensitivity, asthenia, muscle weakness, gastro-intestinal disturbances, sensitivity to thyroid preparations and unfavorable response to salt deprivation after three to four days, were considered of great diagnostic importance. Such criteria are still satisfactory. There can be no question that the salt-deprivation response has subsequently proved to be a valuable diagnostic tool[354, 362] in primary adrenal insufficiency. Stephens[459] has clearly shown a similar unfavorable response in hypopituitary states, some of them coincident with chromophobe adenomas. Such studies have demonstrated serum electrolyte disturbances closely following the patterns defined by Loeb and Atchley[315] for primary insufficiency. The latter workers[312, 315] emphasize certain atypical dissociations in hypoadrenal states: the lack of invariable parallelism between serum electrolyte, blood sugar and nonprotein nitrogen alterations and severe or fatal insufficiency, the extreme sensitivity of the hypoadrenal individual to loss of interstitial fluid. The fact that identical abnormalities have been observed in some of our patients with chromophobe adenomas demands a closer study of these aspects of adrenal function, as revealed in controlled studies.

Observations of general nature

In the face of the torrent of information presently[376, 377] pouring forth with regard to hypophyseal-adrenal-organism relationships our discussion of this problem must appear brief and largely concerned with the development of knowledge in this field which led to interest in ACTH and adrenocorticoids.

Humoral control of adrenal secretions is exercised by the adenohypophysis possibly by the basophilic cells.[287] The output of ACTH may be governed by the demands of the peripheral tissues for adrenal hormones. Thus the administration of corticoids will inhibit secretion of ACTH by the pituitary, presumably through this mechanism.[410] However it is also possible that the adrenal steroids may have inhibitory action on the anterior pituitary directly.

Recently Li and his associates[306] have demonstrated that a substance of molecular weight about 1000, possibly a polypeptide, possesses adrenocorticotrophic effects. Whether this fragment is in fact ACTH or some functionally active component of this molecule which can induce adrenal cortical secretion remains a question. Recent developments indicate that the administration of ACTH or its liberation from the adenohypophysis through the intervention of stress on the intact organism has marked effects on the adrenal gland. Within this gland a sudanophilic substance, which is probably a cholesterol ester, decreases in amount. The concentration of ascorbic acid, cholesterol esters, but not free cholesterol, and either neutral fats or phospholipids likewise are diminished. The sudanophilic substance and the cholesterol esters are presumed to participate structurally in the formation of adrenosteroids.[410] Further, it now appears that ACTH itself assists in the synthesis of corticoids of the adrenal gland. Experiments by Haynes, Savard and Dorfman[230a] indicate that in adrenal slices ACTH increases the incorporation of C^{14} from acetate-I-C^{14} into hydrocortisone as well as augmenting the output of formaldehydogenic steroids.

The importance of a wide variety of stressful conditions in inducing the liberation of ACTH, and consequently adrenal steroids, has been emphasized. The means by which these disparate stimuli concentrate their effects on the pituitary system are presumed to be either neural or humoral. As mentioned previously, some authors believe the hypothalamus is a receptor station for the nervous excitation produced by the variegated alarm stimuli. The hypothalamus may respond by secreting a hormone which finds its way into the general circulation and finally reaches the adenohypophysis and leads there to the production and/or release of ACTH.[261] Others discount the universal importance of such a relationship and suggest rather that the release of ACTH may be due to direct pituitary stimulation by epinephrine.[320] Another theory is based on the demand for corticoids created in the periphery by many types of threats to the organism. The peripheral utilization of the adrenal hormones creates a deficiency of these in the circulation. The lowered blood concentration of corticoids either induces a liberation of ACTH directly or removes the inhibitory influences exerted by these compounds on the adenohypophysis. Numerous reviews discussing ACTH and pituitary adrenal relations have been published.[5, 6, 376, 377]

In addition to the effect of ACTH, other pituitary secretions are said to stimulate the production of "mineralocorticoids" by the adrenal. Selye[424] has discussed the influence of a somatotrophic factor (STH), believed to be similar to the growth promoting hormone, which causes adrenal output of the doca-like steroids. The evidence adduced is indirect in that the administration of STH, an electrophoretically homogenous protein, produces the renal hyalinois syndrome in unilaterally nephrectominized rats on a 1 per cent NaCl fluid intake. This syndrome is similar to that observed under analagous conditions after the administration of doca itself. The renal syndrome is intensified by ACTH and cortisone in both instances. Other parallelisms are drawn as well. Selye believes that STH is responsible for activating the adrenal secretion of mineralocorticoids, ACTH of glucocorticoids. Although the evidence is inferential and based on morphologic changes, this author's speculations are supported by a tightly linked succession of experiments.

The adrenal cortex, even during pregnancy,[187] undergoes atrophy following hypophysectomy. The specific interpretation of this atrophy has not been thoroughly consistent. Perla[367] and Deane and Greep[118] have considered only the fasciculata to be involved. Whereas the latter authors have identified cortical steroid substances in both fasciculata and glomerulosa, Bennett[39] earlier could find none in any except the fasciculate zone. The final clarification of this point is of considerable interest because Houssay and his collaborators[252] as well as others[33] have reported that hypophysectomized animals seldom develop the electrolyte imbalances characteristic of adrenal insufficiency although they show striking alterations in carbohydrate metabolism referable to adrenal cortical deficiency. The persistent glomerulosa may provide a source of mineralocorticoids in the hypophysectomized animal. Swann in 1940[463] suggested that the adrenals of hypophysectomized rats secrete sufficient salt and water hormone to maintain life though perhaps not enough to effect resistance to certain stresses. On theroretical grounds, he was inclined to assign to the fasciculata the task of elaborating the carbohydrate-regulating factor. This important thesis has not thus far been confirmed. Deane and Greep's observations, while supplying the anatomic mechanism for such a dissociation, are subject to more than one interpretation, considering the known multiplicity of cortical steroid factors.

Electrolyte balance

It was not until 1933 that the changes in serum electrolyte pattern, so striking in adrenal deficient animals, came to be appreciated. Early reviews[52, 226] mentioned alterations in carbohydrate metabolism, lymphoid tissues, plasma volume and blood flow, decrease in basal oxygen consumption, basal temperature and blood pressure. Loeb, Atchley, Benedict and Leland[316] issued the first unequivocal statement about the now familiar serum electrolyte and nonprotein nitrogen disturbances in adrenalectomized dogs. They described a decrease in serum sodium, chloride and plasma bicarbonate, with concomitant elevation of serum potassium and nonprotein nitrogen.

The assumptions that some specific adrenal cortical factor for which sodium chloride cannot entirely substitute[312] is essential to adequate maintenance of electrolyte balance and that the electrolyte changes in experimental adrenal insufficiency might reflect in part a renal factor[316, 477] have been the stimulating origins of numerous experimental studies which will be summarized in the following sections.

Body fluids and water balance

Swingle and his collaborators[464-466, 469] have presented convincing evidence for the proposition that under some circumstances adrenalectomized animals are inadequately equipped to redistribute body fluids from the cellular compartment to the depleted extracellular spaces and vascular bed. They have consistently maintained that adrenal cortical extract acts by mobilizing water and salt from the cellular compartment

to facilitate hemodilution and reestablishment of electrolyte equilibrium. The mechanisms by which such changes could be effected are
purely speculative. Silvette, as early as 1934[435] demonstrated that the
water content of muscle and liver tissues (not specifically cells) of
adrenalectomized animals was markedly increased over normal. He
observed a concomitant decrease in tissue chloride. This author also
maintained that such a state was not prejudicial to the well-being of
the animal and could likewise be produced by many other procedures
not directly related to adrenal cortical lack. It has been repeatedly
emphasized that in the adrenalectomized animal there is a disproportionate retention of potassium which may, in part, be responsible for
the neuromuscular symptoms noted in this deficiency state. Doca effectively restores the disturbed electrolyte pattern.[313]

Renal function and adrenal insufficiency

The observation of Loeb and his collaborators[316] that diuresis with
increased sodium and chloride loss follows bilateral adrenalectomy, has
been repeatedly confirmed. They suggested that the adrenal gland
might well maintain regulatory functions over both sodium metabolism
and renal function. Except for the contrary view of Swingle et al.,[466]
other workers[188, 224, 226] have presented substantial evidence that the
kidney is unquestionably one effector of both electrolyte and fluid
disturbances associated with adrenal insufficiency. Disturbances in renal
tubular function during insufficiency have been demonstrated by several methods.[194, 222] Talbott[472] has investigated renal status in human
hypoadrenalism. His observations demonstrated that renal plasma flow
and glomerular filtration are decreased and that the filtration fraction
is strikingly diminished. Although the administration of doca did affect
these it did not restore glomerular filtration to normal. Moreover, in the
normal individual sodium clearance is not affected by this mineralo-
corticoid. In a different though related vein, studies[328, 346] stimulated
by the observation that fasting pregnancy ketosis is abolished in adrenalectomized rats[326] have established the occurence of an increased renal
threshold for ketone bodies in adrenalectomized animals.

Whether or not a neurophypophyseal or, more accurately, an
antidiuretic factor enters into the mechanism of altered renal function

as suggested by Martin and his collaborators[338] will be discussed in a subsequent section.

Crisis and irreversible adrenal insufficiency

Hartmann and Winter in 1933[227] noted that certain animals died in adrenal insufficiency in spite of intensive therapy with adrenal cortical extract. Himwich and his co-workers[246] shortly thereafter observed that low serum electrolytes, as such, were not invariably associated with such crises, an observation confirmed by numerous clinical and experimental observations, although disputed by Gilman.[198]

Speculations concerning the causes of crises have been many and varied. Swingle and his group[467, 468] at first suggested failure of blood-diluting mechanisms and later, possible capillary atony. Cleghorn et al. in 1939[82] wrote an extensive review of such theories and reported their own observations. One of their prefatory remarks was that crises can occur without hemodilution and without severe changes in serum electrolytes. They listed potassium toxicity, failure of fluid-mobilizing mechanisms (with irreversible fluid loss into the gastro-intestinal tract) and edema of the lungs as relatively frequent, hypoglycemia as uncommon. They likewise stressed a decline in reflex excitability of the heart, with bradycardia and heart block as an occasional factor. Cardiac failure from compensatory overwork or potassium accumulation with its resultant capillary dilatation, stasis and fluid loss were associated possibilities. Some of the mechanisms assumed to operate are not definitely established but the main presuppositions are generally agreed upon. The problem of critical irreversibility is probably one of degree rather than of kind.

Stress and the adrenal glands

The sensitivity of the adrenalectomized organism to salt deprivation is familiar. Suffice it to say that this is one stress which appears to challenge the functional integrity of the adrenal cortex in a specific way. Ingle and his co-workers[137] early noted increased energy output, running time and endurance of normal animals primed with adrenal cortical extract, though hypoglycemia occurred simultaneously. The extreme sensitivity of adrenalectomized rats to histamine[529, 530] was also observed in hypophysectomized rats.[368] The degree of hypersensitivity roughly correlated with the extent of adrenal cortical change, and was almost completely abolished by adrenal cortical extract. Evidence was subsequently presented[395] that a specific adrenal cortical factor, presumably not the salt and water or carbohydrate-regulating factors, might be responsible for this action.

Cold intolerance of hypophysectomized rats has been thought to be largely a manifestation of adrenal insufficiency, possibly contributed to in small measure by secondary gonadal failure, but little influenced by secondary thyroid deficiency.[28] Horvath[250] noted both subnormal basal heat production in adrenalectomized rats and their failure to respond calorigenically to decreased environmental temperature as normals did. He had no conviction concerning the specific mechanism of this disturbance.

Pressor factors

The rapid and progressive drop in blood pressure in the totally hypophysectomized toad, noted by Houssay and his group,[251] was not observed after anterior lobe removal alone. These workers, however, reported no histologic changes in the adrenal cortex of the toad subsequent to anterior lobe removal. In the adrenalectomized dog there is increased susceptibility to any threat which places a strain on the circulation.[467] Adrenal cortical extract may consistently maintain its pressor effect independently of serum electrolytes, hemoconcentration or fluid distribution. In hypophysectomized rats,[298] normal blood pressure cannot be completely maintained with adrenal cortical extract, doca or growth hormone. In adrenalectomized rats, however, normal or even supernormal blood pressure levels may be attained with doca alone, although this is rarely the case with supernormal levels. These observations would again suggest that the pressor action of the adrenal cortex is only one subsidiary factor in blood pressure maintenance and that doca, effective as a pressor agent in the presence of as yet unidentified pituitary factors, loses that effect after hypophysectomy.

Summary

The precise nature of the changes in the adrenal cortex incident to pituitary deficiency is not fully clarified. Only the toad shows intact adrenal glands following anterior lobe removal. The evidence to date would suggest that the zona fasciculata suffers most conspicuous atrophy and that if consequent disturbances in adrenal function do occur they are more marked in the sphere of carbohydrate metabolism than in others.

Concerning mechanisms and manifestations of adrenal hypofunction (exclusive of carbohydrate metabolism) it is reasonable to state that the disturbances in electrolyte and fluid balance are the result of two factors: (1) Alteration of renal function primarily referable to the tubules and (2) shift of extracellular fluid to the cellular compartment. The first mechanism is apparently antecedent to the second. Crisis may well be a manifestation of the operation of these factors, aggravated by a variable cardiac component.

The organism in adrenal insufficiency, whether primary or secondary, poorly combats stresses of many and varied types; these may include cold, hemorrhage, shock and salt depletion. Finally, one must hesitate to ascribe exclusive responsibility to the altered adrenal cortex in explaining the hypotensive phenomena subsequent to hypo- or apituitary states.

GONADS

Many clinical studies have affirmed that disturbances in gonadal function are frequently associated with hypopituitary states. Such disturbances reflect a loss of trophic influences of the normal anterior pituitary gland over the affected gonadal structures. Smith[443] in early animal studies, could discover no corpus lutea or follicles in one ovary of the hypophysectomized rat. The opposite ovary appeared normal if extirpated subsequent to a series of injections of anterior pituitary extracts. This significant observation as well as others relating the adenohypophysis to eugonadism have been amply confirmed.[187, 440, 446] Evolving from this work, it has been generally appreciated that implants of anterior pituitary gland substance are able to stimulate interstitial gonadal elements and accessory reproductive structures.[149] Subsequent investigations have indicated that there are three primary gonadotrophins secreted by the anterior pituitary: (1) FSH (follicle stimulating hormone), (2) LH or ICSH (luteinizing or interstitial cell stimulating hormone) and (3) prolactin or luteotrophin. These have complex relationships with each other and with the primary gonadal hormones.

The pituitary gonadotrophins have been chemically purified to a high degree. FSH and LH appear to be glycoproteins and function both individually and synergistically. FSH induces growth of graafian follicles and spermatogenic tissue.[72, 207, 430] LH is related to progressive follicular development, luteinization, and to growth and stimulation of ovarian and testicular interstitial tissue.[159, 168, 169, 305a] These results have been verified[78, 208] in both normal and hypophysectomized animals. Prolactin, a simple protein, is the third gonadotrophin. It induces glandular hypertrophy of the mammae primed by estrogens, initiates lactation, apparently maintains the corpora lutea in a functional secretory state, and stimulates hormonal secretory production by the Leydig cells of the testes.[15, 46, 511a]

Although the cellular origin of these hormones within the pituitary is uncertain it is known that basophilic cells of the adenohypophysis show intracellular vacuolation following castration,[4, 160] while at the same time the output of FSH increases. It is thought, therefore, that this latter hormone is secreted by the basophils and that the modifications in appearance of these cells indicate a morphologic change consequent to oversecretion. In accord with these observations estrogens have been shown to inhibit the pituitary production of FSH. Castration, by removing the restraining influence of the estrogens, presumably permits an increased output of FSH with consequent "exhaustion" changes in the basophils. The cellular origin of the other gonadotrophins is not indicated even by such inferential evidence although the carmine type acidophilic cell is said to secrete luteotrophin.

The fluctuations in gonadotrophic content (FSH and LH) of the female rat pituitary[297] exemplify their relationship to the sexual functioning of the animal. The gonadotrophins rise to a peak shortly after birth and decrease slowly until the onset of puberty, at which time there is a sudden precipitous decrease. A low pubertal content is recoverable during active sexual life in spite of increasing pituitary size. Finally, there is a marked increase in potency coincident with involutional ovarian failure. These data have been interpreted as suggesting that the maturing gonads actually metabolize pituitary gonadotrophins at highest rates during the periods when the pituitary content is simultaneously lowest. Thus their accumulation in blood stream or pituitary gland or their appearance in the urine is prevented by their utilization in the periphery.

It is probable that other endocrine glands affect the gonadotrophin content of the pituitary but there is little direct evidence except for the observation that a slight decrease occurs following thyroidectomy.[457] The complex interplay between the gonadotrophins and the peripheral sex hormones may be illustrated by the following mechanism[150] assumed to operate in the menstrual cycle: FSH in association with small amounts of LH evokes follicular development to the stage at which estrogen is liberated in amounts sufficient both to inhibit further production of FSH and augment the release of LH and prolactin by the pituitary. Under the influence of these latter hormones luteinization and ovulation occur. Progesterone, from luteal cells, then may partially inhibit the adenohypophyseal output of LH and prolactin. Diminished ovarian estrogen formation at this time once again permits the secretion of FSH and the cycle resumes.

The relationship of testosterone to the pituitary is similar to that of the female gonadal hormones. Its actions are directed toward the development of secondary sex organs and, in lesser degree, to spermatogenesis. When small doses of testosterone propionate are implanted intratesticularly the hormone maintains only regional spermatogenesis in hypophysectomized rats. Under these conditions the maintenance of accessory sex glands requires far greater doses.[134] In larger amounts it is inhibitory to the adenohypophysis. Its effect is to depress the secretion of gonadotrophin and it is similarly inhibitory to the testis itself.

The difficulty in presenting general schemata for the actions of trophic and primary sex hormones arises from the synergistic, antagonistic, and inhibitory effects which these hormones have upon each other and upon their cells of origin.

Significant urinary excretion of the gonadotrophins in humans has been found to occur after the age of 11 years in females and 14 years in males. In the normal female there may be a peak of urinary excretion of gonadotrophins about the middle of the menstrual cycle. Pregnanediol excretion[491] is at a maximum 24 to 48 hours following ovulation. The gonadotrophin peak occurs immediately before the pregnanediol peak. Although this suggests that the increased output of gonadotrophin is related to ovulation, some[508] have taken issue in view of the occurrence of several accessory gonadotrophic excretory peaks which could not be correlated with increase of estrogen or endometrial state.[236] The gonadotrophin excreted in functioning females, menopausal females, castrates, and functioning males has been identified mainly with FSH. However, especially in males, traces of LH have been detected by bioassay. The methods for determining trophins are unsatisfactory and the units vary depending on the test employed. In general, castrates, non-menstruating menopausal females,[237] and sexually active males and females have comparable decreasing gonadotrophic titers in the order presented. In cases of hypogonadism secondary to pituitary deficiency the gonadotrophic urinary content is decreased while in those with primary gonadal failure normal or elevated amounts of trophins are excreted.

Further experience annotating the inhibitory effect of testosterone on pituitary secretion of gonadotrophins was reported by Catchpole and associates.[72] They noted increased urinary excretion of pituitary gonadotrophin in men with testicular insufficiency and were able completely to inhibit this excretion by injections of testosterone propionate. The effect occurred quite promptly and persisted for ten months during therapy. Following completion of a three month course of such injections they observed a gradual rise in urinary gonadotrophin titer beginning within the first two weeks.

An important index of pituitary activity is the urinary content of androgens and 17-ketosteroids. These excretory products are found in both males and females increasing in concentration from birth to adulthood. With the approach of senility there is a notable decrease in the values of both these groups of compounds. The organs from which the androgenic metabolites and precursors of 17-ketosteroids are presumed to evolve are mainly the testes and the adrenals and secondarily, if at all, the ovaries. The influence of various endocrinopathies on the output of androgens and 17-ketosteroids can be inferred from table 2. In relation to the present study it is worthwhile emphasizing that in pituitary insufficiency both androgens and 17-ketosteroids are appreciably lower than normal and somewhat lower than in primary Addisonian disease. Although the chemical relations of the urinary products to the primary secretions have been established in some cases, the complexity of this field is beyond the range of the present discussion.

TABLE 2—*Summary of Androgens and 17-Ketosteroids in Human Urines**

Males			Females		
	% of adult male levels			% of adult female levels	
Status	Androgens	17-keto-steroids	Status	Androgens	17-keto-steroids
Boys—5 yrs.	3	5	Girls—5 yrs.	5	5
10 yrs.	10	10	10 yrs.	10	15
14 yrs.	20	50	14 yrs.	25	60
Old men	15	30	Old women	25	—
Castrated Men	40	17	Eunuchoid	33	—
Eunuchoid	40	—	Ovariectomized†	50	100
Addison's disease	50	38	Addison's disease	70	36
Pituitary Insufficiency	3	5–10	Pituitary Insufficiency	—	10
Hyperthyroidism	50	80	Cushing's Syndrome‡	40	163
Myxedema		57	Hyperthyroidism	10	60
Interstitial cell			Myxedema	—	16
tumors of testes		10,000	Chorionepithelioma	—	100
Seminoma		150	Hydatiform mole	—	100
Teratoma of testes		133	Hirsuitism without		
Macrogenitosoma			tumor	100	200
prepubertal boys		100	Adrenal cancer	4000	20,000

* After Dorfman.[129]　　† Callow.　　‡ Basophilism without adrenal tumor.

Conclusions

It is established that the pituitary gland exercises a direct trophic influence over the sex organs. The excretion of increased amounts of pituitary gonadotrophins is one acceptable evidence for gonadal deficiency. By inference we may assume that the excretion of clearly subnormal amounts in the presence of gonadal deficiency is presumptive evidence of pituitary deficiency in this sphere. Castration is associated with only a partial reduction in urinary excretion of total neutral 17-ketosteroids, more marked in males than females. Such excretory levels are of little diagnostic significance unless radically reduced. They then mirror a convincing reduction in elaboration of active hormonal precursors by the gonads and particularly by the adrenal cortex.

The effects of ventrolateral hypothalamic structures on gonadal function and structure have previously been summarized.

METABOLISM OF CARBOHYDRATES

Clinical remarks

Except for studies such as that of John in 1925,[275] where the precise basis of pituitary dysfunction was in most instances unclear, hypopituitary states with Simmonds-like syndromes[175] or chromophobe adenomas[113] are consistently associated with increased sensitivity to administered insulin. In similar states where anterior pituitary destruction is extensive[146, 432] low fasting blood sugars are common. So common is this that the contrary, frank diabetes, is worthy of special note.[157] There is not, however, such agreement concerning observations of glycosuria or oral tolerance responses. Eidelberg[138] as well as Davidoff and Cushing[113] have agreed with reservation that increased tolerance is a manifestation of hypopituitarism. Exceptions have been noted (as in the studies by Anders and Jameson[11] and Davidoff and Cushing themselves) but in these cases there were not infrequently evidences of fugitive hyperpituitarism.[11, 14, 18] Nonetheless careful inventories in large series of Simmonds' disease[73, 146] where fugitive hyperpituitarism would scarcely be considered, have disclosed a certain number with delayed blood sugar falls following oral ingestion.

In hyperpituitarism of acidophilic type observations are uniformly in accord. The evidence for decreased insulin sensitivity is satisfactory[113, 166] and diabetes is a relatively frequent accompaniment.[113] Such diabetic states are more variable than in clinical pancreatic diabetes and at times are perhaps even spontaneously reversible. Partial removal of an acidophilic tumor has been noted to increase insulin sensitivity and decrease blood sugar levels.

The conclusion of Mayer et al.[342] that pituitary hypertrophy is a factor of little importance in clinical diabetes mellitus is debatable. It is evident that visual field changes (their criterion) are usually associated with hypertrophy of a degree not uniformly reached even in acromegalics, and that patients with field defects from such cause might be expected to be segregated for special studies quite promptly. Undoubtedly some of the confusion in interpretation is matter of terminology alone.

Finally, it is possible from the histologic standpoint to adapt the pituitary changes noted by Kraus in diabetes mellitus[290] to whatever thesis is proposed concerning the anterior pituitary gland's role in disturbed carbohydrate metabolism. These pituitary changes include decrease in number and size of eosinophils, alteration in cytoplasmic characteristics of basophils, and presence of so-called fetal cells.

Structural framework of experimental studies

Extensive reviews of theories and facts concerning carbohydrate metabolism have traced the gradually expanding knowledge of this problem from 1920 to the present. The first such review was made in 1931 by Houssay and Biasotti[257] who established the lines for further study. The alleviation of pancreatic diabetes by hypophysectomy suggested a contributory role of the pituitary in carbohydrate metabolism. A dual action of the anterior pituitary gland was postulated (1) directly on tissues to stimulate the production of sugar as well as to retard its consumption when insulin was lacking; (2) indirectly through pancreas, liver and nervous system. Observations of the effects of anterior pituitary substance suggested that anterior pituitary deficiency might well reduce endogenous protein metabolism.

In 1936 a subsequent review by Houssay[253] considered in more detail the important metabolic characteristics of the pancreatectomized-hypophysectomized animal mentioned above. Elevation of respiratory quotients, sometimes to normal levels was subject for considerable speculation. Alleviation of the diabetes of the phlorhizin-diabetic animal by hypophysectomy was also mentioned, though prolonged studies were impossible because profound and rapidly fatal hypoglycemia intervened. Tuberal lesions and thyroidectomy were considered to provoke no changes in pancreatic diabetes. The role of the anterior pituitary gland in controlling endogenous protein conversion to glucose was stressed again shortly afterwards by Russell[401] whose basic conceptions concerning the direct role of the anterior pituitary in conservation of tissue carbohydrate reserves centered in the belief that adenohypophyseal secretions inhibited oxidative carbohydrate combustion.

Houssay, in 1942,[254] dismissed the neurohypophysis as a factor of any significance, but considered the participation of hypothalamic structures still unsettled, especially in humans. A growing appreciation of the direct effect of anterior pituitary extract on pancreatic islets themselves was clearly reflected in this review. Soskin[449] (also Houssay[256]) particularly emphasized the role of the liver as the prime reactive mobilizer of glucose. The endocrine activators of the liver were classified primarily as of insular or contra-insular nature by Soskin. He considered the contra-insular effect to be exerted by anterior pituitary, thyroid and adrenal glands. This was manifest primarily in alterations of liver glucose output and in primary insulin deficiency operating independently of blood sugar levels. Later Houssay's broad synthesis of available information[256] stressed the twofold function of an hormonally mediated equilibrium acting both on the liver to control the amount of glucose delivered to the blood, and on the tissues, the consumers, to control its peripheral metabolism.

At this time it is pertinent to survey some of the observations which have allowed elaboration of these general concepts. An attempt will be made to present studies concerning absorption, storage, transport and utilization of carbohydrates; particular attention will be given to the roles played by anterior pituitary, adrenal and thyroid glands in these activities.

Absorption of glucose, maintenance of fasting blood sugar levels and insulin sensitivity

It is generally agreed[258, 405, 451] that the absorption of glucose from the intestinal tract is decreased in hypophysectomized animals, an exception being the toad.[258] Whether or not hormonal agents produce direct effects on phosphorylation mechanisms necessary for such absorption is not established.[451] Soulairac[451] has stated that intestinal absorption of glucose is markedly increased by extensive bilateral hypothalamic lesions when these are associated with hyperphagia.

Fasted, hypophysectomized animals fail to maintain satisfactory blood sugar levels[233, 252, 253, 406] though the significant alleviation of this tendency by previous high-fat diet has been demonstrated by Samuels and his co-workers.[406] Houssay, in 1936,[252] stated that he had never seen spontaneous hypoglycemia in dogs with extensive tuberal lesions alone.

The uniform tendency to insulin hypersensitivity in hypophysectomized animals is clearly established.[231, 233, 253, 257, 447] It likewise seems to be diminished by previous adjustment of the hypophysectomized animal to a high-fat, low-carbohydrate diet. The evidence suggests that such sensitivity is a direct result only of anterior lobe deficiency[233] (with its peripheral endocrine concomitants), and is independent of hypothalamic neurovegetative control by way of the infundibulum.[56]

Adrenal glands and carbohydrate metabolism

The appreciation of the part played by the adrenal glands in carbohydrate metabolism has slowly evolved in the past fifteen years. It is probable that the medullary component is of secondary importance in this connection, although impairment of this division was at one time believed to be responsible for the appearance of hypoglycemic convulsions in hypophysectomized animals.[54, 318] The proportionate role of the adrenal cortex is less controversial.

Britton and his co-workers[54] have shown that the adrenal cortex (through the now recognized glucocorticoids) plays a central role in the maintenance of liver and cardiac muscle glycogen and a somewhat less important one in maintenance of skeletal muscle glycogen. Thus, as would be expected, the adrenalectomized–depancreatized animal survives longer than the depancreatized animal with intact adrenals.[318, 324] In the former the metabolic routes of dietary proteins which are directed toward carbohydrate formation are partially blocked due to the lack of glucocorticoids. The ability to reinstate, in significant measure, this altered diabetic state with adrenal cortical extract is postulated on the basis of clinical and animal studies.[324, 476] Large doses of adrenal cortical extract have maintained normal or supernormal blood sugar levels, normal liver glycogen and near-normal muscle glycogen in hypophysectomized animals.[93] The conclusion that adrenalectomy modifies to a significant degree the diabetic manifestations induced by anterior pituitary extract[325] was long questioned[212, 253] but now appears tenable.[256] Observations of both a clinical[48] and experimental nature[54, 97] make imperative the recognition of a separate adrenal cortical factor for regulation of carbohydrate metabolism, as contrasted, for example, to the salt and water factor. Parenthetically, a plausible theory has been suggested to explain release of cellular potassium subsequent to adrenalectomy, on the basis of inhibition of glycogen formation.[436]

Available evidence indicates that the diabetogenic property of some anterior hypophyseal extracts is only partially mediated through the adrenal cortex.[40, 100] It has been found that anterior pituitary extract in the hypophysectomized rat may maintain muscle glycogen but not liver glycogen. Moreover, hypoglycemia persists. In contrast, ACTH or appropriate adrenal glucocorticoids reverse both the defects caused by pituitary removal.[401] The precise mechanism by which the carbohydrate-regulating factor of the adrenal cortex implements formation of glycogen from endogenous protein is speculative.[54] (See Growth, page 105.)

It has recently been observed[451] that the adrenalectomized rat shows significantly subnormal intestinal glucose absorption which suggests even a broader role of the adrenal glands in carbohydrate metabolism.

Thyroid gland and carbohydrate metabolism

The thyroid gland appears to play a role significantly different from that of the adrenal cortex in the processes of carbohydrate metabolism. Hypophysectomy increases insulin sensitivity in thyroidectomized animals,[253] while thyroxin and pituitary thyrotrophin[241, 450] prevent neither insulin hypersensitivity nor exhaustion of glycogen stores in fasted hypophysectomized animals. Thyroxin, however, may maintain relatively normal blood sugar values during fasting. The thyroid gland plays a much more remote part in the maintenance of liver and muscle glycogen stores than does the adrenal cortex. Thyroidectomy has relatively little effect on pancreatic diabetes,[325] though Houssay[255] in contrast to Lukens and Dohan,[325] has succeeded in inducing permanent diabetes in partially depancreatized animals by prolonged administration of thyroid extract. Houssay does note that the exhaution of carbohydrate stores following hypophysectomy or bilateral adrenalectomy prevents production of such permanent diabetes, though thyroidectomy does not.

Russell's review[402] emphasized that a fundamental role of the thyroid gland is in the maintenance of normal absorption of glucose from the intestinal tract. Thyroid priming increases such absorption to normal values in hypophysectomized rats. That the thyroid may play a relatively minor role in the conversion of protein to glycogen is conceivable. In this regard Soskin and his co-workers[450] have observed an increase in urinary nitrogen following intramuscular thyroxin therapy in hypophysectomized dogs.

Diabetic state induced by anterior pituitary extracts

J. H. Burns[cited in 113] is considered the first to have demonstrated an antagonism between anterior pituitary extract and insulin. It was not until 1937, however, that Young[531] successfully induced permanent diabetes in dogs with daily injections of anterior pituitary extract, though transient diabetic states, similarly induced, had been observed previously not only by him but also by Houssay and his group. The contrast of this diabetic state to that induced by pancreatectomy has been the subject of many subsequent metabolic studies,[128, 325, 337] all verifying both the early transient, reversible or "hypophyseal" phase as associated with reversible islet cell damage and the permanent phase as invariably associated with irreversible islet cell change. The lack of significant alteration in the anterior pituitary gland itself, associated with the permanent phase[337] dovetails well with the subsequent observation that the anterior pituitary gland in rats of inborn diabetic strain[190] is normal. This is in sharp contrast to the changes in human clinical diabetes mellitus already reported by Kraus.

Lukens' contention[323] that the growth and adrenotrophic components of anterior pituitary extract are largely responsible for the observed diabetogenic effect, is amply supported by metabolic studies,[128, 324, 325] which stress gluconeogenesis from protein and suppression of carbohydrate utilization as two prime factors in this form of diabetes. He emphasized the important role of hyperglycemia itself in the production of permanent and irreversible pancreatic islet damage. That sustained hyperglycemia might be a factor in producing such damage was suggested by the failure to produce permanent diabetes in rats[220] (where anterior pituitary extract has only a transient hyperglycemic effect). Dohans and Lukens[cited in 33] have subsequently confirmed this mechanism. After repeated intraperitoneal injections of glucose, they succeeded in producing permanent diabetes, with degeneration of pancreatic islets, in normal and partially depancreatized rats. Likewise Houssay's successful production of metathyroid diabetes[255] even in thyroidectomized animals, would lend further validity to Lukens' contention. Such animals are consistently hyperglycemic during the transient phase. It is of particular interest to note that the diabetogenic potency of anterior pituitary extract does not appear to bear any relationship to its hexokinase-inhibiting potency, as observed by Broh-Kahn and Mirsky.[cited in 33]

Peripheral mechanisms of carbohydrate utilization

By what precise mechanisms insulin and anterior pituitary extract influence peripheral carbohydrate utilization are not completely known, though observations of great importance and interest have been made by Price, Colowick, Cori and Stein.[88, 378] In 1945 this group reported that anterior pituitary extract inhibits the enzymatic conversion of glucose to glucose-6-phosphate. This inhibitory action is effectively counteracted by insulin. Of special interest is their observation that insulin itself does not enhance this enzymatic conversion. Only ratbrain hexokinase failed to show such inhibition. Subsequently they have observed that adrenal cortical extract, while failing to inhibit hexokinase of normal muscle, nonetheless inhibits that of diabetic muscle. There have, however, been reports[455] which disputed these dynamics of hormone-enzyme relationships in diabetes mellitus. In the 1953 Silliman Memorial Lecture, Cori revealed that his laboratory isolated a lipoprotein, present in the blood of diabetics, which is stable at room temperature but not in the cold. This lipoprotein is derived from the anterior pituitary and effectively inhibits the activity of hexokinase and is itself inhibited by insulin. This is a fascinating and magnificently demonstrated display of metabolic interrelationships.

Summary

A re-evaluation of the observations summarized in this chapter makes possible a working reference system to which we will return in interpreting the complex disturbances of carbohydrate metabolism observed in chromophobe adenomas. We are justified in stating that the normally functioning anterior pituitary gland elaborates principles which not only inhibit utilization of carbohydrate stores directly, but also maintain a steady flow of glycogen sources to the liver through mediation of the thyroid and, possibly, the adrenal glands. The anterior pituitary likewise effects an adequate maintenance of glycogen reserves for use in ordinary and stressful situations through the mediation of a factor manufactured by the adrenal cortex.

The elaboration of glycogen from protein sources would appear to be most directly under adrenal cortical influence.

We must hesitate to apply too enthusiastically the data derived from the diabetes induced by anterior pituitary extract to the interpretation of clinical deficiencies. Young himself urged such caution in his earlier papers, and subsequent developments, suggesting that sustained hyperglycemia may be the only common denominator for its production, increase the need for conservative application.

Insulin hypersensitivity is not adequately explained by available data but in hypopituitarism this phenomenon appears to be most closely related to adrenal cortical deficiency.

CALCIUM AND PHOSPHORUS METABOLISM

Clinical remarks

Relatively few observations about calcium and phosphorus metabolism in states of altered pituitary function have appeared in the clinical literature. Starr and Davis,[456] in 1941, reported normal serum

calcium and inorganic phosphorus levels in all 13 patients with hypopituitary states whom they studied. How many of these had chromophobe adenomas, is not stated in their report. Bauer and Aub in the
same year[36] observed normal serum calcium and phosphorus levels in
5 acromegalics. However, they noted increased urinary excretion of
calcium and phosphorus in all 5. The fecal excretory figures were
normal. The magnitude of urinary calcium excretion bore no apparent
relation to the degree of elevation of BMR. Deep x-ray therapy to the
sellar region reduced abnormal excretion in one of their patients but
Lugol's solution produced no alterations in BMR or calcium excretion
in another.

Experimental investigations

Collip, in a survey of the experimental literature to 1942[86]
emphasized that the existence of a parathyrotrophic hormone was by
no means proven. Experimental investigations of this metabolic problem are few. Baker in 1942[29] published the results of a careful histologic
study of the parathyroid glands of hypophysectomized monkeys. He
noted slight questionable atrophy of these glands without any significant alteration in normal cell types or their functional cytoplasmic
constituents. His conclusion was that the pituitary gland exerts conspicuously less trophic influence over the parathyroid, than over the
adrenal, gonadal or thyroid glands.

In summarizing the observations of his group in 1936, Houssay[252] described normal serum calcium and phosphorus levels in hypophysectomized and thyroidectomized dogs, and in those with lesions
of the tuber cinereum. He noted minimum elevation of calcium and
moderate elevation of phosphorus in normal dogs injected with anterior
pituitary extract, but a significant decrease in calcium and moderate
increase in phosphorus following pancreatectomy. In pancreatectomized
animals subsequently hypophysectomized decreased serum calcium
levels persisted but serum phosphorus returned to normal. Houssay also
reported in this review a marked decrease in serum (alkaline) phosphatase following hypophysectomy in dogs. Schaur and Rogoff,[415] in the
same year, observed the occurrence of globular predentin in rats subjected to parathyroid extract therapy, a phenomenon previously ob-

served in adrenalectomized rats. The observations of Houssay's co-workers that anterior pituitary extract produces moderate elevation of serum phosphorus was confirmed by Snyder and Tweedy[448] though these workers noted no significant changes in serum calcium. Gergely, in 1941,[191] observed that in hypophysectomized dogs fasted for 24 hours the calcium concentration of the urine is subnormal; following an infusion containing 5 cc. of 10 per cent calcium chloride, the urinary excretion of calcium is less than in normals. This decrease is not explicable on the basis of the course of the blood calcium curve following infusion. This finding is quite the opposite of Bauer and Aub's in clinical acromegalics. However, in spite of the fact that the latter observers could note no interdependency of the observed changes with BMR elevation, the possible influence of changes in renal blood flow in states of altered pituitary function must be considered in interpreting these data.

Törnblom[483] has suggested that the pertinent hormones of the adenohypophysis and the parathyroid are in some ways antagonistic. He states that the former decreases renal excretion of phosphorus and may decrease slightly the level of serum calcium. Parathyroidal secretion has the reverse effect. The influence of the pituitary may be mediated either through the growth hormone or through ACTH via the adrenal cortex. The parathyroid appears to be relatively independent of the adenohypophysis but it is evident the relationships of both to Ca-P metabolism is only partially appraised.[483] Some[531a] consider the serum inorganic phosphorus level an index of growth hormone activity and find this a useful clinical tool.

Summary

There is insufficient histologic alteration in the parathyroid glands of hypophysectomized monkeys to suggest a direct trophic influence of any magnitude.

Hypopituitary states are not associated with any conspicuous changes in the levels of serum calcium or inorganic phosphorus. There are some indications that anterior pituitary extract may elevate serum phosphorus slightly, though clinical states of acidophilic hyperpituitarism are irregularly associated with such a change. Alterations in renal excretion of calcium have been observed both in hypo- and hyperpituitary states, with increase in the latter, and decrease in the former. These changes have not been convincingly dissociated from concomitant changes in renal blood flow.

HYPOPITUITARISM, GROWTH AND PROTEIN METABOLISM

Nitrogen balance and growth processes

Houssay, in 1936,[252] outlined the influences of the pituitary gland on nitrogen balance. He reported a significant decrease in nitrogen excretion in hypophysectomized dogs and toads, the decrease being even more conspicuous on a protein-free diet. A significant decrease in the usually elevated values of nitrogen excretion in pancreatic and phlorhizin diabetic animals was likewise observed following hypophysectomy. Anterior pituitary extract increased nitrogen excretion as did impure thyrotrophin in these animals. Houssay disclaimed any role of the thyroid gland in these changes. Samuels and his co-workers[405, 407] further amplified these observations. They noted a slow and distinctly subnormal growth increment (10 per cent of normal) in hypophysectomized animals fed by stomach tube. Though intestinal absorption was subnormal in such animals, it was efficient. This group also noted subnormal nitrogen storage (30 per cent of normal), with the deamination of more endogenous protein than in normal animals. Houssay's group found no contribution of posterior lobe or tuber cinereum to the nitrogen sparing effects of hypophysectomy.

Mirsky[347] has suggested that insulin plays a fundamental role in protein breakdown. He states that a permanent increase in the rate of protein catabolism will occur only if the secretion of pancreatic insulin is inhibited or decreased. However, as Houssay's group has demonstrated, hypophysectomy does significantly diminish such insulin-deficient catabolism. Thus the insulin mechanism is neither an adequate nor a complete answer.

Growth hormones and protein metabolism

Growth hormone (GH) has been purified to the extent that it can be identified as an electrophoretically homogeneous protein relatively free of ACTH and other activities.[307] Its administration induces many of the changes noted in eosinophilic adenoma, particularly increase in the size of organs and total growth of the experimental animal. Its metabolic effects, however, are more difficult to unravel. Outstanding is its induction of positive nitrogen balance which is associated with a diminution of NPN, urea and amino acid content of the blood.[221] The retention of nitrogen has been ascribed either to increased anabolism, decreased catabolism of protein, or to both. In keeping with the thesis that the predominant effect of GH is to inhibit degradation of tissue proteins is the demonstration that liver arginase activity is decreased following the administration of GH. This indicates that the final steps of protein catabolism leading to the formation of urea are reduced in rate.[173] GH produces nitrogen retention even in the presence of experimentally produced diabetes mellitus.[42] Moreover the growth promoting faculties of GH are evidently maintained, though reduced, in the absence of adrenals, thyroid and pancreas.[340] In addition to its influence on protein metabolism GH has further important activities, although these may be related to growth and protein metabolism. It appears that GH may suppress the peripheral oxidation of carbohydrates as well as increase the production of ketone bodies, thus suggesting that fats are then utilized for caloric needs in place of carbohydrates[41, 240] and secondarily increasing the turnover of phospholipids.[306] The hypoglycemia which develops in hypophysectomized fasting rats may be ascribed in part to reduction in gluconeogenesis from protein normally brought about by the growth hormone.[221] Certain data, on the other hand, indicate that the diabetogenic action of hypophyseal extracts may be effected by GH. These contrary functions of GH may be the result of impurities in the factors administered rather than physiologic attributes of this particular hormone.

Some have expressed the opinion that insulin is necessary for the action of GH. It is suspected that antipancreatropic elements may exist in growth hormone fractions since GH may inhibit insulin production and decrease the content of insulin in the pancreas.[13, 171] Work by Griffiths and Young indicates that the pancreas does not require the adenohypophysis for secretion of insulin and the administration of so-called pancreatropic factor is virtually ineffective.[211] Whatever action GH does exert on the pancreatic islets is probably not directly antagonistic to other secretions of the pituitary. The fact that stands out, however, is that administration of GH, whether to normal or diabetic animals, produces nitrogen retention. The interrelations of GH, insulin and carbohydrate which may exist normally do not appear essential for the synthesis and storage of tissue proteins.

In an extensive experimental study Hoberman[248] examined the influence of various hormones on the rates of metabolism of proteins and amino acids. From the kinetic data gathered, he made certain inferences which are largely in agreement with prior concepts and may be profitably summarized here. The catabolism of amino acids is depressed by growth hormone and accelerated by adrenocorticosteroids. The inhibitory action of growth hormone on the breakdown of amino acids is not mediated through the adrenals. In depancreatized diabetic animals GH is still effective in diminishing the rate of deaminatory processes. This suggests that insulin is not necessary, although it may be adjunctive to the action of GH. Thyroxine appears to potentiate the effects of GH. With respect to protein synthesis GH has been found to augment this process, but not to slow catabolism directly. Adrenal corticosteroids, on the other hand, increase the rate of degradation of proteins. Since protein synthesis is accelerated in adrenalectomized and hypophysectomized animals so notably sensitive to insulin, the pancreatic hormone is thought to be responsible for this anabolic result. On the basis of these and other findings Hoberman postulates that growth hormone "accelerates the synthesis of protein by inhibiting adrenal-induced inactivation of insulin or by inhibiting those effects of the adrenal corticosteroids which oppose the peripheral effects of insulin."

Gonadal interrelationships

The fact that arrested general growth is associated with testicular or ovarian deficiency is clearly implied in experimental[400] and clinical[490] observations. Testosterone preparations produce significant nitrogen retention[1] which in no way conflicts with the interesting observation of Rubinstein and Solomon[400] that testosterone propionate increases growth inhibition already instituted by castration alone.

Inhibition of a pituitary growth factor need not be postulated to explain this seeming paradox since subsequent studies have established that testosterone initiates epiphyseal closure.

Serum proteins

Goldberg, [cited in 252, 303] Levin and Leathem[cited in 303] and Mosonyi[350] have all reported an increase in serum globulin and a less marked but distinct decrease in serum albumin, following hypophysectomy in dogs, cats and rats. Levin and his co-workers[303] have explained these changes on the thesis that the decrease in serum albumin is a concomitant of adrenal cortical deficit[329] and the increase in serum globulin, a reflection only of postoperative hemoconcentration.

Specific dynamic action of protein

Fulton and Cushing in 1932[185] noted neither significant nor specific alteration in the metabolic response to a protein meal in patients with acidophilic hyperpituitarism, hypopituitarism or mixed states. Goldzieher[203] later confirmed these observations relative to neoplastic pituitary disease processes but considered this response to be strikingly decreased in non-neoplastic hypopituitarism. He felt that thyroid dysfunction played no significant part in this decreased response. He noted a variably increased specific dynamic action in castrate or menopausal individuals. The experimental investigations of Houssay's group[252] are not in complete harmony with Goldzieher's observations. They noted no abnormality in specific dynamic action in 20 hypophysectomized dogs, but recorded a minimum decrease following primary thyroidectomy, with additional slight accentuation after subsequent hypophysectomy.

Since the current belief is that the specific dynamic action of protein is fundamentally a manifestation of the energy spent in absorptive and intermediary metabolic processes, it is not difficult to accept Houssay's observation of slight decrease following thyroidectomy. There are, however, some evident discrepancies in his data which are difficult to explain, perhaps because the phenomenon itself is a hybrid and inconspicuous one.

Summary

The anterior pituitary gland appears to influence the maintenance of nitrogen equilibrium by many mechanisms, of which a few are pertinent in patients with chromophobe adenomas. It affects protein conservation through gonadal mediation yet tends to counteract this conservation through adrenal cortical mechanisms activating tissue protein breakdown for purposes of maintaining glycogen stores. The adrenal cortex itself plays at least a dual role since it is intimately involved in the elaboration or maintenance of serum albumin.

The process of skeletal growth is distinct from that for maintenance of positive nitrogen balance since growth may, in fact, be arrested prior to normal skeletal maturation, in the presence of a positive nitrogen balance. It has been considered preferable to outline those processes concerned with nitrogen balance in the adult rather than with growth itself since chromophobe adenomas occur, for the most part, in mature individuals. Furthermore the information related to growth is so great that it deserves treament only in a more specialized review.

WATER BALANCE AND RENAL FUNCTION

The occasional upset of water balance in hypopituitary states is strikingly manifest in the phenomenon termed diabetes insipidus. It is, therefore, appropriate to review briefly the precise relationship of the deficiency state of the neurohypophyseal unit to this phenomenon before considering alterations in renal function itself.

Anatomic structures and diabetes insipidus

The hypothalamico-hypophyseal tract arises from the cells of the supraoptic and paraventricular nuclei and also from less well defined groups in the tuberal area. The fibers of this tract terminate within the median eminence, the infundibular stalk and process. This system has been shown to be related to the regulation of renal output of water.[162, 283, 284, 372, 492]

Heinbecker and his co-workers[232, 234] have elaborated the fundamental studies of the Ranson school[162] already discussed (see Chapter 2). The former group has reported that permanent diabetes insipidus of maximal intensity follows denervation or destruction of the entire neurohypophysis, including the median eminence. Degeneration of all the cells of the paired supraoptic nuclei as well as those of the rostral third or half of the paired paraventricular nuclei results. As little as 15 per cent of this complex, actively functioning, may prevent the onset of diabetes insipidus. Below this minimum the intensity of the diabetic state increases with decreasing number of functioning neurones. They have maintained that the pars distalis is essential only for maintenance of maximal diabetes insipidus, though they had suggested earlier that the pars distalis was not essential even for this. As supporting evidence, the experiments of Goldzieher and Kaldor[204] are of interest. They noted that during theobromine or novasurol diuresis in guinea pigs, the anterior pituitary becomes hyperemic. The eosinophils decrease in number while the basophils increase. Vacuolation appears in all cells. These workers suggest that the adenohypophysis participates in or is affected by excessive water excretion. It would appear that Von Hann's original contention,[218] that functioning anterior lobe is necessary for marked diabetes insipidus, is true. It is not likely, however, that the anterior pituitary secretes a specific diuretic hormone but rather that it secondarily influences the intensity of diabetes insipidus through its target organs.

Within the supraoptic and paraventricular regions of some mammalian species dilated vesicular spaces are found in close relation to the neurons and their processes. It is possible that these structures, if they are not fixation artefacts, act as osmoreceptors.[492] Changes in their volume may depend on the osmotic pressure of the milieu. Nerve fibers ending in apposition to the spaces may be stimulated by stretch of their walls in accord with volumetric fluctuation of these vesicles. By such a mechanism the osmotic pressure of the blood might activate indirectly the hypothalamico-hypophyseal system. It is postulated that when the osmotic pressure of the blood is elevated, antidiuretic hormone is secreted, thus reducing water diuresis. Water retention then tends to restore the blood osmotic pressure to normal and to remove the stimulus for activation of the neurohypophysis. Whether this mechanism operates in the human has not been determined. One of us (J. N., unpublished observations) has had occasion to study a large series of supraoptic nuclei in the rat. These structures were fixed by the freeze-drying technic, thus avoiding usual fixation artefacts. Widely dilated vesicles, such as described by Verney,[492] were rarely if ever seen in these specimens. The intimately interlacing capillary mesh forming the bed of these nuclei did, however, show evident volumetric changes after brief exposure of the animal to low temperature. Because the supraoptic nuclei are so extensively vascularized such changes as these might well produce local pressure effects which could serve as one stimulus for local neural activation or secretion.

The cellular source of antidiuretic hormone is not known, although the pituicytes have been implicated in its formation.[498] The hormonal target organ is the kidney. The antidiuretic hormone acts on the distal part of the nephron to enhance the active reabsorption of water and possibly on the other tubular segments to decrease the absorption of sodium chloride. The glomerular filtration rate is unaffected directly by antidiuretic hormone (ADH). Shannon[428, 429] has shown that during dehydration the electrolytic and fluid shifts of dogs in the normal and insipidus state take a similar direction and that excretion of a hypertonic urine is possible in the latter under special conditions. This suggests that although ADH is an important hormone in renal regulation it is not essential for the active absorption of water in the distal segment. This observer has emphasized that the ratio of the function of glomerular filtration to proximal tubular reabsorption of electrolytes and water is of prime importance in the rate of water excretion. The reabsorption of water in the distal tubule may be an active process influenced by ADH but the need for this hormone at this stage depends on the type of urine with regard to its formation rate and concentration of solutes. If ADH acts both to decrease the absorption of sodium and augment that of water it serves to preserve intracellular fluid in the last analysis.

Thyroid gland and diabetes insipidus

Houssay in 1936[252] reported the observation that anterior pituitary extract of high thyrotrophic potency induced polyuria in the normal dog but not in the thyroidectomized dog. Heinbecker and his group[234] more recently have reported that thyroidectomy immediately terminates the transient diabetes insipidus of the dog with median eminence still intact. Thyroidectomy, according to them, depresses but does not eliminate the diabetic state following complete denervation of the neurohypophysis. Parenteral or oral thyroid preparations increased urinary output in their animals with transient or permanent diabetes insipidus.

Adrenal glands and diabetes insipidus

The several studies of Britton, Corey and Silvette,[53, 94, 95] Winter, Ingram and Gross[268, 520] and of Swann[462] consistently indicate that a relationship exists between diabetes insipidus, the salt conserving hormone of the adrenal cortex, and the level of serum electrolytes. Swann, in fact, has maintained that with low sodium intake diabetes insipidus is almost completely inhibited in the permanently diabetic animal. Britton, Corey and Silvette have demonstrated the antagonism between the salt conserving factor of the adrenal cortex and antidiuretic posterior pituitary preparations. Heinbecker and his coworkers[234] have likewise stated that doca increases the urinary output of the dog with permanent diabetes insipidus. Such fundamental agreement has not often been reached in the elucidation of mechanisms related to neurohypophyseal disturbances.

Renal function and the hypo- or apituitary animal

The effects of secondary hypoadrenalism on renal function have been discussed as also the evidence for the conclusion that the renal threshold for ketone bodies is elevated in hypopituitary states.

White, Heinbecker and Rolf[514, 515] have observed a decrease in renal plasma flow and a significant decrease in diodrast tubular mass in hypophysectomized dogs. Thyroidectomy alone produces a moderate but not comparable decrease in renal plasma flow.[cited in 33] These changes occur four to six days after hypophysectomy, hence are not thought to be related to adrenal cortical or thyroid factors. The validity of such an inference is questioned. Loss of pitressin-forming tissue has no relationship to these reported changes. They report the interesting observation[515] that increase in inulin and diodrast clearances and in diodrast tubular mass sometimes occurs two to three days after manipulation of the anterior lobe of the pituitary gland.

Summary

Certain disturbances in renal function attend apituitary states, among them decrease in renal plasma flow, perhaps associated with thyroid hypofunction, and decrease in both excretory and reabsorptive tubular function, at least partially referable to concomitant hypoadrenalism.

The condition of permanent diabetes insipidus ensues almost uniformly when the neurohypophysis (including median eminence) is completely denervated or destroyed. A functioning anterior pituitary gland is essential for maintaining the conspicuously abnormal rates of fluid turnover in this condition both through its probable trophic influence on the salt conserving factor of the adrenal cortex, and likewise through its direct trophic influence on the thyroid gland.

PIGMENTARY DEPOSITS AND HYPOPITUITARISM

Clinical remarks

Lisser and Escamilla,[146, 310] in two exhaustive studies of Simmonds' disease, have reported skin pigmentary deposits in one-quarter of their clinical cases. They made no specific note of mucous membrane pigmentation. German[193] reported no skin or mucous membrane pigmentation in 100 chromophobe adenomas of Cushing's series and the Lahey clinic group[531a] report none in a larger series. This contrasts with Davidoff's finding of pigmentation in 46 per cent of acromegalics studied. The conspicuous absence of pigmentation in those with chromophobe adenomas is noteworthy, as also the relatively high incidence of pigmentation in Simmonds' disease, where normal or relatively normal posterior lobe tissue is almost the rule.

Experimental investigations

Houssay[251] records the appearance of cutaneous pallor and melanophore contraction in the toad following removal of the posterior lobe and pars intermedia, thus extending the similar observations of Smith[442] in hypophysectomized frog larvae.

In a recent conference on pituitary-adrenal function a precise summation of observations with regard to pigmentation in both clinical and experimental states indicates that an explanation of this phenomenon is not yet formulated.[6]

V

THE MATERIAL AND INITIAL
SYMPTOMS

SOURCES AND CRITERIA FOR INCLUSION

This study is based upon a critically selected series of 117 patients with chromophobe adenomas admitted to the Neurological Institute of New York or the Medical Services of the Columbia-Presbyterian Medical Center, from 1929 to 1948. The histologic material was prepared and made available by the Department of Pathology, Division of Neuropathology, College of Physicians and Surgeons, Columbia University.

The cases are classified as follows: (1) 52 patients with clinical investigation and histologic verification of tumor; (2) 26 patients with clinical investigation including air study (pneumoencephalography and/or ventriculography) but without histologic confirmation; (3) 39 patients with clinical investigation alone. In addition to these groups, a total of 34 tumors removed at operation from patients whose studies were not adequate for inclusion in the clinical portion of this report, were examined from a histopathologic standpoint and the results incorporated in Chapter 9, Pathology.

A total of 6 patients are included in the above series even though they satisfy all the criteria for fugitive hyperpituitarism of acidophilic type; 18 patients with at least minimal x-ray traces of skeletal overgrowth are likewise included above. These two groups are separately

evaluated in Chapter 9 to determine the incidence of pertinent metabolic disorders in this group and thus to estimate bias that may have
been introduced into the group as a whole. The inclusion of this latter
group is quite justified in such a report since its usual characteristics
are much more readily identified with those of chromophobe adenomas
than with those of acidophilic adenomas. It is acceptable to consider
it a transitional stage, more closely linked to chromophobe than to
acidophilic adenomas.

Only those cases are included as confirmed by air study in which
well delineated filling defects were demonstrated in the basal cisterns
with or without filling defects in the floor of an otherwise distinct third
ventricle. Deformities of frontal or temporal horns were not accepted
as diagnostic criteria but rather as indications of local extension. The
data from air study were, of course, considered as confirmatory only
in the presence of clear-cut bony changes of characteristic sort[177, 288, 359]
in the sella turcica itself.

The criteria for inclusion of the 39 cases of group 3 were rigid.
They were satisfied only after evaluation of history, physical characteristics, visual field defects, x-ray deformities of the sella turcica
(present in all patients of this series), skeletal changes and, finally, response to deep x-ray therapy. In those instances where the diagnosis
was questioned by any member of the hospital staff (the most frequent
differential diagnostic problems being presented by craniopharyngioma,
intracranial aneurysm, basal meningioma, borderline acromegaly, or
nonlocalized intracranial tumor) the case was included solely after
resolution of the difficulty by appropriate study.

For studies on the influence of tumor size the cases were divided
into those with large, medium and small tumors. The basis for such
arbitrary classification was as follows: *small:* sella turcica measuring
not more than 20 mm. A.P. by 20 mm. in depth; *medium:* sella turcica
measuring between 20 by 20 mm. and 30 by 30 mm.; *large:* sella
turcica measuring more than 30 by 30 mm.

The information from air encephalography and operation was
included for further verification of relative tumor size, where the total
rather than intrasellar growth was considered. Since this classification
is arbitrary and enjoys the doubtful advantage of encompassing the
range, conclusions drawn from its use must be judged as tentative.

Statistical methods

Statistical methods were applied, where indicated, to an evaluation of mean trends, significance of mean differences and error from random sampling. The sigma-probability technic described by Richardson[392] was used for an initial screening of the data relative to tumor size but was amplified by the Chi-squared (χ^2) procedure of Fisher.[164] Where any two groups contained a factor less than five, Yates's correction for continuity in small groups was applied,[164] unless otherwise indicated in the text. The standard error of estimate (Sy) of the concentration of points about a line of regression was derived from Richardson[392] as was the computation of reliability of mean differences and the standard error of the mean.

Special technics or procedures

The following technics and procedures are accorded special note here either because they are not considered as of routine nature or because their proper interpretation presupposes definite criteria:

Thyroid function

Radioactive iodine tracer studies according to the technic of Werner et al.[509] *

Adrenal and gonadal function

The mecholyl tolerance test according to the technic of Perera.[366]

The salt-deprivation test using a modification of the salt-poor diet of Harrop et al.,[223] further described by Nettrour and Rynearson[354] and Parker.[362] The diet used contained less than 1 Gm. of total salt daily. Serum sodium and potassium, blood urea nitrogen, plasma volumes and serum proteins were checked immediately prior to and at the termination of five days of salt deprivation. Fluid balance sheets were maintained. Necessary precautions were uniformly observed in the conduct of this potentially dangerous test. All tests could not be run for the full five days because of intervention of symptoms or signs demanding termination.

Plasma volume according to the method of Gregersen.[209] Plasma volumes were calculated for ideal weight unless otherwise specified.

Total neutral 17-ketosteroids by the Zimmerman colorimetric reaction.[508]

Urinary estrone and estradiol by the fluorometric technic of Jailer.†

---

* Determinations made by Dr. Sidney Werner's laboratory.

† Determinations by Dr. Joseph Jailer.

Urinary estrogen by the castrated rat vaginal smear technic.[506]

Urinary gonadotrophins by the mouse uterine weight method of Levin and Tyndale.[508]

Carbohydrate metabolism

The 100 Gm., single dose, oral glucose tolerance test using the technic of Hamman and Hirschman.[217] In most instances the test followed consumption of the standard hospital diet (approximately 175 Gm. CHO daily) for a minimum of three days. In some instances (a majority of those described in table 12) the test was preceded by a diet containing 300 Gm. carbohydrate daily for three days. The normal maximum limits of response to oral glucose were derived from several competent studies.[174, 178, 217, 499]

The intravenous glucose tolerance test according to Lozner et al.[322]

The insulin tolerance test according to Frazer et al.[174]

SPECIFIC OBSERVATIONS

Sex incidence of chromophobe adenomas

If there is a significant difference in the incidence of chromophobe adenomas in the two sexes, it is of some importance to confirm that difference. As suggested in the section concerning pathogenesis of these tumors, hormonal factors of gonadal origin are widely implicated as a possible mechanism of tumor production.

Our data indicate a definite though not striking preponderance of such tumors in the male; of a total 117 cases studied, 60 per cent, or 70 cases, were male. A similar preponderance in the male is suggested in the studies of Starr and Davis,[456] Frazier and Grant[177] and less impressively in German's analysis[193] of 100 chromophobe adenomas of the Cushing series. A recent analysis of 164 patients with probable chromophobe adenomas[531a] suggests no preponderance in either sex (81 in women, 83 in men).

In Simmonds' disease,[434] on the other hand, females show a distinct preponderance over males, a fact which is not surprising when one considers the close relationship of the puerperium to this illness.

A casual examination of the data in table 3 would lead to the impression that large pituitary tumors are more common in the male, medium and large more common than small tumors in the female. We have submitted this impression to statistical analysis and discover that we are not justified in concluding that such a distinction exists, the variations being within a quite normal distribution range for data of this magnitude. Unfortunately there are no similar observations available in the clinical literature with which we might verify this seeming trend.

TABLE 3—*The Incidence of Chromophobe Adenomas in Relation to Estimated Tumor Size*

	Total No. of Cases	Male		Female		Statistical data $\chi^{2\dagger}$
		No.	% of total	No.	% of total	
Large	56	37	66	19	34	
Medium	45	25	56	20	44	Between large and medium 1.16*
Small	16	8	50	8	50	Between large and small 1.37*

* No significant difference, large and medium, large and small.

† When the sigma probability technic was used, all cases fell within a 2:1 probability range relative to the incidence of sex.

Age incidence of chromophobe adenomas

The peak incidence of chromophobe adenomas between the ages of 31 to 50 years is matter of unquestioned agreement in previous clinical studies.[177, 193, 239] Our data suggest that more specific information is obtainable by analyzing age incidence for each sex separately. Our results are presented in figure 27. The age of onset, as indicated in this figure, must necessarily be somewhat later than the actual onset of tumor growth itself because the tumor has already attained considerable size when significant symptoms appear. Peaks of incidence appear in the age groups 41 to 45, and 51 to 55 for the female, in age groups 31 to 35 and 41 to 45 for the male. It is of importance to decide whether these peaks deviate significantly from a hypothetic linear trend which reflects no relationship of age to incidence. For the females of our series the equation of such a straight line trend is: Y equals 5.22. For this equation Sy, i.e., the standard error of the estimate, equals

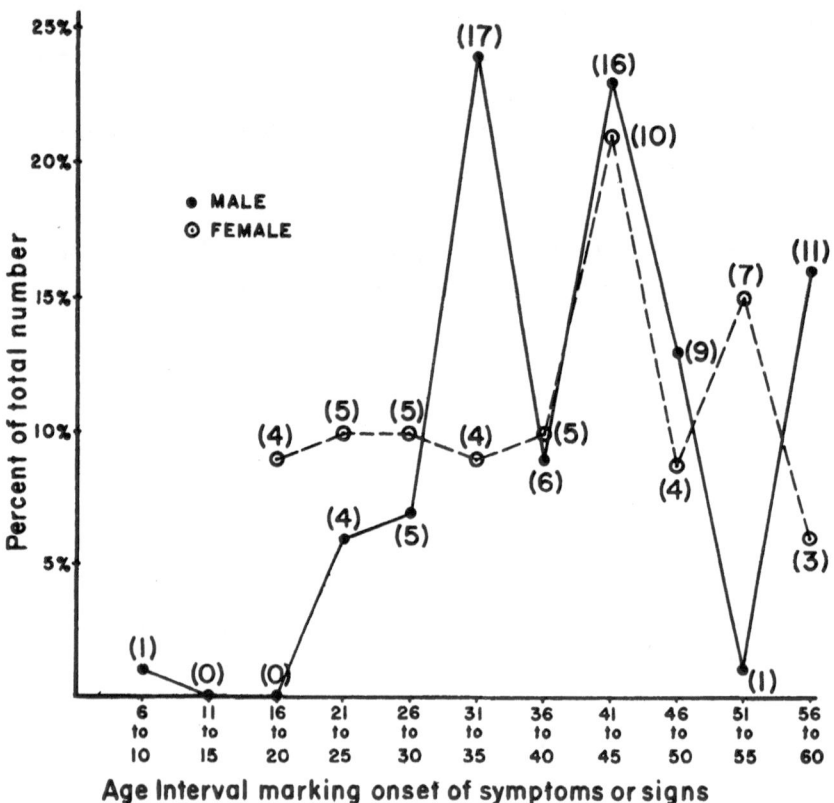

Fig. 27—Age of onset of symptoms in chromophobe adenomas by sex. Numbers in parentheses indicate numbers of patients.

1.98. Only the incidence at the age grouping 41 to 45 falls outside the 5 per cent probability range.

In the males of our series the equation of a similar linear trend is: Y equals 6.36, with Sy equal to 5.9. No peaks, as recorded, fall outside the 5 per cent probability range though those at the age groups 31 to 35 and 41 to 45 years are at the extreme of this range.

Summary

Chromophobe adenomas are somewhat more common in males than in females. It is possible that large tumors are relatively more common in males than in females.

There is a significant maximal incidence of chromophobe adenomas in females within the age group 41 to 45 years. In the male possibly significant maxima in incidence occur in the age groups 31 to 35 and 41 to 45 years.

SYMPTOMATOLOGY

The regional anatomy and physiology of the hypothalamicohypophyseal axis represent the basic cloth into which a variable and subtle pattern of disease has been woven. The neurologic symptoms are derived from disturbances in the structures we have discussed. The nature of the symptoms, their frequency, the order of their presentation are characteristics which usually distinguish chromophobe adenomas from other parasellar disturbances and compose a clinical entity.

Initial symptoms

Of the many symptoms which parade the course of this tumor any one may, on occasion, lead in the introduction of the syndrome. Visual symptoms, however, were foremost among the usual presenting symptoms. A significant defect in this major sensory system is soon impressed upon the patient while comparable disabilities of a subjectively less disturbing sort may pass unnoticed or be tolerated. The incidence of visual disturbances as an initial complaint equaled that of all other introductory symptoms combined. Moreover, in those instances where diminution of visual acuity and/or visual field were not the primary events they later accompanied the other presenting complaints. Deficiencies in sexual function and headache constituted the other two numerically significant groups. Aside from these major categories the remaining rarer symptoms were widely distributed through physiologic systems.

The following data indicate the distribution of the presenting symptoms: *defect in visual acuity and/or field,* 62 cases (47 per cent); *headache,* 26 cases (20 per cent); *sexual dysfunction,* a total of 22 cases (17 per cent) with the following symptoms: amenorrhea (15 cases) and impotence (7 cases). The *remaining symptoms* were distributed among 21 cases (16 per cent) as follows: palsies of EOM, 4;

hypoadrenalism, 3; drowsiness, 3; asthenia, 2; seizures, 2; polydipsia and polyuria, 1; alopecia, 1; personality disturbance, 1; gaze palsy, 1; hemiparesis, 1; visual hallucination, 2 (one of these visual hallucination cases apparently manifested illusory rather than hallucinatory disturbances).

The mean age of onset in patients with visual symptoms was 42 years and the duration of symptoms prior to medical examination six years. When half or more of the visual field was affected and/or visual acuity reduced to 20/100, 20/200 or less the visual defect was termed severe. Impairment less marked than this was termed moderate. The pre-existent duration of symptoms in cases with severe visual impairment was longer than in those with moderate involvement, 4.7 years in comparison with 3.5 years. The prognosis as far as the reversibility of the visual impairment and the general outcome was less favorable in the severe than in the moderate cases. Age of onset bore no relationship to the development of particularly severe visual symptoms. Finally, the size of the tumor did not correlate with the degree of visual impairment.

The symptoms of sexual dysfunction make an interesting contrast with those due to visual disability. The mean age of onset of initial symptoms in the cases with amenorrhea as the presenting finding was 25.5 years and the duration of symptoms antecedent to examination was 12 years. The size of the tumor in these cases was not related to the duration of the interval between amenorrhea and the initial examination. The cases of impotence were too few for significant comparison. However, in both sexes the prognosis was uniformly good in terms of the general outcome. Data with regard to the return of menstruation and potency following radio- and surgical therapy were not adequate for generalization, although both functions were reestablished in several instances.

Those patients complaining of headache as an original symptom began their clinical illness at a mean age of 37 years with a latency prior to investigation of five years. The intensity of this symptom was indeterminable since an objective evaluation is not easily realized. The prognosis with regard to the degree of headache, therefore, could not be assayed but in this group as in others the general outcome was related inversely to the size of the tumor.

The disparaties in the age of onset, pre-existing duration of the initial symptom and prognosis between patients with visual defects and those with sexual dysfunction deserve attention. The age of onset of the initial symptom was 37 years in the females of the former and 25 in those of the latter group. The duration from the appearance of the initial symptoms to the time of medical attendance was five years in the cases with primary visual disturbances and twelve years with amenorrhea. There is no reason to assume from inspection of the data that the size of the adenomas vary between the individual classes. The distribution of small, moderate and large tumors was almost identical in both. Moreover, visual defects uniformly accompanied the sexual symptoms at the time of examination so that suprasellar extension was present in both groups. The question arises whether the origin of the pituitary tumor is different in these two types of case. It is possible that the patient with initial visual disurbances without sexual abnormalities may have a neoplasm that reaches a suprasellar location rapidly and causes damage to the optic pathways while at the same time affording a natural decompression to the pituitary gland itself. The assumption made in this event is that the finding of amenorrhea is due primarily to pituitary and not hypothalamic involvement. The origin of the tumor in these patients might be from the superior pole of the pituitary gland. On the other hand, the diaphragmatic restraints might be less formidable and permit ready suprasellar extension.

The lack of correlation between tumor size and the apparent intensity of the visual symptoms is surprising. One would expect larger tumors to be more drastic in their effect. The standards for tumor size may be inadequate for this determination although they seem satisfactory in indicating the general prognosis. The prognosis in cases, viewed indiscriminately, as far as initial symptom is related to tumor size, was favorable in 40 per cent of those patients with large tumors and in 90 per cent of those with small tumors. To a great degree the prognosis reflects the extent of reversibility of visual impairment. Moreover, the degree of visual damage may depend less on tumor size than on the tumor's persistent compressive presence, its invasiveness and its firmness.

In addition, the size of the tumor was not related to the duration of amenorrhea. This might be anticipated if tumors that initiate the train of symptoms of sexual dysfunction arise well within the sella. Compression of normal anterior lobe tissue may be reflected in sexual dysfunction at an early stage of neoplastic expansion. The contrary view that early hypothalamic compression may be the cause of amenorrhea and impotence is not supported by our data. Since the incidence of tumors of all sizes is similar both in cases with visual and sexual defects and since interference with vision arrives at a late stage in the course of amenorrheic patients, the suprasellar extension in the latter symptom category cannot be marked in the initial stages.

There can be no final resolution of the arguments presented in view of the number of complicating neurologic signs found at initial examination. Although the patient may not complain of symptoms which arise from the accompanying disorders, their existence prior to investigation is not necessarily a brief one. However, it seems reasonable to accept the sequence of symptoms as described by the patient as valid.

VI

NEUROLOGIC SIGNS AND SYMPTOMS

In reviewing the individual symptoms and corresponding signs found in the neurology of this syndrome characteristic and articulated groupings are sought for, in order to recognize the mechanisms which produce the symptoms and to facilitate diagnosis. The following discussion is concerned first with single symptoms and then with their natural colligation.

VISUAL SYMPTOMS

Although there are many and important symptoms observed in cases of chromophobe adenoma, diminution of visual acuity and limitation of visual fields assume primary place. Visual acuity was measured by test charts and graded reading material. The results reported here are those of maximally corrected acuity. Visual fields were tested by means of a tangent screen one or two meters from the patient. A white test object of two or eight millimeters was used routinely; in this manner a visual field of about thirty degrees was explored. Less frequently perimetric examination of the peripheral field was undertaken. Occasionally more elaborate investigations of visual field defects were carried out.

In the usual case the patient outlined a nondescript story of gradually decreasing ability to read or view with former clarity. Eighty-nine of the 117 patients were unaware of the degree or location of field cuts. There were 5 who recalled that the bitemporal areas were partially defective. In 6 patients of this series negative central scotomata, scintillations and flashes of colored light, illusions or photophobia centered attention on disturbed visual function. In the presence of these more dramatic introductory symptoms there were no particular gross findings in the remainder of the examination or at operation to indicate extraordinary location of the tumor. In contrast to the findings of others[505] hallucinations were not found as an effect of pressure on the optic nerves or anterior portions of the optic tracts. One patient with homonymous hemianopia complained of hallucinations which were associated with seizures preceded by a gustatory aura. Involvement of the temporal lobe and optic tract in this region was found.

To add to the delay before clinical emergence of the syndrome, the onset of visual symptoms was almost uniformly gradual. In those instances where the advent was acute, a history of slowly progressive visual impairment was recalled. In 6 of the 7 rapidly progressing cases primary optic atrophy was definite and fairly advanced at the time of admission. In 2 patients trauma and prolonged exposure to sun, respectively, appeared to induce sudden symptoms, perhaps a result of edema and expansion of the tumor with marked compression of the optic tracts. In the others, spontaneous hemorrhage into a cystic tumor or swelling of the tumor were associated with rapid failure of vision. Only 1 patient with a sudden onset had neither primary optic atrophy nor a history of decreased visual acuity. Here an unexpected extravasation of the contents of a cystic chromophobe adenoma into the subarachnoid space caused an aseptic meningitis and sudden blindness.

Five patients (4 per cent of the series) had no evidence of impaired visual acuity; the nature of field defects and the changes in visual acuity are reviewed in tables 4 and 5.

Criteria for serviceable vision may be defined rigidly, but in practice judgment of visual impairment must include consideration of the individual's adaptibility, as well as his occupation and avocations. Generalizations cannot include these factors without introducing unwieldly amplifications. With these qualifications in mind, the following three classifications can be established.

Group I: Visual acuity, 20/100; 20/100 minimum. Visual field, 15 degrees minimum diameter in horizontal meridian.

Group II: Visual acuity, 20/100; blind, minimum. Visual field, 15 degrees minimum diameter in horizontal meridian.

Group III: Visual acuity, 20/200; 20/200 or worse. Visual field, 15 degrees or less in horizontal meridian.

TABLE 4—*Nature of Field Defects in Patients
with Chromophobe Adenoma*

Symptom-Field Defect	% Neurological Institute Presbyterian Hospital	% Henderson-Cushing[239]	% Davidoff[114]*
Bitemporal hemianopia	57.0	65.0	70.0
Blind in one eye and temporal cut in other	19.0	10.0	15.0
Homonymous hemianopia	3.0	10.0	7.0
Temporal in one eye	3.0	3.0	2.0
Inferior altitudinal or central scotoma	—	7.0	1.0
Temporal in one eye, central scotoma in other	4.0	—	—
Blind in one eye, no defect in other	—	—	1.0
Blind in one eye plus constriction	4.0	—	—
Constriction—bilateral	2.0	—	—
Bilaterally blind	4.0	3.0	2.0
No defect	4.0	2.0	2.0
Number of patients	117	260	91

* Tabulation of this series is slightly condensed.

Groups I and II may be considered to include patients with functional vision, all other variables acknowledged as potential limitations. Of the total of 101 patients who attained the state of visual acuity ascribed to these two groups, 71 possessed equally satisfactory visual fields. Therefore, 70 per cent of the patients with visual disturbances could expect a reasonably gratifying outcome if the effects of optic compression could be halted at this stage. The remaining patients required such therapeutic intervention as would reversibly alter the visual insufficiency.

TABLE 5—*Visual Acuity and State of Visual Fields in Patients with Defective Vision**

Range of visual acuity				Number = %	Visual fields	
					Satis-factory	Unsatis-factory
Group I					*Group I*	
$\frac{20}{20}$	$\frac{20}{20}$	$\frac{20}{50}$	$\frac{20}{50}$	28		
$\frac{20}{50}$	$\frac{20}{50}$	$\frac{20}{50}$	$\frac{20}{100}$	15	39	5
$\frac{20}{50}$	$\frac{20}{100}$	$\frac{20}{100}$	$\frac{20}{100}$	1		
Group II					*Group II*	
$\frac{20}{100}$	$\frac{20}{100}$	$\frac{20}{50}$	$\frac{20}{200}$	27	32	15
$\frac{20}{50}$	$\frac{20}{200}$	$\frac{20}{100}$	$\frac{20}{200}$	2		
B†	$\frac{20}{50}$			15		
B	$\frac{20}{100}$			3		
Group III					*Group III*	
$\frac{20}{200}$	$\frac{20}{200}$			1		
B	$\frac{20}{200}$, or worse			4	0	10
B	B			5		
			Total	101	71	30

* The patients are divided into three groups in accord with the degree of initial involvement of vision.
† B = blind.

It is characteristic to observe a progressive decline in vision in untreated cases. Modifications in the rate of interference with visual ability are toward accelerated impairment of this function. Spontaneous remissions have been reported, perhaps as an effect of displacement of the tumor and consequent decompression of the optic tracts, but none occurred in this series.

Although extensive and frequent examinations of visual defects have been performed on a number of the patients presented here, the total data is insufficient and not of the type to relate to the development of the field changes.

The optic nerve is a centripetal extension of retinal ganglion cells and as such represents fibers of a higher order neuron; in effect it is a brain tract with an extra-axial location. Prolonged and substantial pressure on this pathway produces degenerative changes of the nerve fibers and retrograde degeneration of the retinal ganglion cells. The optic papilla loses its normal pinkish hue and becomes pale and atrophic. The duration and extent of the compressive effects of pituitary tumors required to produce clinically recognizable optic atrophy are not definitely known but a few weeks of adequate pressure is all that is needed to realize detectable ophthalmoscopic signs.

Since the degeneration of a significant number of optic nerve fibers may occur without visible ophthalmoscopic findings, it is surprising that only 5 per cent of those with visual difficulties had no evidence of primary optic atrophy. As with many other areas of the nervous system, where reserves are limited, functional disabilities may be more apparent than structural alterations as a result of crucially located but minor defects. However, there may be an explanation for the high correlation between primary optic atrophy and visual disturbances. In most of the patients, visual acuity was noticeably affected. This may indicate that fibers originating in paracentral and central retinal areas have been involved. Since these fibers constitute a large percentage of those feeding into the temporal part of the papilla, atrophic changes in them are likely to be visible on ophthalmoscopic examination. When the effects of pressure are felt by fibers arising from other retinal areas atrophy of the papilla becomes more widespread.

It has been said that local vasoconstriction contributes to the atrophic appearance of the optic papilla in cases of chromophobe adenoma. Although this may be true in their early development, those cases with a year or more of optic changes have concomitant and significant structural defects in the nerve fibers sufficient to account for pallid discs. The waxy tone of the optic papilla believed to be a feature of pressure atrophy by chromophobe adenomas, has not proved to be notable or novel.

When the autonomic innervation of the eye is not directly affected in the sellar syndrome, the occurrence of anisocoria indicates the laterality of more pronounced visual loss. Dilatation of the pupil has been found to be ipsilateral to the greater visual defect in three-fourths of the 21 cases in which the condition of the pupils was expressly mentioned. However, the situation may be reversed so that this sign, although reliable, is not infallible.

There are several possible reasons for the association of pupillary dilatation and visual defect. Special sensory fibers carrying impulses which initiate the pupillary response to light may be injured by pressure of the tumor against the optic nerve, chiasm or first part of the tract, and the constrictor response to stimulation by light so diminished. This explanation supposes that the pupillary diameter of each eye is partially governed by appreciation of the intensity of the sensory stimuli impinging on the corresponding retina. When the pupil is dilated more light reaches the retina and a greater surface of retina is stimulated. This may compensate for the diminution in functional macular and paramacular retinal area. The retina excited is no longer the most sensitive central area and although cortical perceptive centers may receive contributions from the rods as well as the cones located peripherally a more diffuse image is formed centrally as a result.[7] The relatively fixed pupil and the associated reduction in visual acuity probably tends to diminish the perceptions of the details of the stimulus. This unorganized type of stimulation does not lead to satisfactory central perceptive definitions.[286]

The kinetics of pupillary reactions in instances of visual defects has not been adequately reported in this series. The correspondence between diminution of visual acuity and decrease in the reactivity of the light reflex has been noted and is, as expected, very high where visual acuity is severely affected, but not striking in other circumstances. However, if the light source used to elicit the reflex is directed onto the blind retinal areas, there may be very little or no pupillary response. This is well known and has been of service in corroborating the defects found on field examination.

In the finer differential diagnosis of the source of visual inter-ference there are certain generalities which assist in localization. These may be summarized as follows. In lesions involving the optic nerve one eye usually is affected unless the genu of the crossing nasal fibers of the other eye is implicated near the chiasm with the corresponding development of a junction scotoma. Defects of both nasal and temporal fields of one eye without invasion of the fields of the other eye results from pathology confined to one optic nerve. Optic atrophy and pupil-lary abnormalities may accompany the field defects. In lesions of the chiasm the fields of both eyes are usually involved; the field cuts are not frequently homonymous, although such a defect is possible. Atrophy and pupillary changes may be present. Fixation in this case and in the following situations may or may not be impaired. Infra-geniculate tract lesions are associated with homonymous hemianopia and incongruous fields. Optic atrophy occurs and pupillary abnormal-ities such as may develop in lesions more distally placed are possible, namely, anisocoria, paresis of light reflex and hemianopic pupillary response to light. Suprageniculate lesions are rare in association with parasellar and sellar tumors. Here the fields are congruous and homonymously hemianopic. Central vision is spared, optic atrophy does not occur and pupillary abnormalities are absent.

In general, routine examinations by means of ophthalmoscope, visual acuity tests and field studies suffice to develop a pattern of the visual defect. Investigation of visual fields under conditions of dim light and with colored objects are of assistance since the decreased definition and intensity of the stimulus tends to reveal defects in otherwise border-line performances.

There were only 7 instances, representing six per cent of the total, in which papilledema was noted. Two of these cases had minimal evidence of edema; only 1 had a cavernous sinus syndrome. In the others the tumors protruded subfrontally, filled part of the basal cisterns or shouldered into the third ventricle. In 6 of the 7 cases the develop-ment of papilledema cannot be ascribed to occlusion of a cavernous sinus, even if this is pathogenically important in some cases. More anteriorly directed pressure or spreading edema of the brain due to the effects of the adenoma growing into the hypothalamus and partially obstructing the third ventricle may be independent causes for papilledema in cases of chromophobe adenoma. Evidently the capacity of the basilar regions is adequate to accommodate most tumors without causing compression of the brain. Moreover, there may be sufficient play in the basal vessels to permit their deflection without critically narrowing their diameters.

The occurrence of papilledema in patients with general or local increase in intracranial pressure is not explained satisfactorily by the concepts advanced. Currently, mechanical obstruction to the return of retinal venous blood or perineural cerebrospinal fluid is thought to be the most important predisposing cause of plerocephalic edema. In the case of chromophobe adenoma, lateral expansion may retard venous flow through the cavernous sinus and elevate intraocular venous tension. The existence of well developed anastomoses between the ophthalmic and the facial veins vitiates the importance of cavernous sinus obstruction in the production of papilledema in such cases.[133] It is possible for the tumor to obstruct circulation from the retina by direct compression of the ophthalmic vein and optic subarachnoid space. Chromophobe adenomas also may cause a block in the ventricular system. The resulting hydrocephalus may lead to impairment of centripetal flow of retinal blood and perineural cerebrospinal fluid. In animals, elevation of intracranial pressure and intracranial venous tension or obstruction of the retinal venous return do not cause papilledema with regularity.[104] Therefore, other explanations for papilledema have been advanced. Lowering the retinal arterial pressure can produce edema when the ratio of arterial to venous pressure becomes less than about three to one. However, there is no definite clinical counterpart in these cases to this experimental observation.

A further theory introduces the idea that as a result of increased intracranial pressure transudation within the brain occurs, and modifies the colloidal state of the brain substance, a change which extends forward in the optic nerve. The effect of optic atrophy may so alter the physicochemical characteristics of the optic nerve that the edema of the brain is not transported anteriorly within the nerve. This may be one of the reasons for the infrequency of plerocephalic edema in cases of chromophobe adenoma.

Headache

Headache is a common but rarely dominating symptom in the sellar syndrome. In the present series, headache occurred in 78 of the 117 patients. As was noted in the discussion of initial symptoms, visual disability and headache are among the most common complaints. The incidence of large tumors was twice as great in patients with the symptom of headache as in those without headache. However, this symptom can occur with tumors of all sizes and in many locations. The data with regard to the exact anatomic deformations produced by chromophobe adenomas are incomplete. In operated cases, the surgeon rarely recapitulated for the record with sufficient detail the extent of the neoplasm in relation to surrounding structures other than optic nerves and hypothalamus. If mechanical influences are one of the prime determinants for causation of headache the finding of a higher incidence of large tumors in the cases with headache is in apparent harmony with this hypothesis.

In view of the location of most tumors in the middle fossa and in relation to the anterior part of the circle of Willis it is not surprising to find that only 9 of the 78 instances of headache are occipital in origin. Of these cases only 1 had definite extension into the posterior fossa. The other 8 records do not indicate any unusual spread of the tumor, but it is not impossible that the traction induced by the neoplasm was felt by the arterial and venous vessels innervated by the ninth and tenth nerves within the posterior fossa. Under these circumstances the projection of headache on the surface would tend to be occipital.

About one-third of anterior headaches were unilateral. Those which occurred in the orbital area manifested a high correspondence between the side of the more marked or complete visual loss and the headache, but data concerning unilateral headaches in other cephalic regions with respect to observations at operation of the predominant laterality of the tumor were insufficient. It is probable that unilateral headache in cases of chromophobe adenoma has a significance equal to that in other intracranial tumors, designating the side of greater local involvement.[527] By the time the patient comes under observation, the extension of the tumor may produce a complicated neurology making it difficult to unravel the origin of the headache in relation to involvement of particular structures even with full information at hand. For example, extension into the cavernous sinus does not appear to be associated with a predictable localized headache, despite the fact that this is at some variance with the experimental facts.[527] In these cases the invasion of the sinus was known to be accompanied by extension into other areas and the headache could no longer be identified with involvement of the cavernous sinus alone.

Of the 117 patients in this series, 78 presented headache symptoms, some complaining of headaches in more than one location at different times. The total number of complaints came to 89. Locations and incidence of these 89 complaints are as follows: 28 frontal, 17 related to orbit, 14 temporal, 9 occipital, 6 vertical, 2 generalized and 13 unlocalized. This unlocalized category consists of those whose descriptions did not designate the specific site of headache.

Usually, headache was gradual in onset and moderately severe. Although the intensity was difficult to judge an approximate estimate of its degree can be made on the basis of the amount of interference with normal activity caused by this symptom and the stress which the patient places upon it. Intermittency of occurrence was the rule, but a few headaches were continuous over the span of months and even years. Paroxysms of headache were noted occasionally but could not be attributed to any particularity of the syndrome. Aggravation or relief of the headache by changes in posture were observed only in 1 case. There were 9 instances in which nausea and vomiting were notable accompaniments of the headache. Increased intracranial pressure was not found in this group nor was the third ventricle particularly impressed. Nausea and vomiting may occur when there is traction or displacement of the great vessels of the base. Such a mechanism may exist in these cases. In this series an acute onset of a very severe headache with nausea and vomiting was found only in the presence of an important event such as extravasation of a cyst or sudden edematous or hemorrhagic expansion of a chromophobe adenoma.

Headache responded in a manner which seemed dependent on regression of the tumor as a result of therapy. Although the data is not clear in this regard, spontaneous relief of headache and a course at variance with other symptoms have been observed. Ordinarily this symptom is so subjective in evaluation both for the patient and the examiner and depends so greatly for definition of its mechanism on precise and clear-cut situations and recording that one can more readily state its occurrence than describe its significance or pathogenesis.

In attempting to correlate the data with the observations of Wolff and his collaborators[527] and also of Northfield,[357] Pickering[371] and others the headache of pituitary tumors as in the case of other intracranial expanding masses may be due to the effects of traction or displacement of pain sensitive structures. The responsive areas involved with parasellar tumors include primarily the dura of the anterior two-thirds of the base of the skull, the lining of the air sinuses, the arterial vessels of the circle of Willis and perhaps the larger venous sinuses in the parasellar area. Branches of the fifth cranial nerve innervate these structures in their supratentorial location. The mechanical distortion produced by an adenoma has been seen to be exerted on similar structures of other regions, such as the basal dura and venous sinuses of the posterior fossa and the posterior portion of the arterial circle, which are supplied by the ninth and tenth nerves.

Inflammation as well as mechanical or electric stimulation of these sensitive areas may evoke painful responses. In this connection, a meningitic complication of pituitary adenoma may account for a limited number of acute headaches. Direct pressure on a sensory nerve such as the ophthalmic branch of the fifth is an occasional source of pain. There are probably other factors which lead to headache in the presence of an expanding intracranial lesion, but those mentioned have been carefully investigated and full treatment of the problem may be found in a pertinent monograph by Wolff.[527]

Extraocular nerves

In a previous chapter certain general aspects of the effects of chromophobe adenoma on the third, fourth and sixth nerves have been discussed. The incidence of involvement of these nerves is about 17 per cent of all cases. In the event of involvement of a single nerve, the third was predominantly affected. Evidently the proximity and accessibility of this nerve to sellar tumors overrides the importance of the precavernous length of the sixth, which is somewhat more inferiorly placed within the sinus and not in direct route of expansion. However, when the mechanical effects of the expanding lesion were more extensive the third and sixth nerves suffered equally. Because palsy of the superior oblique is so frequently diagnosed mistakenly or entirely overlooked the findings of trochlear injury are not useful for comparison. It is usual to observe only partial interference with the function of these nerves. This is noted especially in the case of the third nerve, where incomplete paresis of isolated muscles or of pupillary kinetics may exist.

The regions at which tumor pressure was exerted were surmised from associated neurologic findings, pneumoencephalographic and operative reports. The intracavernous segment of the oculomotor nerve was directly involved in one-third of the cases. In another third there was pressure probably against the nerves in the cavernous sinus. Finally, displacement of the nerves at the precavernous intervals or at the superior orbital fissure was noted. While it was possible to approximate the region at which the pressure occured, the actual location of injury to the nerves may have been projected to their points of binding.

In several instances the occurrence of an infective meningitis as a result of erosion into the sphenoid sinus or the rupture of a cyst and a consequent aseptic meningitis caused inflammation of perineural and neural elements, with the sudden development of ocular palsies.

Abnormalities of pupillary reactions were observed in association with palsies of the third nerve. Involvement of the oculomotor components in cases with paresis of the reflexes of light and/or accommodation was noted in only a few patients. Reduction in pupillary responsiveness to light was most frequently the result of visual impairment. There was no evidence of involvement of sympathetic innervation to the eye although presumably this may occur in the presence of injury to the pericarotid plexus or to the center within the hypothalamus. Intra-axial disturbances of pupillary functions were not evident, unless hippus could be so considered. Hippus was found only in the presence of marked visual defect. An increase of the physiologic fluctuations in pupillary diameter depends in part on an upset of balance between the reflex functions concerned with the reaction to light and the adjustments required by fixation. Hippus is noted infrequently in this syndrome although here difficulties in fixation are characteristic. It is possible that the light reaction is similarly, though subclinically, affected and the equilibrium between it and the fixation process is maintained at a lower level of function.

Two cases with the finding of gaze palsy had neoplastic extensions into the subfrontal regions as demonstrated by pneumoencephalographic and operative observations. In gaze palsies one must distinguish which type is present. Kestenbaum[281] has introduced a rather categorical division of gaze palsies that depends on the ocular responses to command (schematic movement), to an object appearing in the visual fields suddenly (optically elicited movement), to following movements and to vestibular reflexes. In these cases the gaze palsies were associated with extension of the tumor into the frontal region where the relevant tracts which descend from this lobe were implicated. Schematic movements were principally affected. When there was an extensive reduction in the field of vision an apparent palsy based on ocular inertia was noted occasionally. This has been ascribed in part to the demonstration in following and optokinetically oriented movements.

Nystagmus in sellar syndromes is most generally the result of diminished visual acuity and/or palsies of extraocular muscles. In the former event the nystagmus is related to faulty fixation and in the latter it is directly dependent on the inability of paretic muscles to sustain an ocular position. However, 4 of the 10 cases in which this dyskinesia was observed did not exhibit any muscular weakness or interference with fixation. Vertical, rotary horizontal and horizontal second and third degree nystagmus were noted. In 2 of these cases the adenoma was confined to the sella; in the others extensions into the third ventricle and frontal regions were observed. Unless the effects of these confirmed small tumors of the pituitary confined to sellar and perhaps the lateral parasellar areas were experienced remotely, somewhere in the system associated with the posterior longitudinal bundle, it is difficult to explain vertical and rotary nystagmus occurring in the presence of normal fixation and ocular movements.

In the absence of paresis of the medial recti convergence and fusion deficiencies were believed to be the consequence of severely impaired vision with unstable fixation.

Extra-axial extension

After adequate evidence that a sellar syndrome has been present for some time, symptomatic progression of an adenoma into frontal, parieto-temporal or peduncular areas may occur. These extensions can generally be considered avoidable complications which usually impair the functioning of the patient irreversibly as well as add to the difficulties of therapy. Viewed in this manner the fact that one-fourth of all the patients had unequivocal signs of involvement of frontal, temporal, parietal or peduncular regions indicates either a delay in the patients' seeking advice or a delay in the consulting physician's diagnosis.

The motor symptoms most commonly remarked were paresis of the extremities, clumsiness of the hands and ataxia of gait. From a review of the data it is apparent that the tumors which induced such effects were almost exclusively large. Indeed they were usually too extensive to permit selective localization of the structures involved or estimation of the neural mechanisms disordered. It is probable that the fibers which enter the internal capsule en route to and from the frontal or temporoparietal lobes are compressed or rendered ischaemic, either within the centrum ovale or near the capsule itself. Their dysfunction produces either fragments or all of the picture of an upper motor neuron lesion, essentially the result of conductive defects in the cortico-spinal, cortico-bulbar, cortico-cerebellar tracts.

In several cases the peduncles were directly affected by the pressure of a tumor. Occasionally signs of an extrapyramidal syndrome were found, i.e., retropulsion and tremor. There was one illuminating instance of extension of an adenoma to implicate the brain stem and cerebellum within the posterior fossa. Symptoms and signs of a cerebellar and pontomedullary lesion were present.

In association with the motor symptoms of frontal and tempo-roparietal involvement were defects in symbolism both in language and performance. Sensory deficits were rarely found.

Evidence of hypothalamic compression was notable in this group with motor disabilities. Symptoms referable to neural systems other than those already described as related to the hypothalamus were not seen; in fact, there were as many cases with marked hypothalamic compression without motor disabilities as there were with these complaints. These data may indicate that involvement of the hypothalamus neither augments already detectable motor difficulties nor initiates them.

The appearance of epilepsy in mature individuals without a suggestive antecedent history is commonly associated with grossly evident intracranial pathology. Somewhat less than 10 per cent of the patients registered this complaint, and in each case marked compression of frontal, temporal or hypothalamic regions by a large pituitary tumor was found. Whether the tumor initiates the convulsive phenomenon at its site of pressure or whether its effect is produced by disturbances somewhat remote from the actual region of compression is difficult to judge. The mechanisms of production of epilepsy by expanding lesions are unknown. It is assumed that pathologic cortical ganglion cells at the periphery of the pressure cone may give rise to an extraordinary outburst of neural activity which is transported to other anatomically related areas by means of transcortical, subcortical or projectional interconnections.[330] The pulsatile electrical activity of ganglion cells which exists in isolated cortical slices undoubtedly depends on intracellular chemical events.[293] It is probable that consequent to the effects of pressure a disturbance in the chain of these events leads to neuronal hyperirritability and temporal conditions suitable for the genesis of an epileptic discharge. In part, the further passage of this discharge depends on the receptivity of the units to which it spreads.

The type of seizure has a certain localizing value.[365] For example, when parts of the temporal cortex are fired by the effects of compression, complex patterns,[364] represented in several of these cases as psychical and uncinate fits with hallucinations, may occur. Excitation of other cortical regions produces less organized but still recognizable motor or sensory patterns. These characteristics were observed in this series as well.

The finding in one patient of akinetic seizures with diaphoresis and flushing was noted to be associated with pressure on the hypothalamus. However, in other instances of equally intensive hypothalamic compression, seizure states did not occur. Akinesis may be thought the result of excitation of inhibitory mechanisms of cortical or subcortical origin. The infrequency of seizures in the event of hypothalamic distortion and probably associated transmitted compression to the thalamus should be remarked. Recent work has advanced the thesis that the thalamus and other subcortical regions, either independently or through the cortex, may be a contributory source of epileptic discharges. Moreover, the thalamo-reticular system is believed to have great influence over the electrical activity of the cortex.[230, 272, 396] The low incidence of seizures in cases of chromophobe adenoma suggests that these tumors may not affect the subcortical structures to a sufficient degree or in a manner which could provoke paroxysmal dysrhythmias and clinical seizures. However, the fact remains that a few pituitary tumors which exert pressure on cortical or subcortical areas may induce seizure states of almost any definition.

Observations with regard to the mental and affective states of these patients were inadequate. Psychologic symptoms resulting from the effects of tumor, dysendocrinism and the patient's reaction to the situation of illness and economic deprivation require a most expert differential analysis for meaningful interpretation. Nevertheless, readily detectable intellectual and personality changes were obvious in a quarter of the patients. These could be divided broadly into two types: one arising from frontal lobe involvement and the other occuring in the presence of hypothalamic compression, alone or in conjunction with an extension of the tumor into the frontal lobes. Emotional lability, confusion and apparent difficulty in recall were predominant in the former, whereas impairment of consciousness ranging from somnolence to stupor was more outstanding in the latter instance. For the most part these symptoms were dealt with ineffectually. As a counterpart to the physical basis of therapy and before one is able to evaluate the extent of reversible injury, psychologic rehabilitative measures should be included in the therapeutic regimen.

Miscellaneous

Olfaction may deteriorate due to the effects of compression of the olfactory tract or invasion of the nasal passages by tumor. The former situation is probably more common than the 5 per cent recorded in this series. In fact this comparatively low incidence is more likely the result of the inadequacy of the testing methods than a reflection of the frequency of olfactory nerve involvement. The olfactory tract extends from the cribriform plate caudally along the inferior surface of the frontal lobe to end at the olfactory trigone, anterosuperior to the tuberculum sellae. It is shielded by the optic nerve and anterior cerebral vessels, but is exposed in some degree to suprasellar growths pressing upwards and forwards. Perhaps the yielding environment and the play along its length diminish the possibility of injury to the olfactory tract.

The trigeminal nerve was affected in less than 1 per cent of this series. It lies along the lateral wall of the cavernous sinus, reaching this location by passing from the frontal aspect of the pons across the tip of the petrous bone and under the free edge of the tentorium cerebelli to enter the sinus. It extends forward below the nerves to the extraocular muscles and external to the internal carotid artery, which partially protects it from an expanding adenoma. The second and third components, which have a short, inferiorly situated, intracavernous course, are scarcely ever affected. The first division, somewhat more vulnerable by virtue of its position and length, is also rarely involved. This nerve, the ophthalmic, supplies sensory fibers to the orbital and supraorbital area. The finding of decreased corneal sensitivity is the usual fragmentary evidence of interference with the first branch of the fifth, but diminished sensibility to the modalities of pain and touch in the entire area of its innervation may occur.

Multiple cranial neuropathy is noted very occasionally when the adenoma assumes a more invasive character and metastasizes locally in the middle and posterior fossa.

At the present time invasion of the paranasal sinuses is a less common event than in the early period, during which adenomas were treated more conservatively and at a later stage in their course.[100] A history of impairment in the function of smell and epistaxis should serve to initiate investigations of the nasal passages and sinuses. Local nasal examination and x-rays of the sinus are most helpful in this regard. By virtue of the adoption of the transfrontal operative approach limited opportunity to detect downward extensions of the tumor is afforded. In 1 of the 3 cases of nasopharyngeal extension recorded here a suprasellar removal and decompression of a pituitary adenoma was successful and great visual improvement was observed. At a later date spontaneous hemorrhage into the nasal projection of this patient's neoplasm occurred. The hemorrhage dissected superiorly and induced mortal disturbance within the hypothalamus. A history of repeated and chronic epistaxis had been ignored. It is possible that a combined transfrontal and intranasal approach might have been therapeutically effective in this case. A further complication of invasion of a sinus is acute meningitis which can occur without apparent antecedent infection or local physical disturbances.

The many symptoms of the sellar syndrome described here form multiple and varying patterns that cannot be rigidly categorized. With this reservation in mind a qualified attempt to identify groups of neurologic symptoms can be made.

Primarily the sellar complex presents visual defects. Further extension of the tumor involves the hypothalamus with consequent drowsiness, modifications in appetites, perhaps sexual dysfunction and thermal changes and an increased susceptibility to operative trauma. Lateral expansion into the parasellar region is associated with a partial syndrome of the cavernous sinus: extraocular muscle palsies, occasionally diminished sensibility of the cornea and supraorbital area and, rarely, exophthalamus and papilledema. Invasion of the frontal and temporal lobes may pass unnoticed, but it is more usual to find signs of an incomplete upper motor neuron lesion, supranuclear cranial nerve palsies, aphasias, seizures and uncinate fits and possibly emotional and intellectual disorders. The findings of diminished olfaction or homonymous hemianopia may differentiate frontal from temporal involvement.

The more acute manifestations of pituitary adenoma are found in the meningitic form in which the rupture of a cystic tumor, hemorrhage from an adenoma into its surroundings or bacterial invasion of the cranial cavity from invaded or eroded nasal sinuses appear to initiate the meningitis. The meningitis not of bacterial origin is usually local, self-limiting and its effects reversible. Dramatic symptoms of an acute sellar form associated with cystic extravasation and edema or bleeding into a tumor may consist of sudden visual impairment, a diminution in consciousness, the appearance of meningismus and signs of pituitary insufficiency. There is little that clinically distinguishes between the sudden rupture of a cyst and hemorrhage into a tumor.

VII

METABOLIC
SYMPTOMATOLOGY

The same group of individuals who are troubled by visual, motor and other neural deficits are further burdened by derangements of metabolic function and balance. It is well to emphasize that the syndromes observed in patients with chromophobe adenomas are compounded of such diverse disturbances. The separate analysis of such defects is a practical necessity but it must not obscure the fact that these are most often co-existent and not infrequently functionally related in the same individual.

THYROID FUNCTION

Symptomatic disturbances

The selection of criteria symptomatic of thyroid disturbance was difficult. Symptoms customarily referable to hypothyroidism were often difficult to distinguish from those more directly implicating the adrenals or gonads in the same patient. The constellation of symptoms and signs used as an arbitrary reference was as follows: extraordinary sensitivity to cold or to rapid changes in environmental temperature in the absence of hypoadrenalism; recent or abrupt changes in body hair exclusive of pubic hair, in the absence of clear-cut gonadal hypofunction; an enlarged thyroid gland or historic and physical evidence of previous thyroid surgery; clinical myxedema of pituitary origin. These criteria leave much to be desired and could justifiably be amplified were we dealing with primary hypothyroidism. However, in a

metabolic study of this complexity it was considered advisable to re-
strict clinical criteria to a minimum.

As indicated in table 6, 18 patients, less than one-fifth of the entire
series, had symptomatic disturbances in thyroid function. Of these, 3
had evidence of past or present hyperthyroidism. Only 1 of the series
was thought to have pituitary myxedema. Asymptomatic thyroid enlargement was noted in an additional 9 patients. Thus 24 per cent of
patients had symptomatic or physical evidence of thyroid dysfunction.
The incidence of symptomatic hypothyroidism was almost identical in
the group with BMR of − 15 or less and in the group with BMR of
− 14 or above. In the latter the trend was clearly toward the minus
side though within the normal range. In contrast, only 1 of 58 patients
with BMR of − 15 or less was noted to have an enlarged thyroid
gland, although 6 of 25 with BMR of − 14 or above had enlarged
thyroid glands. Clearly the level of resting metabolism is an inadequate
biologic index.

Pertinent laboratory studies

1. Basal metabolic rate

A total of 141 satisfactory BMRs were performed on 83 patients
of this series; of this number, 58 had BMRs of − 15 or below consistently throughout the total period of observation. With thyroid
medication BMRs usually returned to normal range. Individual tests
varied rather widely, but the trend was clearly toward decreasing BMR
with progression of the disease process. X-ray therapy or surgical intervention produced no consistent alterations in this trend. The mean
BMR in this group was − 25 and the distribution was essentially of
normal type.

The mean BMR in the remaining 30 per cent of patients, with
BMRs of − 14 or above, was − 6. Only 6 of 141 individual determinations were above 0. Even though only 70 per cent of the total had
BMRs below the lower limit of accepted normal, the series trend was
uniformly toward the minus side.

2. Iodine metabolism

Blood iodine level was determined in 5 patients with BMRs of

TABLE 6—*Thyroid Functional Status*

Status or finding	Incidence			Statistical data				
	No.	Total studied	%	Mean trend — Mean Sigma	Max. Min.	Mean Diff.	σ Error Mean Diff.
1. Symptomatic disturbance	18	113	16				
2. Asymptomatic thyroid enlargement	9	113	8				
3. Symptomatic hypothyroidism in those with BMR − 15 or less	9	58	15				
4. Symptomatic hypothyroidism in those with BMR − 14 or above	3	25	12				
5. BMR − 15 or less (total)	58	83	70	− 25 ± 8.5	− 15 − 44		
6. BMR − 14 or above (total)	25	83	30	− 6 ± 6.	+ 9 − 14		
7. Total serum cholesterol: BMR − 15 or below (aver. values; mg.%)		52		289 ± 68			
8. Total serum cholesterol: BMR − 14 or above (aver. values; mg.%)		26		271 ± 55		18 (7–8) Not Signif.	± 10
9. Total serum cholesterol: normal values (Peters and VanSlyke [369])		174		194 ± 35.6		95 (7-9) Signif. 77 (8-9) Signif.	+ 6.4 + 7.1

− 15 or below, the maximum level being 4.9 gamma, the minimum 2.2 gamma. Thus all were below the conservative low normal level of 5 gamma. Radioactive iodine uptake was especially notable in 2 patients of this group. In one with a BMR of − 17, the uptake was 25.5 per cent, hence well within the usual normal range. In another patient with BMRs ranging from − 27 to − 35, radioactive iodine uptake was at the lower limit of normal, 12.5 per cent, but not within the range observed in primary hypothyroidism (10 per cent or below).

A single blood iodine level in a patient with BMR of 5 was 8.5 gamma, hence well within the limits of normal.

3. *Cholesterol levels*

From 1 to 20 individual total serum cholesterol determinations were performed on each of 78 patients in this series. In the group with BMRs of − 15 or below the mean cholesterol value was 289 mg. per cent. The distribution of values about this mean was normal, the range quite wide. Individual determinations varied widely one from another and could not be correlated with clinical state, BMR or stage of the illness. The mean value, though well below the normal maximum, is significantly higher than the mean for normal individuals.[369] In the group with BMR of − 14 or above the mean value for serum cholesterol was 271 mg. per cent, significantly higher than the normal mean, but not significantly different from the mean value for those with BMRs of − 15 or less.

Discussion

The fact that symptomatic disturbances referable to thyroid dysfunction are relatively infrequent in this study as compared with previous analyses[193] is explicable on the basis of our criteria. Since we have excluded disturbances which must be considered more directly as of gonadal or adrenal origin the implication of the thyroid gland is inconspicuous, at best. In Simmonds' disease Escamilla and Lisser[146] have recorded symptoms referable to hypothyroidism in the majority of their series but the contribution of other endocrine deficits was not considered. They did record the fact that an enlarged thyroid gland was extremely rare in Simmonds' disease, as it is in our series where BMRs were − 15 or below. The thyroid gland is not infrequently enlarged in acidophilic hyperpituitarism,[105] thus suggesting that thyroid enlargement in 6 patients of this series with BMRs of − 14 or above might reflect a fugitive or transitory hyperpituitary state. This thesis is subjected to critical analysis in a subsequent section.

Previous studies of basal metabolic rate in patients with chromophobe adenomas[105, 193, 531a] or with hypopituitary states largely of such origin[456] reveal a high incidence of subnormal rate. Total serum cholesterol was above 200 in 16 of 18 patients with hypopituitarism of neoplastic origin in Starr and Davis's[456] study. It is impossible to reconcile these or our own values with significantly lower trends for serum cholesterol revealed in the early studies of Hurxthal[263, 264] though a recent study by this group[531a] reveals a mean value slightly above the upper limits of normal.

The information given by specific studies of iodine metabolism in this series, though fragmentary, is worthy of note. While the thyroid gland still seems to retain the ability to remove usual amounts of iodine from the blood, even in the presence of conspiciuously subnormal metabolic rate, there would appear to be a defect in maintenance of normal blood levels of iodine (part of which is organically bound iodine). This defect is conspicuous in those with BMR of – 15 or below. No conclusions are, of course, justified by so few observations.

Summary

In spite of the fact that the vast majority of patients with chromophobe adenomas in this series had low normal or frankly subnormal BMRs, less than one-fourth of the entire series suffered from or complained (on specific questioning) of distressing symptoms clearly referable to hypothyroidism. The incidence of hypothyroid symptoms was essentially the same in those with subnormal and with low normal to normal metabolic rates.

Enlargement of the thyroid gland was extremely rare in those with BMR of – 15 or less but was noted in more than one-fifth of those with low normal or normal metabolic rates.

Total mean serum cholesterol, though within the high normal range, was significantly higher in those with chromophobe adenomas than in normal individuals. Mean serum cholesterol level bore no consistent relationship to basal metabolic rate.

The fragmentary data available suggest that in patients with chromophobe adenomas the thyroid gland may still be able to take up iodine more efficiently than in the patient with primary hypothyroidism, though it may metabolize and perhaps incorporate it into organic substances of metabolic importance as inadequately as in those with primary hypothyroidism.

ADRENAL GLAND FUNCTIONAL STATUS

Symptomatic disturbances

The evaluation of adrenal functional status presented more difficult problems than that of the thyroid. Clinical evidences of hypoadrenalism were not reliable. Among symptoms considered as suggestive were apathy, asthenia and excessive fatigue. Postural or stress hypotension (less than 100 mm. Hg. systolic and 70 mm. Hg. diastolic) on physical examination was accepted as a suggestive sign. Diarrhea and vomiting, among others, were included as acute gastro-intestinal disturbances when they occurred in the absence of other demonstrable causes, such as a gastro-intestinal lesion, gastroenteritis or increased intracranial pressure. Abnormal pigmentation of the skin and especially of the mucous membranes was methodically looked for.

By the above criteria symptomatic hypoadrenalism, with or without hypotension, was noted in 29 of 117 patients; hypotension without symptoms, in an additional 13 patients. Thus a total of 42 patients, 36 per cent of the entire series, showed evidence of functional disturbance usually attributed to hypoadrenalism. Diarrhea as a symptom was very unusual and abnormal pigmentation was not noted in any patient of the entire series. Pertinent data are summarized in table 7.

Laboratory documentation of hypoadrenal trends

A considerable number of patients in this series was exposed to stress of nonspecific as well as specific type, the latter designed to bring into focus discrete disturbances in adrenal function. Nonspecific stress was provided, often enough, by the environment itself and included one or more of the following traumatic experiences: exposure to excessive heat with profuse perspiration and uncontrolled salt loss, intensive deep x-ray therapy to the pituitary region, significant and proven extra-pituitary disease of acute type, extra-cranial operation, air encephalography, or finally intracranial surgery in or about the pituitary region. Documentation of hypoadrenalism under circumstances such as are enumerated was provided by analysis of serum sodium and potassium levels, blood urea, plasma volume and protein levels, as well as total urinary neutral 17-ketosteroids. Serum sodium levels below 136 milliequivalents were deemed strongly suggestive of, and levels below 130 mEq. per liter definite evidence of hypoadrenalism, provided such subnormal values did not reflect intercurrent salt

TABLE 7—*Adrenal Functional Status*

Status or finding	Incidence		
	Number	Total studied	%
1. Symptomatic hypoadrenalism..............	29	117	25
2. Hypotension without symptoms...........	13	117	11
3. Total (1 and 2).......................	42	117	36
4. Documented hypoadrenalism under uncontrolled environmental stress: (Group 3).....	15	42	36
5. Documented hypoadrenalism under uncontrolled environmental stress: (exclusive of Group 3)	2	64	3
6. Total with documented hypoadrenalism under uncontrolled environmental stress..........	17	106	16
7. Cardiac (clinical and electrocardiographic) changes noted (Group 6).................	4	7	
8. Positive salt deprivation response..........	4	9	
9. Hypoglycemic episodes (Group 6)..........	5	17	30
10. Insulin hypersensitivity (total)............	6	7	
11. High carbohydrate tolerance (total)	17	80	21

loss through the gastro-intestinal tract itself. The criteria used were those of Loeb and Atchley[315] for primary adrenal insufficiency.

Specific and controlled stress was provided by two technics; the salt-deprivation routine already outlined, and intravenous injection of small amount of insulin. Disturbances in carbohydrate metabolism, more remotely related to adrenal function, were reflected in episodes of symptomatic hypoglycemia, or in abnormally high tolerance for orally ingested or injected glucose.

Pertinent observations are briefly summarized in table 7. It should be noted that documented hypoadrenalism occurred under uncontrolled enviromental stress in only 2 patients with no previous evidence of symptomatic hypoadrenalism, while it was observed in slightly more than one-third of all patients suspected of hypoadrenalism on symptomatic and clinical grounds. A total of 17 patients (16 per cent of the entire series) were proven to have hypoadrenalism under uncontrolled stress. This total includes preponderantly those with disturbances in salt and water metabolism.

Four of 9 patients subjected to salt deprivation showed a response typical for primary hypoadrenalism, except that elevated serum potassium levels were not noted. Elevations of serum potassium were, moreover, not observed in those with documented hypoadrenalism secondary to uncontrolled environmental stress. All of the 4 patients who gave a positive response to salt deprivation had previous signs or symptoms suggestive of hypoadrenalism. An additional 2 patients whose signs or symptoms suggested hypoadrenalism responded in the normal manner to this specific type of stress.

Seven individuals with documented hypoadrenalism were studied electrocardiographically, 4 of whom were studied during adrenal crises. In 2 of the 4, the P-R interval was 0.20 seconds; there was significant bradycardia and low voltage complexes were observed. In 1 of these the P-R interval increased to 0.22 seconds, and voltage further decreased concomitant with deepening crisis. After therapy with doca and salt, the P-R interval of this patient gradually decreased to 0.18 seconds and voltage was elevated. However, venous pressure likewise rose moderately and increasing pulmonary edema supervened. The remaining 2 patients studied by electrocardiogram during crisis revealed no evidence of abnormality, but 1 of the 2 treated with doca and salt developed increasing edema and cardiac enlargement. Three additional patients who had evidence of mild to moderate hypoadrenalism without crisis showed no remarkable changes electrocardiographically, except for suggestive evidence of myocardial damage in 1. Slight enlargement of the heart was noted in another patient with a normal electrocardiogram.

Hypoglycemic episodes appear no more common in this form of secondary hypoadrenalism than in primary hypoadrenalism.[315]

Only 5 of 17 patients with documented hypoadrenalism had confirmed hypoglycemic episodes or abnormally high glucose tolerance. In only 1 instance, however, did the demonstrated hypoglycemic tendency contribute in any way to the symptomatic disturbances noted. In our entire series an abnormally high tolerance for orally ingested or intravenously injected glucose was observed in 21 per cent of patients so tested. Hence the overall incidence of this form of response was not significantly greater than that for disturbances in salt and water balance.

The response to intravenously injected insulin was a different matter. Though only 7 patients of the entire series were tested, 6 of the 7 were abnormally sensitive.

In a few patients in the series total neutral 17-ketosteroids were measured. The appropriate data are summarized in tables 10 and 11, and the values are more extensively discussed in the section on gonadal function. Let it suffice to state here that the level of excreted neutral ketosteroids bore no direct relationship to the presence or degree of documented hypoadrenalism.

Specific extracellular fluid studies made during hypoadrenal episodes under controlled or uncontrolled stress provide provocative observations. The limited data indicate that no single laboratory determination is of such value for the detection of the gravity or imminence of hypoadrenalism in such patients. Plasma volumes were determined one or more times on 11 individuals of the series. Only 1 of the 11 showed any evidence of hypoadrenalism under any circumstances, with a plasma volume greater than 40 cc. per Kg. ideal body weight. This patient, with a plasma volume of 41.6 cc. per Kg., had had severe asthenia on several hospital admissions but with persistently normal to hypertensive blood pressure levels and, at the time of plasma volume determination had a calculated serum sodium of 133 mEq. per liter. In those with plasma volumes below 40 cc. per Kg. body weight the gravity of present hypoadrenalism was directly related to the plasma volume, which provided a most reliable index to the depth of adrenal crisis. Serum sodium levels were a less reliable index of clinical condition; they occasionally remained high even in the presence of deepening crisis, or persisted at a low level in spite of unequivocal improvement in response to vigorous therapy. A significantly low plasma volume (below 35.5 cc. per Kg. of body weight) was not observed in any individual who was not in a grave state. We feel that if plasma volume studies were performed routinely in the process of evaluating patients for operative or other vigorous therapy, the few serious complications attributable to hypoadrenalism occasionally arising under such circumstances could be significantly diminished by the institution of immediate corrective measures.

It is of interest to contrast plasma volume levels found in patients with chromophobe adenomas with those noted by us in several other related diseases. In 2 patients with Addison's disease, under reasonably good symptomatic control and in electrolyte balance, plasma volumes were within the same range as for our controlled chromophobe patients without clinical evidence of hypoadrenalism. In 1 patient with postpartum Simmonds' disease of long standing, the plasma volume determined during a period of moderately severe symptomatic hypoadrenalism (serum sodium 122 mEq. per liter) was 35.0 cc. per Kg. body weight. This value falls well within the range of those with similar hypoadrenalism secondary to chromophobe adenoma. In striking contrast to these observations, the plasma volumes determined at least twice in each of 4 acromegalics ranged well above the upper limit of normal (49 cc. per Kg. body weight). In an additional 2 patients with acromegaly, both women, extreme discrepancies between actual and ideal body weight made comparison difficult. Calculations on the basis of ideal body weight gave values of 64.1 cc. and 61.1 cc. per Kg. body weight for the 2. These values are far above the upper limit of normal. The figures, however, based upon actual body weight, were both below the lower limits of normal. All 6 acromegalics showed progressive weight loss of from 3½ to 7 pounds during the salt deprivation regime. There was no indication of negative water balance in those several instances where balance studies were performed. Comparable weight loss was noted in 3 of 7 patients with chromophobe adenomas subjected to salt deprivation, but interestingly enough, diuresis was not recorded in any, even in those with a distinctly positive response and significant decrease in serum sodium.

Discussion

Asthenia appears to be present in approximately 90 per cent of all patients with Simmonds' disease,[146] hence its relatively infrequent occurrence in our patients with chromophobe adenomas is noteworthy. Hypertension, on the other hand, is as uncommon in Simmonds' disease[434] as in our series. The mean blood pressure in the former disease tends quite clearly toward the hypotensive side.[146] This is not true of the trend observed in chromophobe adenomas.

Disturbances in electrolyte balance, as indicated by response to the Wilder test (which uses urinary chloride excretion as the criterion of adrenal function) have been observed by Stephens[459] in 2 patients with chromophobe adenomas and in 5 of 18 patients with hypopituitarism examined by Starr and Davis.[456] We might safely conclude, therefore, that salt deprivation presents a specific stress which the patient with a chromophobe adenoma is less effectively able to combat than even extraordinary but nonspecific stresses presented by the environment itself. Whether the fact that the female, who appears to have more available extracellular fluid relative to plasma[210] than the male, is better equipped to cope with such stresses more effectively, is not answered by our observations.

We seriously question whether a high carbohydrate tolerance, with or without hypoglycemic episodes, can be safely considered a convincing evidence of disturbance in adrenal cortical function alone. Therefore, we consider such responses in greater detail in a subsequent section on carbohydrate metabolism.

Insulin hypersensitivity is, however, another matter. Only two endocrine structures have been convincingly related to insulin hypersensitivity, the anterior pituitary gland, by inference, and the adrenal cortex, by direct evidence. The evidence available[175, 456] suggests an insulin hypersensitivity in one-half or more patients with hypopituitary states from chromophobe adenomas and other causes. When this material is considered in conjunction with our own observations, it appears probable that more than one-half of such patients are intolerant of this specific stress. This is a slightly higher proportion than those reacting unfavorably to salt deprivation. Dissociations of these two types of functional disturbances are indicated frequently in our series and have also been established by a subsequent intensive study of a small group of hypopituitary patients.[362a]

In patients with secondary hypoadrenalism we noted not infrequent dissociations between the level of plasma volume and serum electrolyte concentration. A possible mechanism for this, which predicates a disturbance in intimate cellular metabolism, has been suggested.[498a]

The absence of diuresis during salt deprivation in those patients with acromegaly is not surprising, since all reacted negatively in all respects to the regime. The progressive weight loss observed in all is, however, puzzling since neither diuresis nor diarrhea was observed. No explanation is apparent. Lack of diuresis in several of the patients with chromophobe adenomas who, in contrast, reacted in a strongly positive way to salt deprivation with striking decrease in serum sodium, is a matter for closer scrutiny. A plausible explanation is that concomitant hypothyroidism, present in each of these patients, obscured any diuretic response because of its probable tendency to decrease renal plasma flow.

Summary

Approximately one-third of all patients with chromophobe adenomas have symptoms or signs suggestive of secondary hypoadrenalism. However, two-thirds of this symptomatic group display a capacity to resist extraordinary stressful environmental traumata without development of frank hypoadrenalism.

An individual whose previous symptoms and signs reveal no hypoadrenal trends will, in all probability, tolerate extraordinary environmental stress without development of hypoadrenalism.

Unphysiologic but controlled strain-inducing procedures frequently bring out latent hypoadrenal trends in patients with chromophobe adenomas. Deprivation of salt may reveal latent disturbances in salt and water metabolism in as many as one-half of such patients, while introduction of minute amounts of exogenous insulin may precipitate hypoglycemia in well over one-half of all.

Abnormally high tolerance for ingested sugar is no more common than significant disturbances in salt and water metabolism and, from a symptomatic standpoint, hypoglycemia induced by any means except exogenous insulin itself, is a relatively infrequent cause of disturbances referable to secondary hypoadrenalism.

Hypoadrenalism and adrenal crisis in patients with chromophobe adenomas are quite similar to primary hypoadrenalism with a few apparent exceptions. Serum potassium was not observed to be elevated in any of our patients at any time, even during deep crisis. Moreover loss of serum sodium precipitated by salt deprivation was not associated with diuresis in the individuals appropriately studied. It is suggested that concomitant hypothyroidism may prevent or obscure such a diuretic response because of its depressant effect on renal plasma flow.

The determination of plasma volume is considered of distinct value as an adjunct to the proper evaluation of the gravity and depth of secondary hypoadrenalism, as it is in primary hypoadrenalism.

GONADAL FUNCTIONAL STATUS

Symptomatic disturbances

Symptomatic disturbances in gonadal function were, of necessity, evaluated separately for males and females in this series. The criteria for males were (1) mild defect with decrease of libido, potency or both, and (2) severe defect with loss of both libido and potency. Physical signs reported include genital atrophy (both penis and testes) with or without symptomatic defect in sexual performance. In females, symptomatic gonadal defects were more clearly defined as persistently irregular menses or amenorrhea. Presymptomatic amenorrhea or menopause occurring at the normally anticipated period, both presumed to be unrelated to the effects of the pituitary tumor itself, are considered under separate categories, as is amenorrhea following bilateral oophorectomy or hysterectomy. In males symptomatic or structural disturbances appearing first after the age of 55 were considered as probably unrelated to the pituitary tumor.

The influence of documented hypoadrenalism and clearly subnormal basal metabolic rate on symptomatic hypogonadism is evaluated wherever possible.

Pertinent data for males is presented in table 8 and for females in table 9. Persistent normal gonadal function was recorded in 17 of the males studied (24 per cent), and in 4 of the females (8 per cent). Symptomatic hypogonadism, directly referable to pituitary tumor effects, was observed in 69 per cent of all males and in 84 per cent of females studied. The remaining few males not included in these categories were thought to have gonadal disturbances not directly referable

TABLE 8—*Gonadal Functional Status: Males*

Status or finding	Incidence		
	Number	Total studied	%
1. Persistent normal gonadal function........	17	70	24
2. Symptomatic hypogonadism*..............	33	70	47
a. Genital atrophy with symptoms..........	10	70	14
3. Asymptomatic genital atrophy.............	4	70	6
4. Total: Groups 2 and 3..................	37	70	53
5. Normal gonadal function where such would normally be anticipated (Groups 1 and 4)†..	17	54	31
6. Documented hypoadrenalism (in Group 5)...	2	13	15
7. Documented hypoadrenalism (in Group 4)...	2	37	5
8. BMR − 15 or less (in Group 5)............	8	11	73
9. BMR − 15 or less (in Group 4).............	22	27	82‡

* Libido decreased without alteration in potentia: 13 of 33 (40 per cent).
† Sixteen patients had hypogonadism not clearly related to tumor effects.
‡ Chi-squared value for Groups 8 and 9 equals 0.36, hence no significant difference is verified.

to the tumor itself. Twenty female patients (42 per cent) had either presymptomatic amenorrhea or a normally anticipated menopause. Slightly less than half of the males with symptomatic hypogonadism showed decreased libido alone, the remainder loss of both libido and potency. Of the 21 females with symptomatic hypogonadism, 6 had irregular or abnormal menstrual periods, while the remainder had persistent amenorrhea.

Documented hypoadrenalism was no more common in males with symptomatic hypogonadism than in those with persistently normal gonadal function and its incidence was approximately the same in the former group as in females with symptomatic hypogonadism referable to pituitary tumor effect.

Frankly subnormal BMRs were obtained in 8 of 11 male patients (73 per cent) with concomitant normal gonadal function. Twenty-two of 27 male patients (82 per cent) with symptomatic hypogonadism or genital atrophy had subnormal BMRs. On statistical grounds we may conclude that our data reveal no significant difference in the incidence of subnormal BMR with and without normal gonadal function. In

TABLE 9—*Gonadal Functional Status: Females*

Status or finding	Incidence		
	Number	Total studied	%
1. Persistent normal, regular menses..........	4	47	8
2. Symptomatic hypogonadism (total)........	21	47	45
3. Symptomatic hypogonadism directly referable to tumor effects.*......................	21	25	84
4. Presymptomatic amenorrhea or normally anticipated menopause....................	20	47	42
5. Documented hypoadrenalism (in Group 3)	2	21	10
6. BMR − 15 or less (in Group 1)...........	1	4	
7. BMR − 15 or less (in Group 3)...........	10	14	71
8. BMR − 15 or less (other than Group 3)....	11	20	54†

* Six of 21 had irregular or abnormal menses, the remainder amenorrhea.
† Chi-squared value for Groups 7 and 8 is 0.95, hence no significant difference is verified. Group 8 is composed largely of those with presymptomatic and normally anticipated menopause.

the female, comparable analyses were not possible because of the extremely small number with normal gonadal function, but there was no significant difference in incidence of subnormal BMR in those with symptomatic hypogonadism directly referable to tumor effects as compared with the group whose symptomatic hypogonadism long antedated or was apparently unrelated to pituitary tumor effects.

Pertinent laboratory studies

Studies of the urinary excretion of hormonal metabolites related directly or indirectly to gonadal function were performed in 12 patients of this series, 7 males (table 10) and 5 females (table 11). Adrenal function status was considered in conjunction with gonadal status in evaluating the significance of these determinations.

TABLE 10—*The Urinary Excretion (24 hr.) of Hormonal Metabolites: 7 Males*

Gonadal status	Adrenal status	Total neutral 17 ketosteroids (mg.)	Pituitary gonado- trophin	Estrogen
Normal	Normal	12		<5 R.U.
Symptomatic hypogonadism or genital atrophy	Not tested	17.5–3.6	<5 m.u.	
Symptomatic hypogonadism or genital atrophy	Adrenal crisis	3.5		
Symptomatic hypogonadism or genital atrophy	Mild documented hypoadrenalism	2.8–4.2	Subnormal	
Symptomatic hypogonadism or genital atrophy	Normal	10.8		
Symptomatic hypogonadism or genital atrophy	Normal	1.2		
Symptomatic hypogonadism or genital atrophy	Normal	2.0 (post operative) 5.0 (convalesced) 2.1–1.1 (after methyl testosterone therapy)	<5 m.u. post- operative)	<5 R.U. post- operative)

In the 1 male with normal function in both gonadal and adrenal spheres total neutral 17-ketosteroid excretion was 12 mg., well within normal limits. Only 1 of 6 males with symptomatic hypogonadism or genital atrophy excreted normal amounts of total neutral 17-ketosteroids (10.8 mg.). This patient had normal adrenal function. The remaining 5 male patients excreted subnormal amounts of total neutral 17-ketosteroids (inconsistently in 1). The total amount excreted bore no evident relationship to the presence or gravity of hypoadrenalism. In 1 of these patients an apparently persistent decrease in excretion of total neutral 17-ketosteroids coincided with a course of oral methyl testosterone. Three patients with symptomatic hypogonadism or genital

TABLE 11—*The Urinary Excretion (24 hr.) of Hormonal Metabolites: 5 Females*

Gonadal status	Adrenal Status	Total neutral 17-ketosteroids (mg.)	Pituitary gonadotrophins	Estrogen
Presymptomatic menopause	Normal	4.2	<10 m.u.	<5 R.U.
Presymptomatic amenorrhea	Atypically positive salt deprivation	29.1		29.4* gamma
Symptomatic hypogonadism	Documented hypoadrenalism	6.6		14.7* gamma
Symptomatic hypogonadism	Normal	2.6		
Symptomatic hypogonadism	Normal	4.6		

* Fluorometric method for estrogens (estrone and estradiol).

atrophy in whom urinary pituitary gonadotrophin titers were determined showed subnormal levels, while 2 of these 3 excreted subnormal amounts of estrogenic substance.

Of the 5 female patients in whom excretory studies were made, 2 excreted total neutral 17-ketosteroids of normal or greater amount. In one patient, a 42 year old woman, amenorrhea had been present for at least fifteen years before onset of the first unequivocal signs of pituitary tumor. She excreted 29.1 mg. of total neutral 17-ketosteroids per 24 hours (rechecked) and 29.4 γ of estrone and estradiol per 24 hours. This patient had a widely ballooned sella turcica and was shown by pneumoencephalography to have an extensive suprasellar mass. Visual field defects were clear and unequivocal and regressed dramatically following deep x-ray therapy. She developed marked hypotension of 88/38, from a previous normal of 140/70, during salt deprivation but maintained a satisfactory serum sodium level, which decreased from 144.1 mEq. per liter to 137.6 mEq. per liter. Plasma volume decreased only slightly during salt deprivation. Her ovaries, uterus, and external genitalia were completely normal on physical examination.

One patient with presymptomatic menopause and normal adrenal function excreted 4.2 mg. total neutral 17-ketosteroids, low normal pituitary gonadotrophin and subnormal estrogenic substance. The remaining 3 women, all with symptomatic hypogonadism, excreted low normal or subnormal amounts of total neutral 17-ketosteroids. The highest level was noted in a woman with documented hypoadrenalism, a paradoxical observation. This particular patient also excreted a normal amount of estrone and estradiol, had had two previous full term pregnancies without labor pains during either delivery but with no evidence of lactation after the second delivery. Physical examination at the time of endocrine study revealed, inter alia, a senile-type vulva with small uterus.

Discussion

Previous analyses[193] of gonadal hypoplasia or atrophy in males with chromophobe adenomas indicate its occurrence in a proportion identical to that in our series. Its incidence in Simmonds' disease, by contrast,[146, 434] is three times greater. No directly comparable published figures for symptomatic gonadal disturbances in the male are available.[176] Henderson,[238] analyzing 93 female patients with chromophobe adenomas from Cushing's series, recorded uninterrupted menses in only 3 of 93 patients studied. Amenorrhea seems to be as common in Simmonds' disease[146] as in our patients with chromophobe adenomas. It should be recalled here that the evidence does not warrant our limiting disturbances in sexual function to alterations in the gonadal structures alone. Significant alterations in sexual performance in male animals as well as disruption of cyclic, rhythmic sexual functions in female animals have been induced by hypothalamic lesions which are associated with no known alterations in anterior pituitary structure, and with no observed changes in gonadal structure.[61]

Talbot and Butler,[471] in an article reviewing observed correlations between total neutral 17-ketosteroid excretion and endocrine status, have suggested that hypopituitary states with retarded sexual development or hypogonadism are never associated with excretory levels over 1.0 mg., this likewise being true for hypopituitary states with fatigue and weakness, and for primary hypothyroidism. They observed, also, that in primary hypoadrenalism low normal or subnormal levels are the rule, the lower limit being 1.0 mg. per 24 hours. In a clinical study Fraser and Smith[175] recorded only one value over 0.5 mg. per 24 hours in 10 patients with Simmonds' disease. Three of these, with diagnosed or questionable chromophobe adenomas, excreted less than 0.5 mg per 24 hours.

Since all of the 11 patients in our series with disturbance in gonadal function or structure excreted more than the minimum amounts of total neutral 17-ketosteroid suggested by Talbot and Butler,[471] it may be that certain minimal gonadal secretory activity persisted even in the presence of hypopituitarism. The fact that 2 of these patients excreted normal or above normal amounts of estrone or estradiol would tend to support such a suggestion, though our data justify no generalizations. It is apparent, from our few studied cases, that symptomatic hypogonadism in combination with documented hypoadrenalism is not necessarily associated with excretion of smaller amounts of total neutral 17-ketosteroids than symptomatic hypoadrenalism alone.

The fact that subnormal amounts of urinary gonadotrophin were recovered from the urines of 3 patients with symptomatic hypogonadism or genital atrophy would suggest a direct relationship between disturbed anterior pituitary function and the observed changes. Recovery of normal amounts of pituitary gonadotrophin from the urine of a patient with presymptomatic menopause, who was, at the time, excreting subnormal amounts of estrogenic substance, suggests that amenorrhea in this woman could not be attributed convincingly to the effect of her pituitary tumor.

Summary

Persistent normal gonadal function was observed in 31 per cent of males and 16 per cent of females with chromophobe adenomas, in an age group where such normal function would be expected.

Documented hypoadrenalism occurred as infrequently in those with symptomatic hypogonadism or genital atrophy as in those with normal gonadal function or unrelated gonadal dysfunctions.

The incidence of subnormal basal metabolic rate was not significantly different in males with and without symptomatic hypogonadism or genital atrophy. In females the incidence of subnormal metabolism was not significantly lower in those with presymptomatic amenorrhea or normally anticipated menopause than in those with symptomatic hypogonadism directly related to tumor effects.

The relatively large amounts of total neutral 17-ketosteroids excreted in the urines of those with symptomatic hypogonadism, especially in the presence of documented hypoadrenalism, suggest that a certain number of such patients with chromophobe adenomas may continue to excrete definite but subnormal amounts of hormonal substances, elaborated by the gonads themselves.

METABOLISM OF CARBOHYDRATES

The metabolism of carbohydrates in our patients with pituitary chromophobe adenomas has been analyzed in a separate section for several reasons: first, because it is a complex analysis which must be approached from more than one direction, secondly because the interpretation of the changes observed presupposes an appreciation not only of several peripheral endocrine components but also of components possibly furnished by the altered anterior pituitary gland itself. Of the peripheral endocrine components, one has already been considered briefly in the section on adrenal function status. Data recorded there will be evaluated in greater detail in this section. Possible effects of the pituitary tumor itself are considered extensively in the section on pathology but are summarized in this section.

Observations (table 12)

Symptomatic diabetes occurred in 4 patients (3 per cent) of the 117 in this series. All 4 had persistent glycosuria, fasting blood sugars consistently above 140 mg. per cent and, in 2 so tested, diabetic oral glucose tolerances. Two of the 4 required small but regular doses of insulin for adequate control. Obesity was observed in 3 of the 4 and subnormal BMR was present in 2.

The mean postabsorptive blood sugar value for the entire series so tested was 90 mg. per cent, the distribution of individual values about the mean being normal. It is of particular interest to note that this value does not differ significantly from the normal mean postabsorptive blood sugar value of Lozner and his associates.[322] Their normal range is almost identical with the range noted in our patients.

A low or diabetic glucose tolerance was noted in 19 of 80 patients so studied (24 per cent). Those with clinical diabetes were excluded from this group. Such responses were of two general types: sustained high blood sugar for 3 and occasionally 4 hours after the test dose (relatively uncommon); and sustained high blood sugar for a minimum of 2 hours after the test dose, with relatively rapid return to normal levels at the third or fourth hour (common). In all instances blood sugar values exceeded 125 mg. per cent at the 2 hour interval. Repeated tolerances in the same individual, occasionally after long intervals, did not consistently yield a similar response. It was observed that a normal response might occasionally follow a low-tolerance response (or vice versa), but never a frankly high or hypoglycemic type of response. A consistent effort was made to judge repetitive responses in such a way that the true trend is manifest in the classification. The mean postabsorptive blood sugar value for this group was 98 mg. per cent. Individual values varied widely from the observed mean.

Not one instance of documented hypoadrenalism was discovered in this group with low or diabetic glucose tolerance. Six of the 19 with this response were obese, although only 8 of 19 (42 per cent) so tested had BMRs consistently below the lowest limit of normal. The incidence of subnormal metabolic rate in this group is significantly lower than in the group as a whole.

TABLE 12—*The Metabolism of Carbohydrates*

Status or findings	Incidence			Mean trend	
	Number	Total studied	%	Mean	Sigma
1. Symptomatic diabetes	4	117	3		
a. With obesity	3	4			
b. BMR – 15 or less	2	4			
2. 14-hour postabsorptive blood sugar value		167 determinations		90	± 6.8
(Normal postabsorptive blood sugar values: Lozner et al.[322])		60		89	± 9.1*
3. Low or diabetic glucose tolerance (exclusive of Group 1)	19	80	24		
a. With obesity	6	19	32		
b. BMR – 15 or less†	8	19	42		
4. Normal glucose tolerance‡	42	80	52		
a. With obesity	13	42	31		
b. With BMR – 15 or less§	28	36	78		
5. High glucose tolerance‖	17	80	21		
a. With obesity	4	17	24		
b. With BMR – 15 or less	11	15	73		
6. Postabsorptive blood sugar value (Group 3)		37 determinations		98	± 19.6
7. Postabsorptive blood sugar value (Group 4)		82 determinations		87¶	± 9.0
8. Postabsorptive blood sugar value (Group 5)		21 determinations		85	± 7.5

* No significant difference between normal postabsorptive and "abnormal" postabsorptive blood sugar values.

† Exceeds 2 sigma probability of being random sampling error.

‡ Five patients so tested showed insulin hypersenstivity (3 had normal I. V. glucose tolerances).

§ Chi-squared value (Groups 3b and 4b) is 7.0 indicating a significant difference in this factor within the groups.

‖ Insulin hypersensitivity in 1 of 2 so tested.

¶ Difference between means of Groups 6 and 7 is 11.0; standard error of difference equals ± 2.3, hence the difference appears significant.

A normal oral glucose tolerance was noted in 42 of the 80 patients tested (52 per cent). Five of these showed insulin hypersensitivity, and in 3 of the 5 the intravenous glucose tolerance response was normal. This so-called "normal" response was of two general types, each equally common. In one the blood sugar rose in a completely normal pattern, falling slowly to normal levels in 2 hours, never continuing on to frankly hypoglycemic levels even at the fourth or fifth hour. In the other, the response to orally ingested glucose was minimal and flat, values near or slightly below the initial fasting level being observed consistently after an initial slight rise. The characteristic pattern suggested by Soskin,[449] i.e., normal initial rise from low normal levels with rapid return to low normal levels, was frequently noted but was certainly not the rule. Mean postabsorptive fasting sugar in this group was 87 mg. per cent, with normal distribution. The range was similar to that observed in normal individuals. This value is significantly lower than the observed mean in those with a low or diabetic tolerance.

In those with a normal tolerance 13 of 42 (31 per cent) were obese, and 28 of 36 (78 per cent) had subnormal BMRs. Although the incidence of subnormal BMR is significantly higher in those with normal as compared to low glucose tolerance, obesity occurs with equal frequency in each group.

Seventeen of 80 patients tested (21 per cent) showed an abnormally high glucose tolerance. Five of these had associated hypoadrenalism yet, as previously noted, symptomatic hypoglycemia occurred in only 1 of the 5. In the remaining 12 patients without proven hypoadrenalism, symptomatic hypoglycemia was substantiated in none. One of 2 patients, so tested, displayed insulin hypersensitivity, the other a normal response. Obesity was associated with this type of tolerance in 4 of 17 patients (24 per cent) and 11 of 15 so tested (73 per cent) had a BMR consistently below the lowest limit of normal. The mean postabsorptive blood sugar value was here 85 mg. per cent, the distribution and range similar to those in normal individuals. Those with normal tolerance and those with high tolerance make up a homogenous group from the standpoint of associated subnormal metabolism, obesity and mean fasting blood sugar. This combined group differs significantly from those with low or diabetic tolerance in all these respects, except for the incidence of obesity.

Discussion

Our observations confirm the fact that clinical diabetes is quite rare in patients with chromophobe adenomas.[113, 182] However, since Davidoff and Cushing[113] have suggested that such a diabetic state may well be a manifestation of fugitive acidophilic hyperpituitarism we have studied these 4 diabetics for such evidence. In 1 of the 4, with mild diabetes, the BMR was – 4, the blood pressure 200/90. The frontal bone was irregularly thickened in x-ray, but such studies revealed no skeletal traces of acidophilic hyperpituitarism. Surgical biopsy and autopsy specimens of the tumor revealed no evidence of any type of secretory granulation in the tumor cells. The second patient, a moderately severe diabetic requiring daily protamin-zinc-insulin, had a BMR of – 34, symptomatic amenorrhea, normal adrenal function and questionable symptomatic hypogonadism. The only trace of hyperpituitary trend in this patient was x-ray evidence of atrophic, tufted terminal phalanges. The third diabetic, easily controlled with diet and daily injections of protamin-zinc-insulin, had a BMR of – 10, questionable symptomatic hypoadrenalism, acute hypogonadism and no traces of acidophilic hyperpituitarism by x-ray. The fourth patient with moderate diabetes, had consistently subnormal BMRs, a surgically induced menopause, no evidences of hypoadrenalism and no skeletal traces of hyperpituitarism. Thus, questionable signs of acidophilic hyperpituitarism were noted in 2 of the 4.

The interpretation of the mean fasting or postabsorptive blood sugar values noted in our series as a whole, and in the three subdivisions, is a matter of considerable importance since our values strongly support the thesis that the patient with a chromophobe adenoma, though he may display conspicuous irregularity in the management of ingested glucose, does successfully maintain adequate blood sugar levels even after a 12 to 14 hour fast, and, in many other instances, after prolonged operative procedures and severe intercurrent illness. Heinbecker and his associates[231] have observed that the fasting blood sugar level in hypophysectomized dogs is reasonably constant though the diet varies from high fat to high carbohydrate. Watson,[499] and Freeman et al.[178] have shown, in humans, that of all blood sugar specimens taken, those taken in the postabsorptive, fasting state are least variable. An increase in fasting or postabsorptive blood sugar level with increasing age has been urged by Punschel[cited in 370] but such a trend is not revealed in the study of Lozner and his co-workers.[322] The evidence therefore warrants confidence in the mean fasting levels we have reported. In this regard it is important to emphasize the observation that postabsorptive blood sugar levels were quite as well maintained in those with abnormally high glucose tolerance as in those with normal glucose tolerance.

The interpretation of our oral and intravenous tolerance figures is a matter of considerable complexity. To dismiss the variations noted as spontaneous and random is simple but not wise, since one ordinarily replenishes carbohydrate stores by the oral route and the efficient absorption of carbohydrates is a matter of unquestioned physiologic importance. Reliance upon intravenous tolerances alone restricts our ability to understand this pertinent aspect of carbohydrate metabolism in such patients.

The influence of thyroid function upon intestinal absorption of ingested glucose has been discussed in the section on physiology. Our data suggests that the incidence of subnormal metabolic rate is significantly lower in the group with low to diabetic tolerance. If increased glucose absorption is to be considered a significant factor in these patients we would expect them to show evidence of increased thyroid activity and not, as we have observed, of normal or low normal activity. On the other hand, a hypothyroid factor is strongly suggested in those with normal or high oral tolerance.

The preceding diet is still another factor to be considered in interpreting tolerance responses. A high carbohydrate diet not only tends to produce increasing tolerance for carbohydrate but also tends to depress BMR. At the same time it favors the deposition of peripheral fat, to the detriment of liver and muscle stores. It is for this reason that we have analyzed the incidence of obesity (including recent abnormal deposition of fat) in the three tolerance groups. Evidently its incidence is almost identical in the three groups. Thus our data fail to reveal an influence of previous conditioning diet on the responses observed.

We have considered the possibility that a low or diabetic glucose tolerance may reflect the presence of transitional or borderline acidophilic hyperpituitarism. Study of histologically proven cases has given no conclusive data: Analysis of the metabolic disturbances in one group with skeletal traces of acromegaly, as compared to another where such traces were absent (see table 19) indicates that the glucose tolerance response is highly variable in the former group. However, the incidence of low or diabetic tolerances was not significantly higher in those with such traces. The trend was, if anything, in the direction of higher tolerance, not lower tolerance. We may, of course, be dealing with minimal acidophilic hyperpituitarism, so slight that it is unassociated with any skeletal overgrowth, yet sufficient to produce a subtle disturbance in one aspect of carbohydrate metabolism. Such an interpretation is speculative. The presence of significantly higher mean fasting sugar with significantly lower incidence of subnormal metabolism in this tolerance group, though it fits the scheme well, is in no sense confirmatory.

Summary

Four patients of the 117 in this series had confirmed diabetes. In only 2 of the 4 could any evidences of acidophilic hyperpituitarism be discovered.

Though the tolerance for ingested glucose was abnormal in one-half of patients so studied, being abnormally high or abnormally low in approximately equal proportion, postabsorptive blood sugar levels were normally maintained in most instances. The added stress of prolonged fasting, operative procedure or severe intercurrent infection was rarely associated with significant hypoglycemia, even in those with high tolerance.

A low or diabetic tolerance was no more common in those with skeletal traces of acidophilic hyperpituitarism than in those without such traces. However, mean fasting blood sugar was significantly higher and the incidence of subnormal BMR significantly lower in those with low or diabetic tolerance than in those with either normal or high tolerance.

Observations previously analyzed (see section on adrenal functional status) indicate that the patient with a chromophobe adenoma is capable of coping effectively with his endogenous insulin in most instances, although he is almost uniformly hypersensitive to minute amounts of exogenous insulin.

INTERRELATIONSHIPS BETWEEN ENDOCRINE AND METABOLIC DEFICITS

The statistical incidence and interrelationships of metabolic and endocrine deficits just discussed have been based largely on adequate investigations in only one or a few of the spheres considered. There is, therefore, always the possibility that such figures may not reflect the true integrated picture. To test this possibility we have separately analyzed the clinical and laboratory studies in 17 patients of this series in whom conclusive and adequate investigations have been carried out for assaying thyroid, adrenal, gonadal function and carbohydrate metabolism. These observations are summarized in table 13.

The incidence of thyroid hypofunction in this small group is 88 per cent; of symptomatic hypogonadism, 71 per cent (3 of the 17 had disturbances in gonadal function not directly related to tumor effect); of documented hypoadrenalism, 47 per cent; and of symptomatic hypoglycemia or abnormally high tolerance for glucose, 35 per cent. These relative figures have been compared, statistically, to the overall figures of incidence previously determined. Only the incidence of documented hypoadrenalism is significantly different from the recorded incidence for the entire series. The small sample is, in other respects, representative of the entire series.

The significantly higher incidence of hypoadrenalism within this small group warrants special comment. Of all the endocrine deficits occurring in patients with chromophobe adenomas, hypoadrenalism is of most serious import and most directly threatens not only the functional efficiency but also the life of the patient. It will be recalled (see table 7) that the overall incidence of documented hypoadrenalism is 16 per cent while its incidence in those with premonitory symptoms or signs is 36 per cent. Within the group we are presently discussing, premonitory symptoms or signs were recorded in 11 of the 17 patients (65 per cent). Even though we weight the relative incidence of docu-

TABLE 13—*Interrelationships between Endocrine and Metabolic Dysfunctions in 17 Patients with Chromophobe Adenoma*

Case	Sex	Age of onset	Duration of symptoms	Endocrine-metabolic disturbances			
				Hypo-thyroid	Hypo-glycemic	Hypo-adrenal	Hypo-gonad
1	M	46	13 yrs.	Yes	Yes	Yes	Yes
2	M	41	3 yrs.	Yes	Yes	Yes	Yes
3	F	31	4 yrs.	Yes	No	Yes	Yes
4	M	34	4.5 yrs.	Yes	Yes	Yes	No
5	M	60	5 yrs.	Yes	No	Yes	Yes?
6	M	43	2 yrs.	Yes	No	Yes	Yes
7	M	46	7 mos.	Yes	Yes	No	Yes?
8	M	49	1 yr.	Yes	Yes	Yes	No
9	M	49	11 yrs.	Yes	Yes	No	Yes
10	F	41	2.5 yrs.	Yes	No	No	Yes
11	M	32	2 yrs.	Yes	No	No	Yes
12	M	35	2 yrs.	Yes	No	No	Yes
13	F	40	3 yrs.	No	No	Yes?	Pre-sympto-matic
14	M	41	1 yr.	Yes	No	No	No
15	F	57	6 yrs.	Yes	No	No	Pre-sympto-matic
16	F	42	1 yr.	Yes	No	No	No
17	F	21	6 yrs.	No	No	No	No

mented hypoadrenalism, it still remains probably significantly higher here than in the group as a whole. We are justified in concluding that hypoadrenalism occurs somewhat more frequently than our overall figures would indicate, irrespective of premonitory signs or symptoms of such disturbance.

Concerning the magnitude and range of endocrine and metabolic disturbances, it is obvious from table 13 that no correlation exists between age of onset or total duration of symptoms, and magnitude or type of endocrine and metabolic deficit. For example, case 2, with a tumor which gave symptoms for only three years, showed endocrine and metabolic deficit in all four spheres, while case 17 with symptoms for six years, showed no detectable deficits in any metabolic sphere.

The disturbances observed were analyzed with reference to relative tumor size and presence or absence of hypothalamic compression and revealed no correlation between tumor size or hypothalamic compression and type or range of metabolic deficit.

The interrelationships of endocrine and metabolic deficits in this small group are of particular interest. Two patients, both males, showed functional deficit in all four spheres of activity. Of the 7 patients showing deficits in three spheres, all except 1 were males. Three of these 7 had normal tolerance for glucose and sustained ability to maintain normal blood glucose levels in the presence of thyroid and adrenal deficit. Two had no evidence of hypoadrenalism (disturbance in salt and water balance or symptomatic hypoglycemia) but had abnormally high tolerance for glucose, and showed both gonadal and thyroid deficit. Two had normal gonadal function in the presence of adrenal and thyroid deficit. One of these 2 died during an adrenal crisis.

Three of the 17 patients had functional deficits in only two spheres, thyroid and gonadal in both instances. Both maintained adequate postabsorptive blood sugar levels, displayed normal response to ingested glucose and showed no evidence of hypoglycemia at any time.

Of the 4 individuals with functional deficit in only one sphere clearly related to the effects of the tumor, 3 were deficient in thyroid function; 1, atypically, in adrenal function. The latter patient, case 13, has been described in detail on page 161. Were it not for the fact that acute hypotension of striking degree developed on the third day of salt deprivation in this woman, one would be tempted to consider the reaction related in no way to adrenal function. However, the fact that her blood pressure had previously been quite stable at high normal values and that repeated blood pressure observations during the period of hypotension gave alarmingly low figures, suggested that the event was more than coincident. Her blood pressure, moreover, returned slowly to previously observed normal levels following termination of the salt deprivation routine.

Another woman, with a relatively small tumor, gave no evidence of functional deficit in any sphere. Visual field changes were minimal in this patient but the sella turcica showed distinctive abnormalities, measuring 16 mm. in depth, 19 mm. in A. P. diameter. Pneumoencephalography in this patient gave no evidence of extrasellar extension of the pituitary tumor.

Summary

The relative incidence of endocrine and metabolic deficits in patients with chromophobe adenomas, as stated in the preceding clinical sections, is probably truly representative with the exception that disturbances in salt and water metabolism, referable to adrenal cortical function, may occur somewhat more commonly than our overall analysis would indicate.

The proportionate impact of separable endocrine hypofunctional states on discrete metabolic functions, as discussed in previous sections, is satisfactorily confirmed.

Neither the range nor severity of metabolic deficits in patients with chromophobe adenomas can be correlated with age of onset of tumor symptoms, total duration of tumor effects or presence of hypothalamic compression. Possible correlations with tumor size are considered in greater detail in the next section.

INFLUENCE OF TUMOR SIZE ON ENDOCRINE AND METABOLIC DISTURBANCES

Implicit is the assumption in previous representative studies[100, 193] that associated endocrine hypofunctional states are a result of compression of remaining normal anterior pituitary remnants by the adenoma, the magnitude of disturbance reflecting the degree of compression. This logical assumption, supported by a wealth of pertinent experimental evidence, has provoked only one fragmentary clinical investigation designed to test its validity directly. In this study Henderson,[238] who analyzed gonadal dysfunction in the patients of Cushing's series, concluded that sexual dysfunction occurs only when the sella turcica has become considerably expanded by an adenoma of chromophobic or acidophilic type. His data were interpreted as indicating that at least in females hypogonadism becomes more frequent as the tumor enlarges.

We have analyzed the influence of relative tumor size on all of the previously noted endocrine and metabolic irregularities. Our criteria for small, medium and large tumors have been previously stated. Clinical data are summarized in table 14.

Symptomatic hypothyroidism was observed in approximately equal percentages of those with large, medium and small tumors. Subnormal metabolic rate was equally common in all three groups. Mean serum cholesterol values did not vary significantly with tumor size. It should be noted, in passing, that the mean serum cholesterol varied inversely with BMR only in the group with large tumors. This limited evaluation of thyroid function indicated no significant difference in functional status between those with large, medium and small tumors.

Symptomatic hypoadrenalism occurred with equal frequency in the three groups. Such variations as were observed were within the limits of usual random sampling variation. When asymptomatic hypotension was included as an evidence of hypoadrenalism, the incidence was noted to be questionably lower in those with medium than with large or small tumors. The incidence of documented hypoadrenalism did not, however, confirm such a difference within the groups.

The incidence of symptomatic hypogonadism in males did not differ significantly in those with large, medium and small tumors. The last tumor group was so small that statistical comparison was impossible. In the female, the small sample defect again made significant conclusions impossible. We are justified in stating only that the trend revealed by our data is similar to that indicated in Henderson's[238] study, i.e., that symptomatic hypogonadism appears in females with increasing frequency, the greater the expansion of the sella turcica.

TABLE 14—*Influence of Tumor Size on Endocrine and Metabolic Dysfunctions*

Status or finding	Large Tumors No. or value	Of total	%	Medium Tumors No. or value	Of total	%	Small Tumors No. or value	Of total	%	Statistical data*
1. Thyroid function										
a. Symptomatic hypothyroidism	6	55	11	7	43	16	2	15	13	Chi²(L, M)† 0.6
b. BMR − 15 or less	28	37	76	21	33	64	9	13	69	Chi²(L, M) 1.2
c. Mean serum cholesterol (BMR −15 or less)	282 σ ±73	17		286 σ ±54	15		306 σ ±78?	8		No sig. diff. (L, M, S)
2. Adrenal function										
a. Symptomatic hypoadrenalism	16	56	29	8	45	18	5	16	31	Chi²(L, M) 1.6
b. Symptomatic hypoadrenalism or hypotension	23	56	42	12	45	27	7	16	44	Chi²(L, M) 2.3
c. Documented hypoadrenalism under stress (of Group 2b)	7	23	30	5	12	42	3	7	43	Chi²(L, M) 0.44
d. Total with documented hypoadrenalism	8	50	16	6	41	15	3	15	20	

* For one degree of freedom, the Chi-squared value for 5 per cent probability is 3.84, for 10 per cent probability, 2.7.

† L is large, M is medium and S is small.

TABLE 14—Continued

Status or finding	Large Tumors			Medium Tumors			Small Tumors			Statistical data*
	No. or value	Of total	%	No. or value	Of total	%	No. or value	Of total	%	
3. Gonadal function										
a. Symptomatic hypogonadism or asymptomatic genital atrophy: Male	20	31	65	14	19	74	3	4	75?	Chi²(L, M)† 0.45
b. Symptomatic hypogonadism: Female	9	9	100	7	9	78	5	7	71	Chi² not applicable
4. Carbohydrate metabolism										
a. Low or diabetic tolerance (excluding clin. diabetics)	6	38	16	9	29	31	4	11	36	Chi²(L, S) 2.2 Yates' correction not applicable
b. Normal tolerance	24	38	63	11	29	38	5	11	46	Chi²(L, M) 4.2 Chi²(M, S) 0.35 Chi²(L, S) 0.49
c. BMR −15 or less in Group 4b	18	21	86	5	10	50				Chi²(L, M) 2.9
d. High carbohydrate tolerance	6	38	16	9	29	31	2	11	18	Chi²(L, M) 2.2

* For one degree of freedom, the Chi-squared value for 5 per cent probability is 3.84, for 10 per cent probability, 2.7.
† L is large, M is medium and S is small.

Experimental studies would indicate, however, that disturbances in menstruation may be of nonendocrine origin since such irregularities can be produced by lesions of the ventro-lateral hypothalamus alone.

The tolerance for ingested glucose varied significantly more in those with medium tumors than in those with large tumors, though the incidence of normal tolerance response was not significantly different in those with large and small, or medium and small tumors. Whether the variations from normal in those with medium tumors favor a high tolerance is not conclusively established by our data, though they suggest that low tolerance may be somewhat more common in those with small tumors, high tolerance in those with medium tumors. Subnormal BMR is somewhat less common in those with medium tumors and normal glucose tolerance than in those with large tumors and similar tolerance. In spite of these minor variations in glucose tolerance the responses are, in general, surprisingly uniform.

Summary

No significant differences in the incidence of thyroid or adrenal hypofunctional states are noted in those with large, medium and small chromophobe adenomas.

In the female symptomatic hypogonadism becomes somewhat more frequent the larger the tumor, but such a trend is not confirmed in the male. It is seriously questioned whether the observed change in frequency may not be a manifestation of hypothalamic as well as gonadal endocrine dysfunction.

Tolerance for ingested glucose is of normal type in a significantly higher number with large than medium sized tumors. The observations suggest that low tolerance is somewhat more common in those with small tumors, high tolerance in those with medium sized tumors.

It is concluded that when a chromophobe adenoma of the pituitary gland has attained a size just sufficient to warrant its recognition and diagnosis, disturbances in endocrine function (at least in the spheres of thyroid, adrenal and gonadal activity) are as likely to be present as in one with a tumor of large size.

MISCELLANEOUS OBSERVATIONS

The endocrine and metabolic disturbances described in the preceding clinical sections are those usually considered to be intimately related to altered anterior pituitary function. Other more indirect trophic disturbances of the pituitary gland, reflected in changes of parathyroid function, protein metabolism and cardiovascular and renal functions, are rarely investigated clinically. Our own pertinent data are fragmentary and presented here for the sake of completeness. In some respects they reflect the efficient manner in which patients with chromophobe adenomas maintain a homeostatic state.

Metabolism of calcium, phosphorus and alkaline phosphatase

We must rely on mineral and enzyme blood levels and on x-ray studies to give us our only information about parathyroid function in this study. There is, to date, no accepted method of placing a specific and controlled strain on this glandular system.

Serum calcium, inorganic phosphorus and alkaline phosphatase levels, as well as skeletal and soft tissue x-ray studies, are available for 22 patients of this series. The data are summarized in table 15.

All the serum calcium levels are within the normal range (9.0 to 11.5 mg. per cent), although 2 of the 16 studied had levels below 9.5 mg. per cent on at least one occasion. Five of 14 patients had serum inorganic phosphorus levels below 2.9 mg. per cent (normal range 2.9 to 4.5 mg. per cent) on at least one occasion. Alkaline phosphatase levels in 11 patients studied were all within low normal range and bore no consistent relationship to the levels of serum calcium or inorganic phosphorus. X-ray studies in those with correlated serum calcium, phosphorus, or alkaline phosphatase levels did not reveal changes suggestive of hypoparathyroidism. In 5 patients, x-ray changes occasionally noted in hyperparathyroidism were observed. It is unfortunate that serum mineral or alkaline phosphatase levels were not determined in any of these, since it is therefore impossible to draw any conclusions about their significance in terms of parathyroid function.

TABLE 15—*Observations Pertinent to the Metabolism of Calcium and Phosphorus: 22 Patients*

Serum Ca (mg. %)	Serum inorg. P. (mg. %)	Alkaline phosphatase. (Bodansky units)	Roentgenographic studies (excluding abnormalities of sella turcica)
11.4	3.0	2.9	Sclerosis, body of 12 D. vertebra
10.7	3.2	3.4	Osteoarthritis, dorsal spine.
—	3.4	2.9	—
10.1	3.9	—	
9.5	—	—	Dorsal scoliosis
9.8	3.2	1.6	Normal*
10.1	2.5	2.3	—
9.8	—	—	Tufting, terminal phalanges. Bones "coarse"
9.1	2.5	—	—
10.2	4.3	3.7	Normal*
10.2	2.9	3.4	
10.5	2.5	—	
—	4.2	—	Slight tufting, terminal phalanges
9.6	4.8	4.3	
10.6	3.8	4.1	Normal*
10.0	3.1	2.7	Normal*
9.5	2.4	3.1	Normal*
10.8	3.4	—	—
10.1	2.6	2.6	Normal*
10.9	—	—	
9.0	—	—	—
9.9	—	—	
—	—	—	Cholelithiasis, renal calculi, thickened cranial vault, questionable rheumatoid arthritis
—	—	—	Calcification of supraspinatus and subdeltoid bursae
—	—	—	Atrophic appendic. joints, mult. humeral spurs. Two cysts-lt. lat. femoral condyle. Mild dorsal kyphoscoliosis.
—	—	—	Area of decreased density—pareital bone. Intervertebral disc calcification (D 11–12)
—	—	—	Renal and prostatic calculi, glenoid calcification. Vertebrae normal. Sella turcica recalcified after deep x-ray therapy.

* Vertebral column, skull, extremities and thoracic cage studied in the majority.

One additional patient, not included in table 15, had bilateral cataracts, but no pertinent laboratory studies.

The possibility that the x-ray and clinical changes noted above in 6 patients may be one manifestation of borderline or transitory acidophilic hyperpituitarism has been considered. Tufting of the terminal phalanges is analyzed in detail in the chapter on pathology. Of the 6 patients with atypical findings, 3 were examples of unalloyed hypopituitarism. Hypertension of minimal to moderate severity was noted in the remaining 3, 1 of whom was nephritic. No usually acceptable evidences of acidophilic hyperpituitarism were noted in any.

Summary

Serum calcium and alkaline phosphatase levels were within normal range in all patients with chromophobe adenomas so studied, the latter levels being consistently low normal.

Approximately one-third of patients studied showed subnormal serum inorganic phosphorus levels on at least one occasion.

No confirmatory evidences of hypoparathyroidism were noted in any patient.

Six patients in the series revealed clinical or x-ray abnormalities sometimes associated with hyperparathyroidism. None of these revealed any abnormalities suggestive of borderline or transitory acidophilic hyperpituitarism in any other sphere, though hypertension of variable severity was present in 3 of the 6.

Serum protein elements

No systematic evaluation of liver function was attempted in our series although previously described changes in insulin sensitivity, blood glucose maintenance and possibly even alkaline phosphatase are partially influenced by liver function. A close relationship also obtains for the maintenance of serum protein levels reported in this section.

Levels of serum albumin and globulin were determined in 15 patients of the series. The data are summarized in table 16. Correlative observations on gonadal, adrenal and renal status are included.

Three of 15 patients had subnormal serum albumin (normal range 4 to 5 Gm. per cent) on one or more occasions. In 2 of the 3, the subnormal value occurred immediately after intracranial operation and in both instances rose to normal during convalescence. In the remaining patient the value rose to normal coincident with oral

Table 16—*Serum Proteins in 15 Chromophobe Adenoma Cases*

Serum Protein (Gm. %)		Gonadal status	Adrenal status	Renal function
Albumin	Globulin			
5.1	1.6	Presymptomatic amenorrhea	Atypical hypoadrenalism	Normal
4.9	1.9	Normal	Normal	Normal
3.3 (post-op.)	1.4 (post-op.)	Hypogonadism (moderate)	Adrenal crisis twice	Normal
4.7 (convalesced)	1.9 (convalesced)			
4.8	1.9	Hypogonadism	Hypoadrenalism (mild)	Normal?
4.9	2.0	Normal	Normal	2 plus albuminuria PSP: 45%
4.9	1.8	Hypogonadism	Severe adrenal crisis	2 plus ketonuria during crisis PSP-45%
4.8	2.2	Hypogonadism	Normal	Normal
3.8	2.5	Hypogonadism	Hypoadrenalism	NPN: 20–39
3.9	2.5			PSP: 45%
4.0–4.3 (With methyltestosterone)	2.9–2.2 (With methyltestosterone)			
4.7	3.3	Hypogonadism (mild)	Hypoadrenalism (questionable)	Normal
5.0	2.3	Hypogonadism (moderate)	Normal	Normal
4.9	2.4	Hypogonadism (minimal)	Hypoadrenalism	Normal
5.3	2.0	Hypogonadism (minimal)	Normal	NPN: 42–32
5.7	2.2	Normal	Normal	Normal
5.1	1.8	Normal	Adrenal crisis	Normal
3.8–3.7 (Immed. post-op.)	2.5–2.2 (Immed. post-op.)	Hypogonadism (moderate)	Hypoadrenalism (questionable)	Renal calculi Arteriolosclerotic kidney (nephrectomy)
4.2 (convalesced)	1.9 (convalesced)			
4.4–4.6 (With methyltestosterone)	1.8–2.1 (With methyltestosterone)			

methyltestosterone therapy. Though hypoadrenalism was suspected or established in all 3, as was symptomatic hypogonadism, 6 additional patients, in whom hypoadrenalism was suspected or confirmed (confirmed in 4), showed normal serum albumin levels, 2 of these during convalescence from crisis.

Serum globulin levels were within normal limits (1.5 to 3.0 Gm. per cent) in all except 1 case where the level was determined immediately after intracranial operation.

It is of interest to note that total protein, in this group, exceeded 8 Gm. in no instance. Six determinations on 3 patients with acromegaly exceeded 8 Gm. in every instance.

Summary

Total serum protein values in a limited number of this series revealed little deviation from normal though they were consistently lower than in 3 acromegalics.

Subnormal albumin, exclusive of that subsequent to operative blood loss, was observed in only 1 patient with documented hypoadrenalism. Even in this instance normal levels were later observed during therapy with methyltestosterone.

The disturbances in serum albumin so consistently observed in animals after adrenalectomy appear to be rare and inconspicuous in patients with chromophobe adenomas who may, at the same time, have clear indications of adrenal cortical defect.

The type of symptomatic hypogonadism characteristic of those with chromophobe adenomas is not correlated in any way with disturbances in serum protein, even in the presence of concomitant hypoadrenalism.

Cardiovascular function

Observations discussed in this section were made during routine physical examination, chest x-ray or fluoroscopic examination, or during special study indicated before institution of intensive therapy. Mecholyl sensitivity tests are included here rather than in the section on adrenal functional status because the manifestations of positive response are largely in the realms of central and peripheral cardiovascular function. Significant electrocardiographic changes have already been discussed. Except for these no remarkable nor consistent electrocardiographic abnormalities were noted.

Blood pressures were recorded in 112 of the 117 patients of this series. A total of 29 (27 per cent) were hypertensive (above 150 mm. systolic, 100 mm. diastolic, or both) either consistently or during certain periods of study. Acute hypertensive episodes occurring during operative procedures have been excluded. Of the 29, 2 had long standing hypertension with known, symptomatic, renal involvement. In the remaining 27, (24 per cent of the total), no relation to kidney disease could be established. The majority of these had both systolic and diastolic hypertension of sustained type. Definite enlargement of the heart by physical examination, x-ray and fluoroscopy was noted in 8 cases.

Three of the 29 with hypertensive trends had documented hypoadrenalism. In 2 of these a previous hypotension had been replaced by sustained hypertension coincident with (or as a result of) prolonged treatment with doca and salt. One patient suffered an acute cerebrovascular accident despite previously decreased doca medication.

Hypertension with hypoadrenalism is so unusual a combination that the third case above, in whom hypertension of systolic type appeared without doca therapy, warrants special mention. This individual, a 52 year old white male, was observed from 1935 to 1947 and was admitted for hospital study three times during that interval. He had a large chromophobe adenoma with progressively increasing hypothyroidism, severe asthenia necessitating admissions on two occasions, loss of libido and potency early in the course of illness and insulin hypersensitivity on third admission. During the last admission, for asthenia, his calculated sodium was 133.3 mEq. per liter, hematocrit 33.6 per cent, and plasma volume 41.6 cc. per Kg. body weight. Salt deprivation routine was not considered advisable under the circumstances. This patient, when first examined in 1935, had a blood pressure of 110/60. On re-admission in 1942, blood pressures were all in the neighborhood of 135/80. On his final admission, when hypoadrenalism was considered, blood pressures varied from 150 to 170 systolic, from 70 to 75 diastolic, and were uniformly unstable. No systolic levels below 150 were noted on repeated examinations during various times of the day. EKG was normal. The x-ray of the chest revealed a questionably enlarged heart. It should be emphasized that this patient received no hormonal therapy of any type during the entire course of his illness.

Hypertension was associated with obesity in 9 of 27 patients, with diabetes of persistent type in 2 of 27. Of the 16 hypertensives studied by air contrast for indications of hypothalamic compression 15 showed such compression. In two-thirds of these the anterior hypothalamic structures seemed to be most severely compromised. It is important to note that all those who were hypertensive, without renal changes, were over 40 years of age.

Acetyl-beta-methylcholine, 2.5 mg., was administered subcutaneously to 4 patients in this series. The procedure and criteria of Perera were followed.[366] Three of the 4 had adrenal crises at some time during the course of illness. In the fourth no evidence of hypoadrenalism was observed at any time, either during salt deprivation or under environmental stress. Only 1 of the 4 had unequivocal hypersensitivity by Perera's standards, this in the presence of documented hypoadrenalism. Another, with borderline hypersensitivity, had no evidence of hypoadrenalism. The remaining 2 were normally sensitive though both had documented hypoadrenalism. Hypersensitivity to mecholyl, in our few cases, was therefore not as consistent as in those with primary hypoadrenalism studied by Perera.

A total of 21 patients in the entire series had significant hypotension, thus the trend toward abnormal blood pressure levels was shown in slightly less than one-half (50 of 112) of all patients with chromophobe adenomas studied. If we remove from the hypertensive group the 2 patients with known renal disease as well as the 2 in whom hypertension appeared with doca therapy, the incidence of hypotensive trends is almost identical with that of hypertensive trends. The latter is probably a part of the aging process operating despite coincident hypopituitarism. The high incidence of hypothalamic compression in those with hypertensive trends is of questionable significance since our studies indicate that 88 per cent of all patients with chromophobe adenomas have evidence of hypothalamic compression.

Summary

Slightly less than one-half of our patients with chromophobe adenomas displayed abnormal blood pressure levels. A hypertensive trend was as common as a hypotensive trend, the majority of those with the former displaying persistent sustained hypertension of both systolic and diastolic type.

All patients with systolic and diastolic hypertension were over 40 years of age.

It was impossible to establish any specific hypothalamic factor as operative in those with either hypotensive or hypertensive trends.

Sustained hypertension appeared in 2 patients with hypoadrenalism during the course of doca therapy.

Sustained systolic hypertension was observed in 1 patient with mild secondary hypoadrenalism, in the absence of any hormonal therapy.

Those patients with secondary hypoadrenalism may not be as consistently sensitive to mecholyl as are those with primary hypoadrenalism.

Renal function

Studies of renal function were performed rarely in patients of this series and the available data cannot be evaluated in the light of experimental alterations.

The excretion of P.S.P. was determined in 11 patients of the entire series. The value was 45 per cent in each of 3 patients with hypothyroidism (1 hour excretion in 2 of the 3), and varied from 54 per cent to 80 per cent in the remaining 8 in whom thyroid function was either normal (in 5) or not determined (2 hour excretion in 5 of the 8). One patient with questionable hypoadrenalism excreted 80 per cent of P.S.P. in 2 hours. Documented hypoadrenalism was present in 2 of the 3 patients with 45 per cent excretion.

Considering the differences in total excretory period, all 11 patients manifested relatively normal renal tubular function, as far as can be demonstrated by P.S.P. No other clearance studies were performed.

Nine of the 117 patients in our series had conspicuous renal abnormalities, 2 with hypertension, 1 with renal calculi. In none were any of the observed changes related to primary or secondary tumor effects.

These observations concerning renal function do not warrant summary or conclusions.

Disturbances referable to hypothalamic involvement

In previous sections we have been describing the changes incident to an enlarging intrasellar mass; it should now be obvious that the posterior lobe of the pituitary must suffer compression and distortion similar to that of the remnant of normal anterior lobe. There is no direct way of determining to what degree loss of posterior lobe tissue contributes to the observed deficits. Experimental and clinical data indicate that this contribution is of little significance. It is possible that posterior pituitary deficit may explain the conspicuous lack of abnormal pigmentation in patients with hypoadrenalism secondary to chromophobe adenomas. German,[193] as a matter of fact, observed no abnormal pigmentation in any of 100 patients with chromophobe adenomas. Such pigmentation has been observed in almost one-half of all acromegalics, according to Davidoff,[cited in 193] and in one-quarter or more of patients with Simmonds' disease.[146, 310] Its presence in Simmonds' disease is especially pertinent since in most such cases a considerable remnant of or a completely normal posterior lobe is noted at autopsy. Some of the peripheral ectodermal and vasomotor changes commonly noted in patients with chromophobe adenomas may be related, in part, to deficient posterior pituitary function. The defects we have described must reflect the effects of total pituitary compression, whatever the contribution of component parts may be.

The hypothalamus is another important structure variably affected by this tumor. It may be disturbed in two ways; first by retrograde degeneration of ganglion cells incident to distortion and thinning of the pituitary stalk; secondly through direct compression by the expanding tumor. Our data allow us to evaluate only the effects of direct compression and distortion.

Observations

In 78 patients of this series clinical studies were sufficiently complete to indicate conclusively the presence or absence of hypothalamic compression. Observations were made either directly at autopsy or operation, or were predicated on the basis of air encephalography. The only cases included are those in which the third ventricle was clearly demonstrated by encephalography, and was shown, moreover, to have either an intact or obviously distorted floor. Anterior hypothalamic compression was considered to be present when the cisterna

TABLE 17—*Hypothalamic Compression: Its Impact on Symptomatic and Metabolic Disturbances*

| | Incidence | | | | | |
| | With compression | | | Without compression | | |
Status or finding	No.	Of total	%	No.	Of total	%
1. BMR – 15 or less*	30	47	64	4	9	45
2. Low or diabetic glucose tolerance†	10	48	21	4	9	45
3. Excited states and/or hyperhidrosis	18	68	26	0	10	0
4. Diabetes insipidus‡	7	68	10	0	10	0
5. Adiposogenital syndrome	8	68	12	0	10	0
6. Autonomic epileptic phenomena	6	68	9	0	10	0
7. Obesity with polyphagia	6	68	9	0	10	0
8. Lethargy, depression or excessive somnolence	18	68	26	0	10	0

* Chi-square value (with and without compression): 0.97.

† Chi-square value (with and without compression): 2.36. (Yates's correction not applicable)

‡ Persistent diabetes insipidus in 3 of the 7. No evidence of hypoadrenalism in any of these 3.

chiasmatic was obliterated and a filling defect was outlined in the anterior portion of the third ventricle. Posterior hypothalamic compression was diagnosed by demonstration of clear-cut distortions of the posterior one-third of the floor of the third ventricle, with or without obliteration of the cisterna interpeduncularis or superior cisterna pontis. Operative data were usually more indefinite than those derived from air encephalography. Significant observations are summarized in table 17.

Of the 78 cases studied, 68 (88 per cent) had demonstrable hypothalamic compression. In 29 of the 68 (43 per cent) compression was generalized. An additional 29 showed anterior compression alone, the remaining 10 (14 per cent) showing posterior compression.

The 10 cases with no evidence of compression were used as a control group. This is admittedly inadequate because of the possibility of variable retrograde cellular changes in supraoptic and paraventricular nuclei in these controls. Within this group there were no instances of so-called adiposogenital dystrophy, diabetes insipidus (except for 1 with questionable transient polydipsia without polyuria postoperatively), excessive somnolence, unusual sweating reactions, obesity with polyphagia or autonomic epileptic phenomena. Subnormal metabolism rate was recorded in 4 of 9 so studied. A low or diabetic type of glucose tolerance occurred, likewise, in 4 of 9.

In the 68 patients with hypothalamic compression, critical evaluation of symptoms revealed no single finding or complex which might suggest the site of compression. Somnolence was somewhat less common in anterior than in generalized compression, but the difference was suggestive rather than conclusive.

In 20 of the 68 cases (30 per cent) there were no symptoms referable to hypothalamic compression.

Subnormal metabolic rate was recorded in 30 of 47 patients so studied (64 per cent), its incidence not differing significantly from the incidence of subnormal metabolic rate in those without compression. A low or diabetic glucose tolerance was noted in 10 of 48 in this group (21 per cent), being questionably lower than in those without compression.

Agitation, attacks of drenching perspiration and occasional hyperthermia (the last occurring usually after operative intervention) were noted in 18 of the 68 patients. An identical number suffered from lethargy, emotional depression and excessive somnolence. Diabetes insipidus occurred in 7. In 4 of the 7 this disturbance was transient or appeared only for a time following intracranial operation. The remaining 3 had persistent and distressing diabetes insipidus, but with no evidence of hypoadrenalism.

The association of obesity, genital atrophy and feminine habitus, making up the syndrome of adiposogenital dystrophy, was noted in 8 of the 68 patients (12 per cent). It is not surprising that the relative frequency of chromophobe adenomas was not suspected in the first two decades of this century if attention was attracted to the pituitary gland by syndromes of such relative rarity as adiposogenital dystrophy and diabetes insipidus.

Autonomic epileptic phenomena or aurae, as manifested in striking changes of pulse rate, blood pressure, drenching perspiration and peripheral vasodilation, were observed in 6 of the 68 patients. Disturbances occurring at or after termination of generalized convulsions were, of course, excluded.

Recently acquired obesity with notable polyphagia occurred in 6 patients.

Summary

Symptoms recognized as of probable hypothalamic origin occurred in 70 per cent of patients with demonstrable hypothalamic compression due to chromophobe adenoma.

Subnormal basal metabolic rate occurred in approximately the same relative number of patients, whether with or without hypothalamic compression.

Low or diabetic glucose tolerance was somewhat more common in those with no hypothalamic compression, the majority of whom had small tumors.

Agitation, hyperhidrosis and occasionally hyperthermia occurred in approximately one-fourth of patients with hypothalamic compression; lethargy, depression or excessive somnolence in an equal number.

Approximately 1 of 10 patients with hypothalamic compression had diabetes insipidus, adiposogenital dystrophy, autonomic epileptic phenomena or obesity with polyphagia.

The type or combinations of pertinent symptoms and disturbances gave no reliable index of the site of hypothalamic compression.

VIII

ADDITIONAL LABORATORY DATA AND DIFFERENTIAL DIAGNOSIS

FORMED ELEMENTS OF THE BLOOD

Reports of hypochromic anemia, relative and absolute lymphocytosis and occasional eosinophilia in hypopituitary states were frequent in the early clinical literature, and were summarized by Hubble in 1933.[260] Several pertinent experimental investigations are of interest in this regard. Corey and Britton in 1932,[92] noted a striking decrease in total leukocytes following bilateral adrenalectomy, in spite of hemoconcentration. A concomitant lymphocytosis was associated with this leukopenia. Adrenal cortical extract completely reinstated the normal cellular relationships, adrenalin only slightly and glucose and saline solutions not at all. Splenectomy exerted no apparent effect on the observed changes.

Dougherty and White[132] reported the appearance of an absolute lymphopenia a few hours following a single injection of ACTH in normal mice, rats and rabbits. This response failed to occur in adrenalectomized animals similarly treated or in intact animals treated with pure protein. Dougherty and White also observed neutrophilic increase following hormonal injection and considered it to be nonspecific. Adrenal cortical extract, adrenal cortical steroids, corticosterone and compound F all gave the typical lymphopenic response, though doca did not.

As a result of the action of 11-oxygenated corticoids there is a dissolution of many lymphocytes contained within lymphoid organs and, secondarily, a decrease in the number of circulating lymphocytes. Conversely, a relative lymphocytosis may occur in the presence of hypoadrenalism. One effect of the breakdown of lymphocytes subsequent to the administration of ACTH may be an increase of beta and gamma globulins in the blood. In part these may constitute antibody protein fractions.[512] However, the original belief that anamnestic responses may occur as a result of ACTH has not been borne out.[161] Dougherty and White's work has been supported as well as attacked but does appear to be reproducible if attention is given to the dosage of ACTH and temporal aspects of the experiments.

Although reticulopenia probably secondary to atrophy of bone marrow may occur, hematopoiesis and the formation of platelets are generally found to be normal following experimental hypophysectomy.[344] It is possible that a diminished production of platelets may prevail, since the usual secondary rise in platelets following splenectomy does not occur. Although no direct effect of pituitary or adrenal on the formation of the cellular elements of blood has been recorded, Crafts[96] published provocative observations concerning the anemia of adult female hypophysectomized rats. He characterizes this anemia as microcytic and hypochromic, associated with erythroid hypoplasia of the bone marrow. A combination of thyroxin, iron and copper reverses all the noted changes; iron and copper are relatively ineffective without thyroxin.

There is usually a marked anemia in Simmonds' disease, probably due to deficient absorption of essential hematogenic factors or to hypoplasia of the bone marrow.[434] Peripheral hormones such as testosterone have an erythropoietic effect, but there are only limited indications that the endocrines are necessary for the formation of red blood cells.[493]

Upon the administration of adrenalin eosinopenia appears. This response has been related to an intact pituitary-adrenal or hypothalamic-pituitary-adrenal mechanism, as adrenalin is thought to stimulate the pituitary, either directly or indirectly, to secrete ACTH. This hormone activates the adrenal cortex to liberate steroids that may cause a decrease in circulating eosinophiles.[380] The administration of ACTH and the extent of the consequent eosinopenic response has been used as an index of adrenal cortical activity. Further evidence for the association of hypothalamic mechanisms and circulating white blood cells has been brought forth by DeGroot and Harris.[118a] These workers have shown that stimulation of the posterior region of the tuber cinereum or of the mammillary body resulted in lymphopenia in rabbits. Destructive lesions of these areas appeared to abolish the lymphopenic response to emotional stress.

A lymphocyte count of 39 per cent or more of the total white blood count may be considered unduly elevated. Forty of 99 cases of chromophobe adenoma in whom blood cytology was studied showed a relative lymphocytosis. The average of the white blood counts of these 40 cases was a total of 6900 white blood cells, composed of 51.7 per cent polymorphonuclears and 41.9 per cent lymphocytes. There were instances where one or more counts exhibited a relative lymphocytosis while remaining serial counts were within normal limits. All the counts recorded in these cases were included in the summation. If only the abnormal counts of the 40 cases were averaged, the lymphocytes represented 44 per cent of the total white blood cells.

Fifteen cases exposed to stressful situations were followed during their course with serial white blood counts. Five of these had normal differentials prior to stress but responded with a relative lymphocytosis during or following stress. Of the remaining 10 with initially abnormal counts, 2 continued to maintain a lymphocytosis during stress whereas the others shifted to a predominantly polymorphonuclear response.

The trend in these counts is similar to that noted in hypoadrenalism and panhypopituitarism.[119] The incidence of secondary hypoadrenalism in this series was 36 per cent. When this is compared with that of relative lymphocytosis, one may be led to suspect that the shift in the differential white blood count may be either the result of undetected or subclinical hypoadrenalism, which is probably more common than realized, or of an admixture of several endocrine deficits. There is no apparent relation between degree or region of neural involvement and the appearance of a relative lymphocytosis. Since the total number of white blood cells falls within normal limits, relative lymphocytosis may be accounted for, in part, by a concomitant minimal depression in the formation of polymorphonuclear cells.

The sudden appearance of eosinophilia in patients with extravasation of the contents of a cystic adenoma into the subarachnoid space has been noted. Although this has been observed previously it is an unusual event. Special eosinophil counts in response to stress have not been done on patients included in this series. Data from other patients seen subsequent to this study and from cases of primary hypoadrenalism indicate that with the one dose method of ACTH a dissociation between the eosinopenic response and the results of the other tests for adrenal function may exist. However, we have had no experience with the three day or prolonged administration of ACTH and its effect on circulating eosinophils as an index of adrenal cortical activity. We have been told that the results of this modification are more reliable but have not reviewed the data in cases of chromophobe adenoma.[391a]

The hemoglobin concentration and red blood count were within normal limits in the majority of the 99 patients adequately studied. Although a mild normocytic hypochromic anemia was observed in several instances of secondary hypoadrenalism, a similar number of other patients without apparent dysendocrinism had depressed hemograms.

CEREBROSPINAL FLUID

The cerebrospinal fluid findings in 63 patients reveal that the general intracranial pressures as determined by lumbar manometrics were normal in all. Reference has been made previously to the following facts: (1) the adenoma is usually located outside the direct pathway of cerebrospinal fluid flow, (2) there is a ready displacement of both tumor and basal brain structures and (3) an expanding pituitary tumor is usually not in position to compromise the communicating orifices of the ventricular system. However, it is equally apparent that local increased pressure such as may obstruct the perineural optic sheath does exist and papilledema may occur in the absence of increased intracranial pressure.

The main change in the content of the lumbar cerebrospinal fluid is an increased amount of protein. Considering values above 60 mg. per cent as abnormal, 25 of the 63 cases had elevated spinal fluid protein, with an average value of 113 mg. per cent. There was a qualitative proportionality between the size of the tumor and the presence of a high protein content. Thus, 16 of the 25 instances occurred in those with large tumors, 9 with moderate and none with small lesions. There was no relation to the extent of hypothyroidism in these cases. The origin of the protein in these cases, which do not include the frank meningitides, may be derived from several sources. Locally, circulatory interference due to an expanding tumor probably increases venous transudation. In addition, inflammatory meninges about a tumor may permit leakage of protein from the meningeal blood vessels. The local reaction of subarachnoid mesenchymal cells to the presence of inflammatory and circulatory changes may be associated with "shedding" of these cells and thereby contribute to cerebrospinal fluid protein. Finally, the effects of severe hypothyroidism and perhaps other endocrine deficiencies may so influence the cells of the choroid plexuses so as to increase their permeability to serum protein.

Aside from the cases in which meningitis or meningismus may occur, increase in the white blood cells of the spinal fluid is very rare. A minimal elevation was noted in only 2 of the 63 fluids examined. However, in the event of a slow cystic extravasation, even though unaccompanied by the clinical sign of meningismus, a moderate pleocytosis is usually found.

RADIOLOGY OF THE SELLAR SYNDROME

The x-ray appearance of the sella turcica and its components in cases of chromophobe adenoma frequently is characteristic. In the absence of either clinical or general roentgenographic signs of acromegaly or aneurysms of the circle of Willis, the diagnosis of chromophobe adenoma can be made with fair certainty by x-ray. The technic employed in visualization of the sella turcica and environs may be found in specialized texts.[360] It is customary to include in the examination anterior posterior, lateral stereoscopic, posterior anterior and a foramen magnum view. Reference to figures 28 to 31 will assist in the demonstration of the common x-ray findings. The dorsum sellae suffers the consequences of either direct pressure by the neoplasm or by the pulsating force of arteries displaced against it by the tumor. It thins and becomes concave forward. Depending on the direction of attack, it may be pushed backward or downward and backward. Increasing translucency and finally virtual destruction of the dorsum may ensue, with consequent loss of the posterior boundary of the sella turcica. The fossa itself deepens as its floor becomes thinned and depressed. Erosion through the floor into the sphenoid sinus may occur. Depending on the predominant laterality of the tumor the floor of the sella turcica may be depressed unequally on either side. Anteriorly, the walls of the sella turcica are involved and may appear concave posteriorly. The anterior clinoids are frequently spared but may appear to be undermined by the forward advance of the tumor. Unremitting and unrelieved pressure by the tumor may destroy most of the landmarks of the central regions of the middle cranial fossa. Moreover, the unusual extensions, such as those to the superior orbital fissure or into the posterior fossa, are associated with specific x-ray findings.

Occasionally, intrasellar calcification may be noted. Without specific clinical or roentgenographic evidence this does not indicate the presence of a tumor. Rarely does the x-ray examination fail to reveal the sellar or parasellar lesion. In the present series this occurred in only 2 cases, both of which were confirmed by direct examination as chromophobe adenomas.

Displacement of a calcified pineal gland may occur infrequently but, beyond indicating the presence of an intracranial tumor, it is of limited assistance without the special primary findings.

There are numerous lesions which may affect the sella turcica in a manner which may be visualized by x-ray. Craniopharyngiomas, granulomas, parasellar aneurysms, malignancies of the sphenoid sinus, nasopharyngeal tumors invading the base of the skull, metastatic

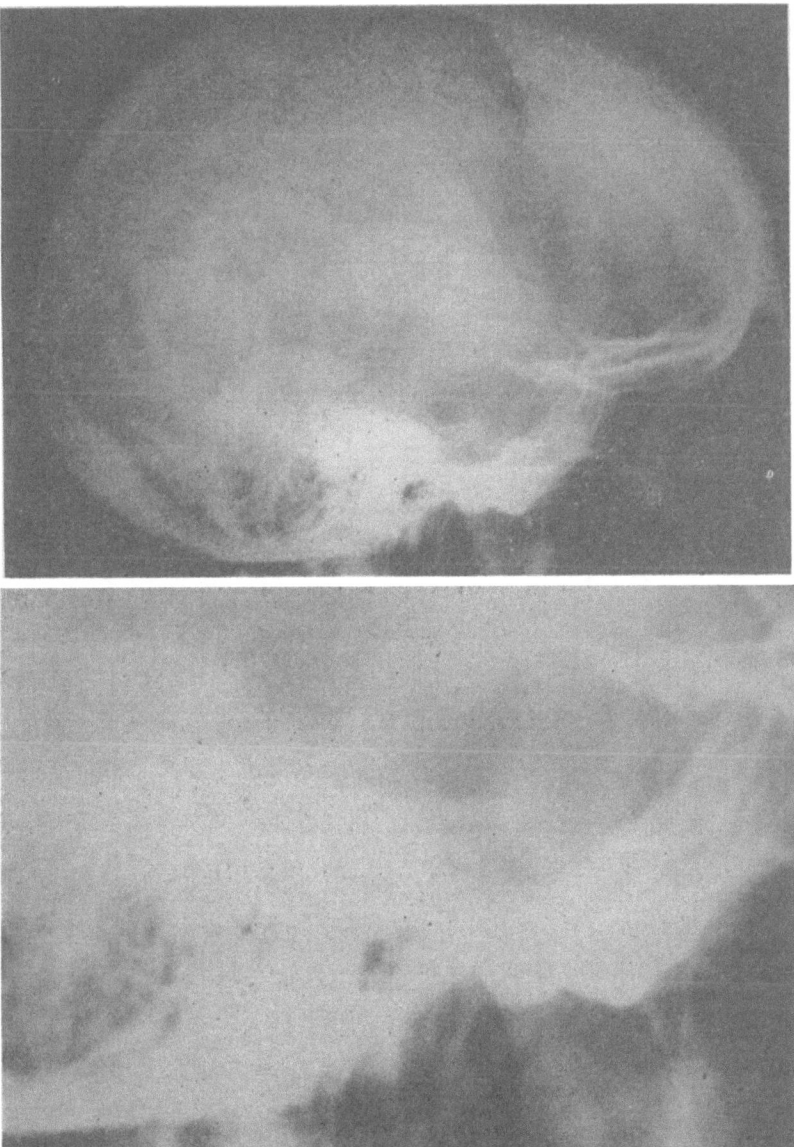

Fig. 28—Lateral view (*top*) and detail (*bottom*) of sella turcica in case of chromophobe adenoma. The characteristic findings are somewhat exaggerated in this reproduction: the depression of the floor, the undercutting of the anterior wall, the loss of the dorsum sellae and the ballooning of the entire hypophyseal fossa. There appears, in addition, calcification of the posterior region of the tumor.

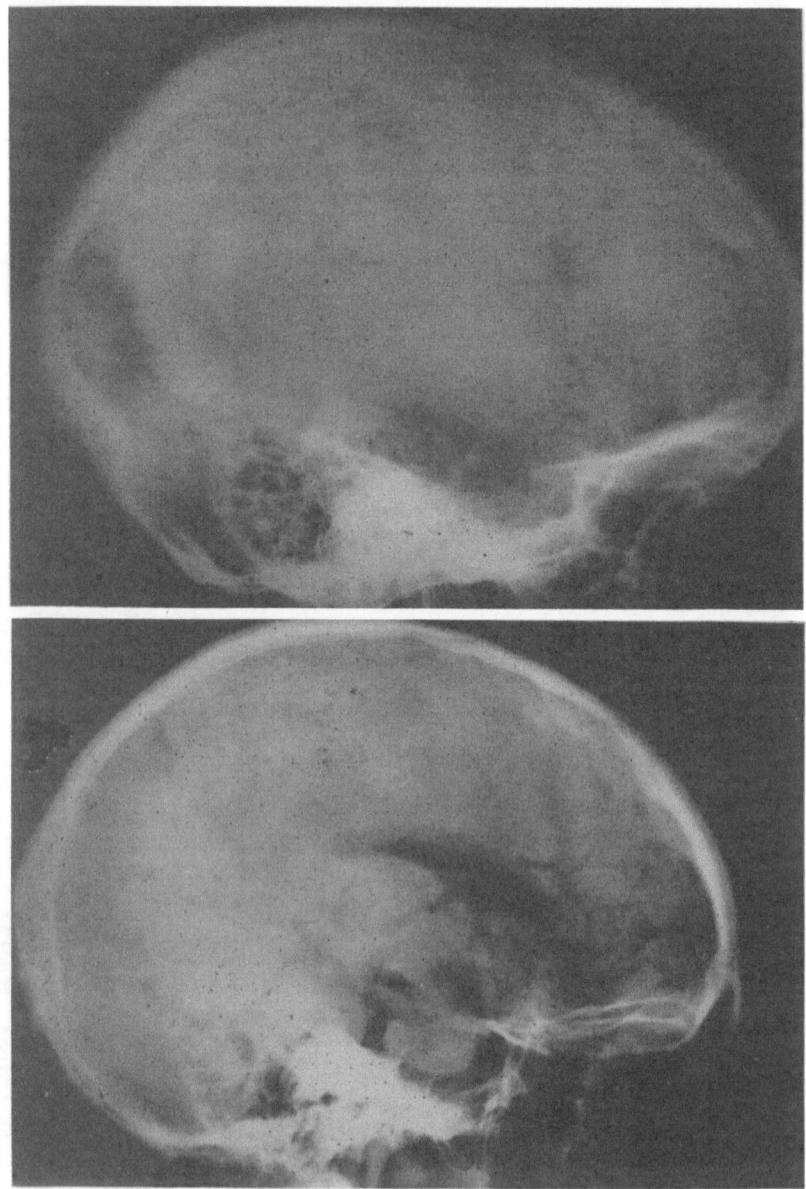

Fig. 29—Roentgenograms of patient with a chromophobe adenoma. See legend on facing page.

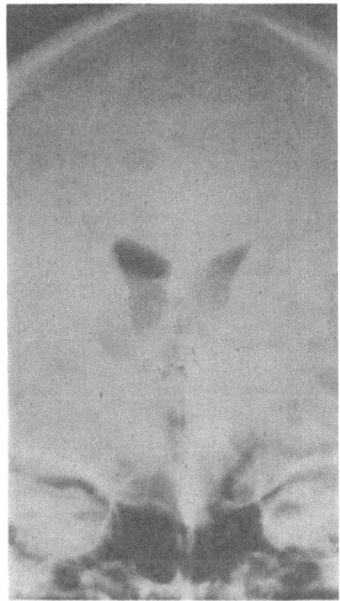

Fig. 29—Series of roentgenograms in the same patient with a chromophobe adenoma. The lateral view of the skull (*facing page, top*) reveals the diminution in normal markings of the boundaries of the hypophyseal fossa. The dorsum sellae is but a fragment of its normal state. The anterior clinoids are indistinguishable and the floor of the fossa deepened. Lateral views (*facing page, bottom*) of the pneumoencephalograph reveal the presence of a suprasellar tumor which extends into the third ventricle. The anterioposterior view (*left*) confirms the existence of encroachment by the adenoma into the third ventricle with lateral displacement of this ventricle. The floor of the lateral ventricle is displaced upward. The sulcal patterns are abnormal.

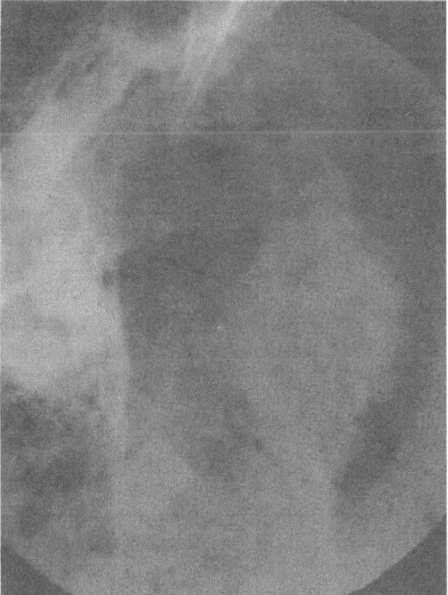

Fig. 30—Projection of a chromophobe adenoma into the basal cisterns and encroachment on the third ventricle. The tumor is well outlined by the air introduced through the lumbar route.

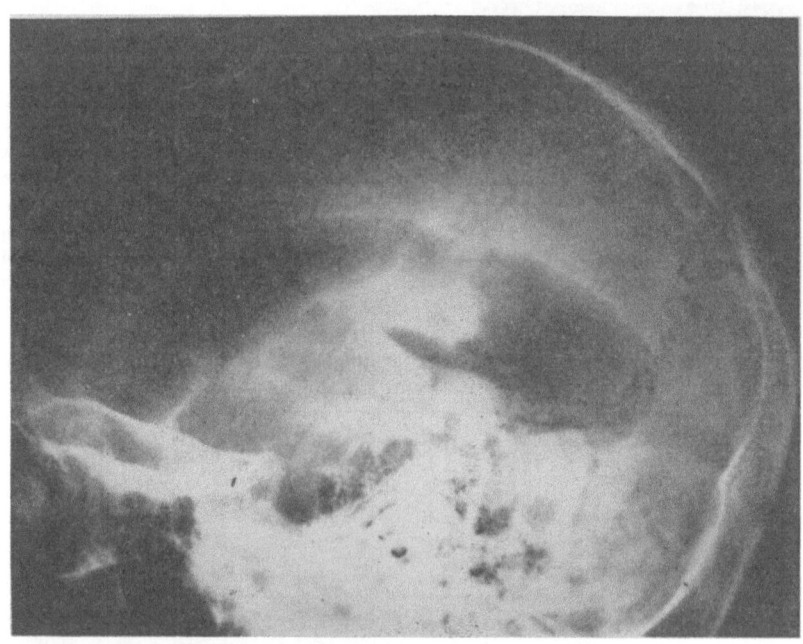

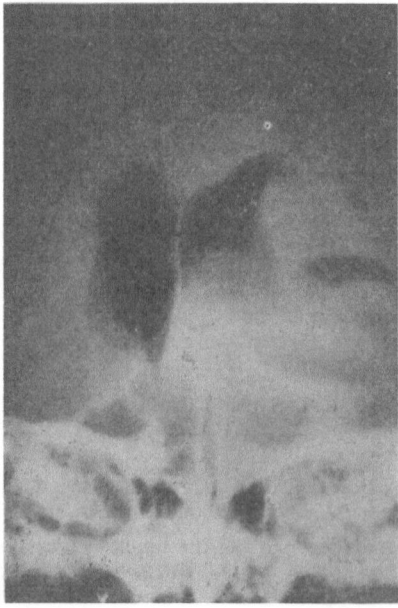

Fig. 31—Lateral (*top*) and postero-anterior (*left*) views of a pneumoencephalogram in a case of chromophobe adenoma.

(*Top*) The lateral ventricles are greatly dilated due to the extension of tumor into the third ventricle with partial obstruction of the ventricular system in front of the neoplasm. The third ventricle is almost entirely occupied by the tumor. The temporal horn is elevated and incompletely filled.

(*Left*) The findings are similar to those mentioned above with the additional observation that the floor of the lateral ventricle is elevated on one side by the expanding mass. There is separation of some of the sutural lines.

osteolytic processes, bone atrophies due to increased intracranial pressures or senility, basal meningiomas—all are representative pathologies which may affect the sella turcica and which may be differentiated from chromophobe adenoma roentgenologically.

Pneumoencephalography, which was performed frequently in this series, is of considerable assistance in confirming the diagnosis of chromophobe adenoma and in outlining the extent of the tumor. It is not usually a necessary examination and may be restricted to those few cases in which plain films of the skull are either debatable in interpretation or atypical. When performed by the lumbar route, the preferred method in the absence of increased intracranial pressure, the basal cisterns and the third ventricle are the regions found to be most commonly affected. Only partial or no filling of the cisterna chiasmaticus, pontis or interpeduncularis may occur. The third ventricle is deformed frequently by the upward extension of the neoplasm which projects against the ventricular walls and invaginates into the ventricular cavity, covered by a thin mantle of hypothalamic tissue. It is remarkable to observe the degree of distortion of the hypothalamus sometimes attained in the absence of definite hypothalamic symptomatology. Forward and upward extensions of the adenoma displaces the frontal horns in about 15 per cent of the cases. Here, too, a lack of corresponding clinical signs may be observed, though less commonly so. Obstruction of either the foramen of Monro or the anterior opening of the Sylvian aqueduct is found rarely. It is associated with dilatation of the ventricular system ahead of the point of involvement. Occasionally lateral projections into the temporal horn are detected.

There were 48 pneumoencephalographic studies attempted, of which 47 were entirely satisfactory. Forty revealed abnormal findings, 7 showing no extrasellar extension. The third ventricle was most revealingly affected in 27 instances. In these the ventricular walls were invaginated either from an anterior or posterior direction, rarely from directly below and sometimes to the point of obliteration of the ventricular cavity. Two tumors projected toward the aqueduct and caused slight dilatation of the third ventricle ahead of the partial obstruction. In one instance there was evidence of moderate blockage of the foramen of Monro. The basal cisterns were only fractionally filled in the 40 cases with abnormal findings. The cisterna interpeduncularis was entirely obliterated in 10 and the cisterna chiasmaticus in 8 instances. The frontal horns of the lateral ventricles were elevated or encroached upon in 6 individuals.

None of the patients included in this series were examined by angiography to establish the diagnosis of chromophobe adenoma. With few exceptions, such as tuberculum sellae meningioma, basal midline tumors are not well revealed by this technic. In some cases angiography reveals that the carotid siphon, a name given to the sinuous intracranial component of the internal carotid artery, is pushed forward by the expanding neoplasm and becomes more angular in appearance. Occasionally when there is ventricular dilatation the pericallosal artery is more acutely curved than normally. Phlebograms may reveal a displacement of the basilar veins in the presence of a chromophobe adenoma.[9a]

Pneumoencephalography and angiography are indicated procedures both as an aid in diagnosis of chromophobe adenoma and as a guide for surgery when the adenoma is presumed to extend significantly into frontotemporal or more remote regions.

ELECTROENCEPHALOGRAPHY

The activity recorded in the electroencephalogram reflects cellular chemical processes and perhaps events occurring at neuronal conductive surfaces. However, the rhythmicity of the discharges, their characteristic frequencies, the apparent indispensability of the fifth and sixth cortical layers for their existence, the effects of other regions of the central nervous system on cortical rhythms and many other factors must be explained to interpret the genesis and significance of the EEG. In the particular instance of a basal tumor such as chromophobe adenoma, the influence of compression on the diencephalon[300] and other subcortical regions[84] might be expected to be revealed. Several observers have claimed that bilateral slow activity may occur in the anterior leads as a result of neoplasm located here.[300] Others have described the appearance of 4–7/sec. waves, theta rhythm, resulting from lesions of the basal nuclei and thalamus, structures which indeed may come within the range of effects from pituitary tumors.[497] In addition to the local processes the supervention of generalized metabolic abnormalities further enlarges the possible variations in EEG patterns. Hypoadrenalism[140, 249, 394] and hypothyroidism[120] tend to slow the EEG and make its patterns less regular.

Although, in general, the EEG speaks clinically in but a few tones, when one considers the combination of the strategic location of the tumor and the induced hypometabolism, the relatively mundane electrical findings reported here are surprising: 24 of 40 patients had abnormal records, 8 of these with focal findings. The remaining 16 cases with normal EEGs were clinically comparable to the group with abnormal findings. The antecedent duration of the disease and the distribution of tumor size were similar. With regard to the latter factor, it was found that the incidence of large tumors was equally great in the cases with normal as with abnormal records. In keeping with this observation is the apparent lack of positive correlation between the presence of elevated CSF proteins and abnormal EEGs.

On closer analysis of the 16 patients with normal patterns, it is striking to note that 8 suffered compression or distortion of the third ventricle to an extent equal to that of the abnormal category. Whether the effects of the upwardly extending tumor were felt in the regions of the basal ganglia and thalamus cannot be surmised, although there was no outspoken clinical evidence of this. In addition, notable compression of the subfrontal cortex was present in 2 cases. There were 2 instances of lateral extension into the cavernous sinus, 1 exhibiting occasional generalized motor seizures, but in neither case were there EEG changes. The remaining tumors were intrasellar.

The abnormal EEGs were divided into two groups: (1) 16 with diffuse abnormalities without lateralizing signs and (2) 8 with focal findings. In the group with diffuse signs all except 2 cases extended into the third ventricle. The remaining 2 involved the subfrontal cortex. The records were moderately irregular, manifesting occasional 6–7/sec. activity, and disorganized patterns in several cases. Bilateral delta waves were noted in only one patient; significant fast activity was seen in another. The 2 instances of subfrontal involvement exhibited moderately irregular EEG patterns.

A review of the 8 patients with focal findings revealed that these were located in the temporal or posterior temporal regions in 6 and in the frontal in 2 instances. In those with temporal foci there was correspondence between the neurologic signs and the slow focal EEG activity in 3, and antagonistic findings in the remaining 3. In the latter homonymous hemianopia and motor weakness revealed that the lesion was actually contralateral to the temporal focus. In the cases of frontal foci one could be accounted for by direct compression of the frontal lobe, while the other was perhaps a transmitted pseudofocus, the result of peduncular pressure where the tumor exerted its main effect.

In several of the cases with abnormal recordings hypoadrenalism and hypothyroidism were observed but their presence was not overtly reflected in the EEGs. Similar instances of hypometabolism were noted in the normal series.

In summary, the findings indicated a substantial proportion of abnormal records without individualized features. The basal location of the adenoma did not appear to produce bilateral slow activity in a significant number of cases in this series. Focal findings were confined largely to the temporal location, but correspondence to neurologic signs was not invariable. The effects of hypometabolism were not clearly evident in this series, but they were undoubtedly muted with respect to the EEG, as they were when directly observed.

DIFFERENTIAL DIAGNOSIS

Differential diagnosis of the syndromes which produce symptoms and signs readily confused with those of chromophobe adenoma should ideally involve recapitulation of a broad segment of medical knowledge. In lieu of this, some of the commoner conditions have been enumerated below, and the procedure for investigation of the sellar syndrome discussed.

The structures in which defects may evoke clinical findings similar to those in chromophobe adenoma are categorized with their main pathologic changes.

1. Visual pathways.

a. Intrinsic: neoplasms, demyelination, vascular changes or trauma of the optic pathways and occipital cortex.

b. Extrinsic: effect of pressure due to (1) tumor of the pituitary, hypothalamus, meninges, pineal gland; (2) granulomas or metastatic invasion of the meninges; (3) aneurysms of the circle of Willis; (4) generalized increased intracranial pressure.

2. Endocrine organs.

a. Intrinsic to the pituitary gland: eosinophilic adenomas, craniopharyngiomas, acute or chronic pituitary insufficiency of non-neoplastic origin.

b. In the target organs: Addison's disease, hypogonadism, hypothyroidism, islet cell tumor of the pancreas.

3. Bone diseases of the sella turcica.

a. Primarily intracranial: chordoma, the demineralization of generalized increased intracranial pressure.

b. Generalized: eosinophilic granuloma or Hand-Schüller-Christian disease, multiple myeloma, metastatic disease.

4. Hypothalamic involvement.

Diabetes insipidus, intra- and extra-axial tumors.

5. General.

a. Psychogenic: anorexia nervosa.
b. Cavernous sinus syndrome.
c. Unexplained nasopharyngeal bleeding.
d. Unexplained disturbances of the frontal and temporal lobes.
Of the many possibilities listed confusion occurs most often with (1) craniopharyngioma; (2) tuberculum sellae meningioma; (3) aneurysm of the circle of Willis; (4) primary hypofunctioning of adrenal, thyroid, or gonads; (5) anorexia nervosa.

The procedure for investigation is resolved into those examinations routinely performed in a patient with symptoms of the sellar syndrome or of an endocrinopathy. Neurologic examination is supplemented by the following:

1. Roentgenograms of the skull.
2. Visual fields (mainly central) and visual acuity.
3. Complete spinal fluid examination.
4. Electroencephalogram.
5. Metabolic studies, such as fasting blood sugar, glucose and insulin tolerance, plasma volume, Na^+ and K^+ determinations in the serum before and after salt withdrawal, eosinopenic response to prolonged administration of ACTH,

assay of total neutral 17-ketosteroids, BMR, radioactive iodine uptake and serum cholesterol.

6. Specific diagnostic procedures, such as pneumoencephalography or angiography, as the situation warrants.

IX

PATHOLOGY

GROSS PATHOLOGY

The gross characteristics and regional pathology of chromophobe adenomas have been studied with exquisite care and technic by Harvey Cushing,[100] Dott and Bailey[131] and Henderson.[239] Our data, derived in large part from a study of operatively removed specimens, offer no additional information concerning the gross pathology of this tumor.

Two previously observed facts are worthy of special note. Dott and Bailey,[131] in an analysis of all pituitary tumors of Cushing's series, noted cystic degeneration in 17 per cent. In this series, chromophobe adenomas compromised 67 per cent of the total. Malignant changes in adenomas are extremely rare,[27, 131] occurring in approximately 2 per cent. Metastasis to the liver has been noted in 1 reported case.[131] In our series the true incidence of cystic tumors could not be assessed. Only 1 patient of the series showed massive regional spread of the tumor without, however, evidence of distant metastases.

ARCHITECTURAL TYPES

Several of the earliest classifications of pituitary tumors now recognized as largely of chromophobe type[49, 398] were unnecessarily complicated. Some pure chromophobe adenomas were listed as probable malignant epitheliomas or sarcomas, while others with prominent stromal background were subdivided as fibro-adenomata or mixed tumors. Cushing,[100] in his first study of 12 chromophobe adenomas, suggested four architectural types that have since been confirmed as representative. These were as follows: (1) loosely packed masses of cells, (2) cells arranged in alveolar pattern, (3) cells oriented about interlacing sinusoids and (4) cells following a papillary glandular structure. Dott and Bailey[131] later simplified and systematized Cushing's classification in their study of 107 chromophobe adenomas. They recognized two general types of tumor; one with normal columnar structure, and one with strumatous arrangement composed of masses of cells with little connective tissue stroma. Subsequently, Bailey and Cushing[24] further subdivided all pituitary tumors into six general types, drawing upon cellular morphology and cytoplasmic components for additional criteria. In this study, the most extensive and well-considered to date, they concluded that chromophobe adenomas composed of narrow columns of cells about numerous vascular sinuses presented a structure most similar to the normal glandular architecture, but were extremely rare.

Observations

Since correlation of histologic structure with type of clinical picture has proved of value in the clarification of some medical problems, a systematic histologic analysis of our material was carried out in the hope that a consistent or hitherto obscure link could be discovered.

A total of 115 separate tumors, removed surgically or obtained at autopsy, were studied. Of these, 86 were adequate for evaluation. In most instances the fixing fluid was 10 per cent neutral formalin solution, but occasionally Zenker's fluid was used. A majority of the specimens were stained with eosin-methylene-blue or hematoxylin-eosin; with one or more connective tissue stains, the most common being Mallory's connective tissue stain or Laidlaw's connective tissue stain; with the cytoplasmic granule stain, azo-carmine; and in approximately one-half, with stains for specific stromal elements, among them Foot-Bielchowsky or phosphotungstic acid.

The 86 tumors were classified architecturally on the basis of the predominant structural pattern observed throughout the tumor. Cell morphology, aggregative characteristics of cell groups and relationships to the stromal and vascular backgrounds were used as criteria for classification. The tumors are subdivided as indicated in table 18, comparing our data to that of Schnitker et al.,[416] who recently have published a histopathologic classification of chromophobe adenomas.

Forty-six of our tumors (54 per cent) were of diffuse type, the tumor cells being relatively small and uniform in size, polygonal in contour, resembling closely-packed liver cells. They were arranged in blocks and continuous sheets in a sparse, delicate reticular stroma, contributed in great measure by the few compressed sinusoids. Such a tumor is represented in figure 32. Careful comparison of many such tumors, stained for structural details, suggests to us—in contrast to

TABLE 18—*Architectural Characteristics of Chromophobe Adenomas*

Total tumors studied	Sinusoidal type		Diffuse type		Papillary type		Unclassified	
	No.	%	No.	%	No.	%	No.	%
86 (Authors' series)	27	31	46	54	13	15	—	—
81 (Schnitker et al.[416])	30	37	46	57	—	—	5	6

Cushing's original contention—that this tumor most closely resembles the normal anterior pituitary gland in architecture. If, as seems probable, such tumors grow largely by amitotic division,[25, 38] then it appears more likely that the clusters and clumps of cells shown in figure 33 would reproduce the cell blocks and sheets of figure 32 rather than columnar architectural patterns revealed in figure 34. The diffuse tumor has lost the normal vascularity of the intact gland because normal existent sinusoids are compressed by the enlarging and expanding cell masses. The architectural characteristics of the columnar or sinusoidal type of tumor, pictured in figure 34, are reminiscent of the embryonic anterior pituitary gland but not of the adult structure.

Twenty-seven tumors (31 per cent) were of sinusoidal type (fig. 34). The individual tumor cells were columnar in shape, with dense ovoid or elongate nuclei in which chromatin was deeply stained

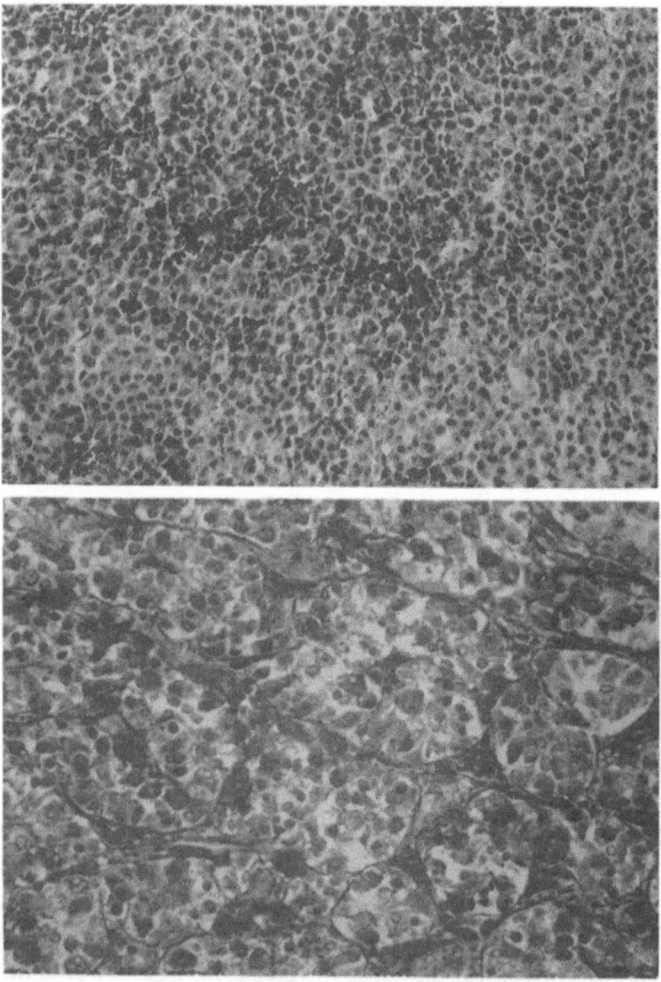

Fig. 32 (*top*)—Section of chromophobe adenoma of the pituitary gland: diffuse type. Note the large blocks and continuous sheets of small, uniform, polygonal tumor cells. The sparse, delicate, reticular stroma is indistinct and relatively avascular. Hematoxylin-eosin stain. Magnification approximately 180 ×.

Fig. 33 (*bottom*)—A section of normal human anterior pituitary gland. Note the delicate, interlacing, sinusoidal channels subdividing clumps and clusters of epithelial cells. Hematoxylin-eosin stain. Magnification approximately 240 ×.

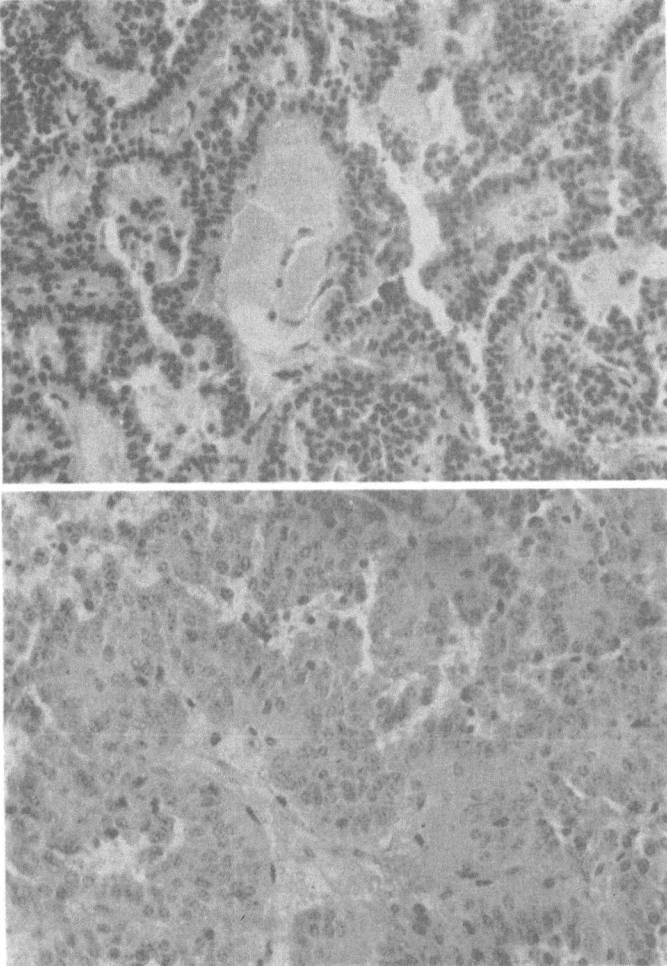

Fig. 34 (*top*)—Section of chromophobe adenoma of the pituitary gland: sinusoidal type. Note the rich network of interlacing and intercommunicating sinusoidal channels whose external walls are composed of elongate tumor cells, one deep, oriented perpendicularly to the sinusoids. Tumor cell nuclei are uniformly dense, the chromatin clumped. Hematoxylin-eosin stain. Magnification approximately 240 ×.

Fig. 35 (*bottom*)—Section of chromophobe adenoma of the pituitary gland: papillary type. Note the dense reticular stroma (left lower center) surrounded by irregularly elongate to columnar tumor cells with abundant cytoplasm and pale ovoid or flattened nuclei. Many tumor processes are three or more cells in depth. Eosin-methylene blue stain. Magnification approximately 240 ×.

and clumped. Cells were arranged perpendicular to the rich network of interlacing and intercommunicating sinusoidal channels. Such channels, with their coronas of radiating tumor cells, were frequently observed in cross section and superficially resembled glandular acini. However, no true acini were found in any tumor.

The remaining 13 tumors (15 per cent) have been classified as of papillary type (fig. 35). They apparently represent a subclassification of the sinusoidal type. These tumors had a relatively dense reticular stroma in which occasional small sinusoidal channels were embedded. Individual cells were elongated, with pale ovoid nuclei and dense abundant cytoplasm. Cell buds or blocks were usually three to five cells deep, and there was conspicuous heaping up of cell masses at the angles of branching strands. Cushing reproduced an example of such a tumor in his monograph.[100] This type is given the dignity of independent classification here because its structure closely resembles that of a papillary adenocarcinoma. Such tumors occasionally have been so diagnosed in the past. The patient, for example, whose operative biopsy is pictured in figure 35 was diagnosed as having such a papillary adenocarcinoma of the pituitary, though some doubt was expressed at the time because of the complete lack of mitotic figures. The patient was still alive and well when last contacted thirteen years after operation and had shown no indication of postoperative tumor growth or extension. A relatively small part of the total tumor had been removed at operation.

One fact of utmost importance must be stressed when considering the data of table 18. Most of the tumors studied were not uniform in architecture. They represented a composite of two or more types imperceptibly merging, one with another, in various regions of the specimen. Our data reflect only the predominant architecture of each specimen, with one exception: three-fourths of the tumors of diffuse type occurred in almost pure form without admixture of other types. The commonest association of the sinusoidal and papillary types was with the diffuse type. Hence, in all tumors studied there was a definite trend toward the diffuse form. Kraus,[289] on the basis of his wide experience in the field of pituitary pathology, has emphasized the occurrence of different architectural types in the same tumor and our observations are in agreement.

We have attempted to establish correlations between the observed architectural types and clinical features in 47 patients in whom such histopathologic studies were made. No apparent correlation in this or Schnitker's series[416] was noted between architectural type and age of onset, duration of symptoms, incidence by sex or total duration of life. The latter investigators did, however, note that the sinusoidal type of tumor appeared to be more radiosensitive than the diffuse type, but our observations do not indicate this to be an important factor.

One evident explanation for the lack of correlation of clinical findings with tumor type is the previously stressed fact that only the diffuse type of tumor is of uniform architecture, the remaining groups being a mixture of two or perhaps all three types.

SPECIFIC SECRETORY GRANULES

The histologic groundwork for the first clear appreciation of the occurrence of specific secretory granules in chromophobe adenomas was established primarily by Bailey,[21] and later by Bailey and Davidoff[25] in several careful analyses of the staining characteristics of pituitary tumor cells. Although Kraus described the transition of a chromophobe to chromophile adenoma in one case in 1926,[289] Bailey and Cushing[24] first defined clearly the transition phases in a meticulous analysis of 100 pituitary tumors. Among these were frank acidophilic as well as chromophobe adenomas. Two transitional groups were distinguished, as follows: (1) 11 tumors (13 per cent of those with pure chromophobe or transitional types) were classified as mixed or minimal transitional, in that occasional acidophilic cytoplasmic peripherally arranged granules could be detected in all; (2) 11 tumors were classified as transitional (Type IV, see below) since their peripheral cytoplasmic limits retained ethyl-violet dye with considerable tenacity although no specific secretory granules could be demonstrated. Thus, of all the tumors in their series previously considered as pure chromophobe adenomas, 22 (26 per cent of the total) represented transitional forms.

Bailey and Cushing then examined the histories and clinical investigations in the groups with transitional forms and in those with pure chromophobe adenomas. In 59 with pure chromophobe adenomas no evidence suggestive of fugitive hyperpituitarism was discovered except for tufting of the terminal phalanges in 2 patients and mandibular prominence without malocclusion in another. Evidences of fugitive hyperpituitarism were found in all 22 cases with transitional tumors. They concluded, on the basis of this study, that it is possible to forecast the microscopic character of the tumor from clinical study.

The correlations noted by Bailey and Cushing are most impressive. The only criticism which might arise is with regard to their Type IV group in which secretory granules are not demonstrated. These authors cited corroborative evidence for such a classification. When they stained such tumors with 1 per cent methylene green solution immediately after operative removal cells of two distinct staining types were seen. Cells of these two types have occasionally been noted by one of us (J.N.) in fixed tumor tissues stained with Mallory's connective tissue stain. Additional supportive evidence is derived from a study of the golgi apparatus of tumor cells. Such studies have generally been restricted to the normal components of the anterior pituitary gland,[3, 155] but Severinghaus[cited in 103] applied this technic to a number of chromophobe adenomas removed by Cushing and reported that cells with eosinophilic golgi apparatus were more common than those with golgi apparatus of basophilic type.

Observations

Of the 86 separate tumors evaluated in the previous section, 59 were stained by the azo-carmine method for secretory granules. All available portions of the tumors were studied systematically under oil immersion in each instance, though none were serially sectioned. Forty-four of the 59 (75 per cent) were composed exclusively of pure chromophobe cells without cytoplasmic granules or atypical cytoplasmic staining characteristics. Twenty-eight of these were studied clinically; atypical features for each are summarized as follows:

Case 18: Cranial vault thicker than normal.

Case 19: Spatulate fingers; slight mandibular prognathism (one brother was a borderline acromegalic).

Case 20: Thyroid slightly enlarged; BMR-4; slight tufting of terminal phalanges.

Case 21: Thyroid enlarged and nodular.

Case 22: Slight enlargement of toes and fingers of two month's duration; questionable acromegaloid facial characteristics.

Case 23: Low glucose tolerance preoperatively; normal tolerance postoperatively.

Case 24: Slight tufting of terminal phalanges.

Case 25: BMR-4; low glucose tolerance (4 hour); irregularly thickened frontal bone; borderline hyperglycemia.

Case 26: Transient glycosuria (past history).

Case 27: Unusually tall; skin thickened.

Case 28: Goiter operation ten years prior to admission; BMR-7 during endocrine study; frontal bone thick.

Case 29: Square, broad hands; BMR-13; x-rays showed no acromegaloid features in hands or skull.

Case 30: Transient glycosuria and hyperglycemia; no evidence of clinical diabetes.

Case 31: X-rays of skull five years post-biopsy were suggestive of acromegalic changes.

Case 32: Hirsutism; BMR-5; low glucose tolerance.

Case 33: X-ray showed cranial vault slightly thicker than normal.

Cases 34 to 45: No atypical clinical features.

Sixteen of these 28 patients with pure chromophobe adenomas showed features suggestive of present or past acidophilic hyperpituitarism, 6 showed minimal evidences of bony overgrowth, 4 had physical findings suggestive of minimal acidophilic hyperpituitarism without x-ray confirmation. Normal basal metabolic rate was noted in 5 patients. Five also showed either low tolerance for glucose or transient minimal diabetic trends. One was discovered to have suggestive acromegalic changes in routine skull x-rays five years after operative biopsy, though none were noted in preoperative films. It is difficult to determine what clinical features should be considered atypical. If broad limits are set atypical features can be seen in more than one-half of those who, as far as can be demonstrated, have pure chromophobe adenomas.

Slight secretory granulation might have been missed in some of the tissues fixed only in 10 per cent neutral formalin. Where the staining technic of Bailey and Davidoff[25] is followed it is probable, as they have suggested, that tissues are only satisfactory after prolonged mordanting. However, the azo-carmine technic used in this study is reliable in formalin-fixed tissues without mordanting.

In 6 of the 59 tumors specifically stained for secretory granules, acidophilic granules were discovered. In none of the 6 were the granules concentrated around the periphery of the cell. They were distributed in a random manner through the cytoplasm, as in eosinophilic cells of the normal anterior pituitary gland. Pertinent clinical data were available in these 6 patients, 5 of whom showed evidences of past or present acidophilic hyperpituitarism. Clinical data on these 6 patients are summarized as follows:

Case 46: Toxic goiter eight years prior to first admission. The acidophilic cytoplasmic granules were rare and diffusely distributed on the first operative biopsy; on the second operative biopsy they were few and densely distributed.

Case 47: Tufting terminal phalanges. The acidophilic cytoplasmic granules were rare and sparsely distributed.

Case 48: Acromegaloid facial features and spatulate fingers with no tufting indicated by x-ray. The acidophilic cytoplasmic granules were few and sparsely distributed.

Case 49: Diagnosed as "fugitive acromegaly"; large hands and feet for twenty-six years without progressive change. On three operative biopsies the acidophilic cytoplasmic granules were (1) occasional and sparsely distributed, (2) of doubtful granulation and (3) of moderate number and sparsely distributed.

Case 50: No acromegaloid trends in history, physical or laboratory studies. Granules were moderate and sparsely distributed.

Case 51: X-ray study revealed a thick cranial vault, enlarged paranasal sinuses, tufting of terminal phalanges and salivary calculus. Granules were rare and densely distributed.

An additional 7 patients were noted to have atypical cytoplasmic details or staining characteristics. These details and characteristics, along with clinical data are summarized as follows:

Case 52: Questionable acromegaloid features and a BMR of -9. X-ray examination showed a thick cranial vault, enlarged paranasal sinuses and marked tufting of the terminal phalanges. The tumor showed pale basophilic tinting.

Case 53: No atypical clinical features. The tumor showed cells with hypereosinophilia, an example of Bailey and Cushing's Type IV pituitary tumor.[24]

Case 54: No atypical clinical features. Cells were markedly basophilic with numerous basophilic vacuoles.

Case 55: Palpable thyroid gland. The tumor showed cells with hypereosinophilia, an example of Bailey and Cushing's Type IV pituitary tumor.

Case 56: No atypical clinical features. Cells were hypereosinophilic, an example of Type IV tumor.

Case 57: Cardiac hypertrophy. Cells were hypereosinophilic, an example of Type IV Tumor.

Case 58: Diabetic glucose tolerance with subsequent transient glycosuria and ketonuria; thick frontal vault; BMR – 6. Cells were hypereosinophilic, an example of Type IV tumor.

In one of the above 7 cases, with no atypical clinical features, the cytoplasm of all tumor cells was markedly basophilic and numerous vacuoles with marked affinity for aniline blue stain were observed. The tumor of another patient with sufficient atypical features to warrant a clinical diagnosis of fugitive acidophilic hyperpituitarism, showed cells with uniform palely basophilic cytoplasm. It is probable that the latter tumor was overstained with aniline blue although such overstaining occurs less frequently with aniline blue than with hematoxylin.[24] This objection does not seem to be valid for the first tumor. Both were stained, of course, with azo-carmine. It is of interest to note, in this connection that Bailey and Cushing[24] observed no beta granulation in more than 200 pituitary tumors studied. Even though basophilic cells are relatively infrequent in the normal anterior pituitary gland, this is surprising especially since, according to Severinghaus[425] not all tumor cells showed an acidophilic type of apparatus. In some the apparatus is of basophilic type.

The remaining 5 patients whose tumors are described above are probably examples of Bailey and Cushing's Type IV tumor. All showed cells with unusual and striking hypereosinophilia, although secretory granules were not demonstrated. Three of the 5 showed features of acidophilic hyperpituitarism.

The data summarized on pages 214 and following do not indicate an impressive correlation between cytoplasmic secretory elements and clinical signs or symptoms. There are several possible explanations for such a lack of correlation. One hinges upon the nature of the histologic examination itself. Serial sections might reveal what random sections fail to reveal, or our staining and fixing technics may be too insensitive to reflect the true secretory state of the cell. A second explanation could be that secretory elements, after having produced their effects in the past, disappear prior to operative biopsy and study. Such an explanation is not necessarily valid because Bailey and Cushing have demonstrated evidences of secretory activity in a considerable number of patients with no evidence of secretory overactivity at the time of histologic study. There is a third possibility that some or many of the clinical findings noted may have no relationship to acidophilic secretory overactivity, either past or present. It remains for future studies to clarify this problem.

Because atypical clinical findings were poorly correlated with histopathologic studies and because traces of acidophilic secretory activity were relatively common, possible distortion of our metabolic data was tested in a series of 60 patients, all of whom had skeletal x-ray studies. Tufting of the terminal phalanges was accepted as the minimum x-ray indication of skeletal overgrowth. Twenty-one of the 60 patients (35 per cent) had phalangeal tufting, the remaining 39 showed no skeletal traces of acidophilic hyperpituitarism. Pertinent data concerning metabolic rate and carbohydrate tolerance for this group are given in table 19.

Subnormal BMR occurred in approximately equal proportion in each group, the difference being statistically insignificant. Carbohydrate tolerance deviated from normal in a significantly higher proportion of those with skeletal traces of acromegaly, but the trend, in this group, was toward high and not low tolerance. We might have anticipated quite the opposite. We are justified in concluding that at the time of study evidence of past minimal acidophilic hyperpituitarism, as far as can be betrayed by skeletal x-ray studies, is associated neither with decreased incidence of subnormal BMR nor with increased incidence of low or diabetic tolerance for carbohydrates.

GENERAL SUMMARY

Slightly more than one-half of all chromophobe adenomas are predominantly of diffuse architectural type. In the remaining one-half, two-thirds are predominantly of sinusoidal type, one-third of papillary type. A majority of tumors of diffuse type are of homogeneous pattern. The remaining tumor types show admixtures of several architecturally discrete components, the most consistent being of diffuse character. It is suggested that the diffuse tumor most closely resembles, in architecture, the normal adult anterior pituitary gland.

Tumors of papillary type superficially resemble the structure of a papillary adenocarcinoma.

TABLE 19—*Skeletal Traces of Acromegaly: Their Relationship to Basal Metabolic Rate and Carbohydrate Tolerance*

	Incidence					
Clinical finding*	With skeletal acromegalic traces: 21 of 60 (35%)			Without skeletal acromegalic traces: 39 of 60 (65%)		
	No.	Total stud.	%	No.	Total stud.	%
1. BMR, − 15 or less.	10	15	67	26	35	79
2. Low or diabetic carbohydrate tolerance.	4	16	26	6	31	19
3. Normal carbohydrate tolerance.	6	16	37	21	31	68
4. High carbohydrate tolerance.	6	16	37	4	31	13

* Statistical data for these four groups, based on the chi-square formula (with and without) is as follows: Group 1, 0.32; Group 2, 0.2; Group 3, 3.94; Group 4, 3.8. Yates's correction was not appreciable for Group 4.

No correlation was established between predominant tumor architectural characteristics and age of onset, duration of symptoms, sex incidence or total duration of life.

In tumors composed predominantly of chromophobe cells acidophilic secretory granules can be demonstrated in approximately 1 of 10 (in 13 per cent, by previous workers). Clinical evidences of acidophilic hyperpituitarism are, with rare exception, discoverable in those with such tumors.

In tumors composed predominantly of chromophobe cells unusual cytoplasmic binding of dye, without discrete granulation, can be demonstrated in another 1 of 10 (in 13 per cent by previous workers). Evidences of acidophilic hyperpituitarism are inconsistently noted in those with such tumors.

In 1 of 59 tumors studied, basophilic cytoplasmic vacuoles were observed. Clinical features indicated no evidence of past or present abnormal secretory activity. One additional patient, whose tumor displayed atypical and questionable cytoplasmic basophilia, had clinical features indicative of borderline acidophilic hyperpituitarism.

Over one-half of patients with tumors showing no secretory granulation or abnormal cytoplasmic features, had either questionable or conclusive clinical evidence of present or past abnormal secretory activity, usually associated with acidophilic hyperpituitarism.

Acidophilic hyperpituitarism of minimal degree, indicated by skeletal x-ray studies, does not influence the trend toward subnormal basal metabolic rate, and is not associated with an increased incidence of low or diabetic glucose tolerance. It would appear, therefore, that bias has not been introduced into our series by the inclusion of patients with minimal acidophilic hyperpituitarism. Either the skeletal criteria used are an unreliable index of acidophilic hyperpituitarism or they are stamps of a past state no longer exerting metabolic effects.

PATHOGENETIC FACTORS

Site and mode of origin of chromophobe adenomas

Data concerning the site and mode of origin of chromophobe adenomas have been derived from a study of small tumors, in which relationships to normal glandular parenchyma are still discernable.

Löwenstein[321] published the first extensive studies on this subject in 1907. He concluded that the tumor anlage is an enormously enlarged chromophobe alveolus of embryonal appearance, seen most frequently in the pituitary gland of the young person, though not in the infant. The tumor probably developed by enlargement of this single alveolus. He discovered such alveoli in the pars intermedia, in the vicinity of the stalk and in the peripheral portion of the pars distalis; he further stated that 7 of 9 adenomas studied arose in the last named region. Kraus[289] later concluded that adenomas of chromophobe, transitional and fetal types usually originate from the middle or basal portion of the anterior lobe. It is difficult to detect any clear distinctions between the fetal adenoma of Kraus and the tumor of sinusoidal type noted by us.

Saxton has recently[409] emphasized the multicentric origin of spontaneous chromophobe adenoma-like lesions in senile rats.

Whatever the site and mode of origin of this tumor may be, such information fails to give us tangible clues to its pathogenesis.

Intrinsic mechanisms of tumor cell multiplication

Bailey and Davidoff[25] and Benda[38] have rarely, if ever, noted mitotic divisions in pituitary neoplasms of benign type, though amitotic divisions were frequently encountered by the former workers. We could discover no mitotic divisions in any of our tumors. This fact may be correlated with the observation[292] that regenerative hyperplasia is minimal in the injured human pituitary gland even though tumor growth potential is great.[299, 321, 502]

In striking contrast is the relative frequency of mitotic activity in anterior pituitary cells of experimental animals. Pomerat[374] and Wolfe[525] noted abundant mitotic figures in both eosinophiles and chromophobes of immature rats, the former reporting a distinct increase in mitotically dividing basophilic cells following castration. Hunt[262] further amplified the observations of Wolfe and Pomerat and concluded that the principal factor inducing mitotic activity in the hypophysis of the sexually mature female rat is directly or indirectly related to the estrous cycle. Greatest activity occurred in the postovulatory phase. A striking stimulation of the mitotic activity of chromophobe cells has been demonstrated in experimental animals after injections of estrogenic substance[117, 374, 422, 425] which, as will be discussed later, is capable of producing chromophobe adenoma-like lesions with remarkable consistency. Saxton[409] has observed many mitotic figures in the spontaneous chromophobe adenoma-like tumors in aged albino rats of the Yale strain. The clear distinction between the mode of multiplication of human pituitary tumor cells and those making up similar but induced experimental tumors must temper our interpretation of such data.

Growth potential of normal pituitary gland

Differentiation and localization of cell types.

In the earliest phases of human gestation only agranular chromophobe cells (termed fetal cells or hauptzellen in early studies) are detected[38, 46] in the adenohypophysis; secretory granules appear either later in gestation or during the first year of extra-uterine life. In the adult, chromophobe cells make up 52.2 per cent, acidophiles 36.8 per cent and basophiles 10.9 per cent of the total according to Rasmussen.[386] Severinghaus[425] has maintained that acidophilic cells are concentrated centrally, basophiles peripherally and that chromophobes are distributed diffusely throughout the anterior pituitary gland. Giroud and Desclaux[199] agree only that the chromophobes are dispersed throughout the anterior lobe. Precisely how the population of granulated cells is maintained and physiologic as well as pathologic fluctuations in their relative numbers effected, is still in dispute.

Growth pattern and relative hormonal potency of normal pituitary gland.

Rasmussen, in 1947,[388] published a careful analysis of the growth pattern of the human pituitary gland from birth to the nineteenth year. He noted that the growth curve of the whole gland is a straight line function with age during this period, the female tending to outstrip the male during the teens. The greatest growth increment is contributed by the anterior lobe in all instances. In this regard it is pertinent to recall that in our series of 14 patients with chromophobe adenomas manifested before the age of 26, 9 were in females (see fig. 26).

The weight of the human pituitary gland does not continue to increase with age in a linear fashion. The reviews of Berblinger,[43] Simmonds[437] and Erdheim and Stumme[145] all indicate a peak weight for the human male pituitary gland during the interval 31 to 40 years. Agreement is not uniform for the female. Simmonds'[437] data indicate the peak during the interval 41 to 50 years. Berblinger[43] shows a peak during the 31 to 40 year interval and Erdheim and Stumme,[145] at approximately the fiftieth year in nullipara. The last authors describe gradually and irregularly increasing pituitary weight to the age of 70 years in the married women. They suggest that this reflects the influence of intercurrent pregnancies.

In figure 26 we see peaks which are probably significant of tumor incidence in the male somewhat before the 31 to 35 year interval, and somewhat before the 41 to 45 year interval. In the female there is a significant peak somewhat before the 41 to 45 year interval. The actual peaks in that figure reflect the age of appearance of significant symptoms, not the onset of the tumor.

Lawson and his co-workers[297] reported in 1939 that the gonadotrophin potency of the normal female rat pituitary gland rises to a peak shortly after birth, then decreases gradually until the onset of sexual maturity, when there is a rapid drop. Low prematurity levels are then maintained throughout the period of normal sexual life despite increasing pituitary size. Their limited study of senile rat pituitaries suggested a marked increase in potency coincident with ovarian failure. A similar study in both male and female rabbits by Bergman and Turner in 1942[44] indicates one peak of potency of total gland gonadotrophin in the female, two in the male (one occurring before the female peak, the other at the same relative time). In terms of gonadotrophic potency per gram of gland, they observed a rather uniform gonadotrophin concentration during the entire reproductive life of the female rabbit following the prepuberal rise. They observed a notable decline at the climacteric. In similar units the male gland showed a slow rise to peak concentration, and then a gradual fall.

When the age incidence of pituitary tumors in our series is evaluated in the light of these known facts about the normal growth potential and hormonal content of the pituitary gland, it appears likely that the chromophobe adenoma is, in truth, a manifestation of normal growth potential, at least at its onset.

The influence of age on normal growth patterns and cellular population.

Rasmussen in 1929[386] reported a significant increase of chromophobe cells and a concomitant decrease of acidophils in individuals over 50 years of age. This observation has been confirmed in man[525] as well as in rats.[343, 524, 525] In rats, at least,[525] the recorded alterations in cellular population are almost completed by the twelfth month of life, where the maximal expected life span of the animal approximates 28 months.

Spontaneous chromophobe adenoma-like lesions occur quite commonly in rats over 12 months of age,[409, 525, 526] although sexual preponderance varies widely with the strain studied. In the human Löwenstein[321] observed small asymptomatic pituitary adenomas in 5 of 9 persons over the age of 37.

Influence of hormonal and metabolic factors on anterior pituitary gland

Cushing, in 1912,[100] suggested that the physiologic epochs of life, that is adolescence and puberty, pregnancy, and the climacterium— bore some ill-defined relationship to pituitary tumors. Dott and Bailey[131] later urged a more specific relationship. They noted that a large number of tumors of chromophobe type were manifest in females shortly after pregnancy or the menopause and were inclined to the view that the physiologic disturbances which these events induce may act as a predisposing factor to adenomatous hyperplasia.

There can be no question that pregnancy, as a physiologic phenomenon in the female, is associated with pituitary changes reminiscent of those noted in chromophobe or transitional adenomas. The classic studies of Erdheim and Stumme,[145] amply confirmed,[38, 43, 46] have shown not only a striking gross enlargement of the human pituitary gland, particularly during the last trimester, but also an increasing total growth increment with each subsequent pregnancy, the changes involving only the anterior lobe. Moreover, the so-called pregnancy cells which contribute in largest measure to the increase in size, are either somewhat atypical chromophobe cells or, as Benda[38] and Severinghaus[425] have been tempted to think, transitional or extremely active acidophils. Erdheim and Stumme[145] noted frank adenomas or adenomatous hyperplasia in approximately 10 per cent of all pregnancy hypophyses studied.

That pregnancy is not a necessary condition for the development of this tumor need scarcely be mentioned. Wolfe,[525] for example, described spontaneous adenomatous changes in 27.8 per cent of old virgin rats and in 29 per cent of old rats previously pregnant. Pregnancy, nonetheless, displays to a striking degree the alterations which are induced in the anterior pituitary gland by or in the presence of an altered endocrine milieu in which placental estrogens probably play a prominent part.

Changes associated with other physiologic epochs[180] or rhythms[205] in a wide variety of experimental animals, are minimal or transient. Reported alterations in cell type or relative numbers associated with significantly decreased thyroid[292, 425] or adrenal[98, 355, 391] function produce little or no enlargement of the pituitary gland, even though both favor a relative increase of chromophobe cells. There is no agreement concerning the nature of induced castration changes[292, 425] in the human menopause.

Experimental production of pituitary tumors

It is now generally accepted that the long continued administration of estrogenic substances may produce enlargement of the pituitary gland, in many instances with formation of large chromophobe adenoma-like lesions in experimental animals[423, 425, 503] as well as in man.[422] Severinghaus[425] has reported that the gonadotrophic potency of such tumorous lesions is markedly decreased. He suggests that estrogenic substance exhausts rather than inhibits pituitary gonadotrophin. That androgens[416, 421, 524] not only produce an opposite effect but may actively inhibit the development of spontaneous pituitary hyperplasia[524] and adenoma formation by estrogens[423] is likewise reasonably well established.

Estrogen-induced tumors differ in several respects from spontaneously occurring chromophobe adenomas of humans. Mitotic figures are extremely common in induced tumors and are equally rare in spontaneous human tumors. However, they are not uncommon in the spontaneous senile adenoma-like lesions of the rat, an experimental animal frequently employed for the production of tumors by estrogens.

Further, the rat tumors induced by alpha estradiol are, according to Selye,[423] associated with both an enlargement of the adrenal cortex and a tendency to a diabetic glucose tolerance. Selye suggested that such tumors may produce adrenotrophic, mammotrophic, lactogenic and possibly diabetogenic factors. Inhibition of somatic growth and atrophy of the thyroid gland and gonads were associated with these tumors. Selye has attributed the adrenal changes to the action of the estrogens on the adenohypophysis but has not eliminated their possible direct influence on the adrenals. In a study of the adult female mouse after prolonged daily injections of testosterone propionate he had previously reported[421] the development of adrenal cortical atrophy with decrease in pituitary weight but no evidence of chromophile degranulation.

Hypothetic scheme for pathogenesis of chromophobe adenomas

It is suggested that a chromophobe adenoma is usually a matured manifestation of inordinately stimulated but normal anterior pituitary growth potential. The precise nature of the stimulant is unknown. Mounting evidence indicates that the initial stimulant is provided by estrogenic substance which is either not normally metabolized or exists in an amount disproportionate to host androgenic substance. Since the male as well as the female produce both estrogens and androgens, the nature and extent of the imbalance or disproportion will be characteristic for the sex as well as for the individual.

X

THERAPY

The attitude toward therapy is best described by Oliver Wendell Holmes's aphorism, "To live is to function." For patients with chromophobe adenoma this means the prevention of irreversible impairment to neural structures. Hormonal substitution may counterbalance deficiencies in hypophyseal secretions but there are no means available for restoring destroyed nervous tissue. The functioning brain stands between one who survives to his own and society's satisfaction and the fumbling incompetent so pathetically insecure in many phases of perception, cogitation and movement.

The program of treatment is shaped about the following principles:

1. Adequate estimation of the extent of the nervous and metabolic defects.

2. Substitution therapy for maintenance as well as for critical periods of the illness.

3. The use of intensive radiotherapy to attain definite goals within a relatively determined time.

4. The use of surgery whenever radiotherapy fails (in terms of the criteria described below) or for certain urgent situations.

5. Effective psychologic and social measures for readjustment of the patient.

The criteria of the effectiveness of therapy are as follows:

Group I: (1) Visual acuity 20/50, 20/100 or better, satisfactory visual fields. (2) No evidence of impaired motor power or coordination. (3) No obvious psychologic defects arising directly from the illness. (4) Treated or untreated remedial endocrinal deficits other than hypoadrenalism. (5) Satisfactorily treated hypoadrenalism. (6) No extraocular muscle defects, or of minor extent if present. (7) No persistence of significant symptoms. (8) Return of individual to former social and economic status.

Group II: (1) Visual acuity with minimum of 20/50, 20/200, with satisfactory fields. (2) An intermediate degree of the criteria covered in Group I above, and Group III below.

Group III: (1) Visual acuity worse than 20/50, 20/200, with or without satisfactory fields. (2) Motor impairment. (3) Uncontrolled seizures. (4) Related psychical defects. (5) Incapacitating untreated endocrinal deficits. (6) Untreated hypoadrenalism. (7) Disabling extraocular muscle difficulties. (8) Major subjective symptoms. (9) Total disability or death.

These criteria were used to categorize the patients both prior to and following therapy. As in other comparative reports, changes in visual symptoms which can be estimated quantitatively with facility, are preeminent in appraising the results of treatment. Nevertheless, neurologic and metabolic evaluations were given significant weight in the estimation of the influence of treatment on the course of a patient's illness.

The goal of treatment is reached when the patient can be maintained in the first group throughout the period of management, which in effect should be co-extensive with his life span. In a general way, the limitations of the type of therapies employed influence what may be expected from treatment. Both radiotherapy and surgery are palliative and restrictive rather than curative. The tumor can be decreased in size and rate of growth, but never completely removed. Since most chromophobe adenomas are slowly growing neoplasms these incomplete measures usually are adequate.

In the present series 110 patients were sufficiently well observed before and after treatment for inclusion in this discussion of therapies. The majority of patients in the treatment series were studied for at least four years. About 5 per cent were followed for one to one and a half years. These latter cases usually had unfavorable therapeutic results.

The initial status of the patient was estimated by the same criteria as for final appraisal and the groupings I to III are identical. Independent of the nature of the therapy employed the results were conditioned by the status of the patient on admission.

TABLE 20—*Influence of Pretreatment Status on Therapeutic Results**

Pretreatment Status		Post-treatment Status		
	GROUPS	I (50)	II (17)	III (39)
	I (34)	26	2	6
	II (49)	23	12	14
	III (23)	1	3	19

* Figures in parentheses represent total number of patients in each group.

A preponderence of cases with large tumors was found in Group III, indicating a trend toward less favorable therapeutic results in cases with large chromophobe adenomas. Tumor size however, is not invariably a dominant influence in the outcome.

TABLE 21—*Tumor Size and Post-treatment Status*

Tumor Size		Post-treatment Status		
		I	II	III
	Small	13	2	2
	Moderate	25	7	8
	Large	14	7	30

RADIOTHERAPY

Although the administration of roentgen therapy was technically similar in most instances, the total amounts varied widely over the course of years as improved methods and schedules were adopted. In the majority of cases the following method of radiotherapy, as described by Dyke,[136] was employed:

Both temporal regions and the forehead are irradiated. The diameter of the portals for the temporal areas is 8 to 10 cm., while the forehead portal measures 6 cm. in diameter and is located just above the nasion. The treatments are given usually on alternating days and only occasionally every day. The amount of each treatment varies somewhat as we have used two techniques. . . . In the one technique 400 r (measured in air without back scattering) was given on alternate days to the three portals. Each area treated received two doses, (800 r) of roentgen rays, a total of six treatments being given in such a series. In the other technique, 200 r (measured in air without back scattering) was applied on alternate days, until each region received 800 r, forming a series of twelve treatments. The physical factors employed are: 200 kilovolts; 0.5 mm. copper plus 1 mm. aluminum filter; 20 inch (50.8 cm.) distance; 8 milliamperes; 40 minutes equals 800 roentgens (international roentgens). This usually results in epilation after about two weeks. The patient receives a rest of five or six weeks after which the series is repeated. If possible, at least three or more such series are given in every case.

At the present time Dr. E. Wood has augmented the amount of radiotherapy administered. In a similar period of time about 3000 r tumor doses are given instead of 2400 r measured in air. Very few of the patients included in this series received this degree of radiotherapy but some 25 patients observed subsequent to this report were treated in this manner. A summary of the results of the treatment follows:

Group I: Thirty-six of the 52 patients in this category were treated solely by x-ray. In these cases the average dosage administered was 2730 r. It was most common for each course of x-ray to consist of an initial 2400 r and, within two months, an additional 2400 r. Further therapy occurred within the same year but may have been extended over the following two or three years. Since there were many divergences from the schedule pattern suggested above, no final circumscribing statement can be made with regard to dosage per year or duration of the interval prior to treatment subsequent to the first two courses. There were 13 failures with x-ray alone, but surgery was successfully accomplished in these cases. Three cases in Group I were operated upon directly, without prior radiotherapy.

The first change in the patient's status usually was recorded in the visual sphere, but neurologic improvement was also observed as a primary occurrence. The first indication of a successful outcome was noted in about one-half of the group by the time 1700 r had been administered (1680 r median, 1710 r average). The remainder appeared to have a more delayed response, the first change occurring at about 3000 r. The distribution of the cases in which the initial change was recorded is shown in table 22.

Group II: The tenor of the findings here is consistent with those of the former category. Eleven patients responded to x-ray without additional therapy. Five required surgery. One was operated upon directly. The average total r administered to the nonoperative cases was 4900 r. It is difficult to assess the importance of this lower x-ray dosage in relation to the results. More striking is the observation that, in those instances where x-ray was used to control the expansion of the tumor, initial improvement was again noted in the vicinity

TABLE 22—*The Number of r Administered to the Time of Beneficial Change*

r administered at time of change	No. of cases*		
	Group I	Group II	Totals
0–400	2		2
500–900	5		5
1000–1400	4	4	8
1500–1900	3	2	5
2000–2400		3	3
2500–2900	9	1	10
3000–3400	1		1
4500–4900	1		1
			35

* Cases from Groups I and II are included in this table. Beneficial changes are noted in a significant number of cases in Group I with the administration of 1700 r or less. In Group II the cases are distributed about a dosage of from 1000 to 3000 r.

of 1750 r on the average, with a range of from 1000–3000 r (table 22). However, there was one patient who, after initial response to 250 r, relapsed and required surgery.

Group III: There were several factors of a general nature which contributed to the failure of therapy in this group. Larger tumors predominated and a longer time elapsed prior to investigation of these patients. In addition, the initial status of the patients was less favorable. It is not possible to distinguish the effects of total irradiation given to these patients since, in most cases, there was an overlap between surgical and radiologic treatments. However, 30 patients received x-ray, before as well as after surgery. The total dosage averaged 6300 r, an amount comparable to that noted in Group I. There was no instance of a significant response to radiotherapy, either within the first 2400 r, or during the entire period of irradiation. Aside from the other influences adversely affecting the outcome in these patients, the chief determinant was the fact that the tumors of this group appeared to be radioresistant. A striking finding was the 30 per cent incidence of cystic tumors (confirmed by the neuropathologist). There were only 2 known cystic tumors in Groups I and II. However, 32 cases were operated upon in Group III and only 20 in Groups I and II, thus biasing the statistics. Unfortunately, analysis of the cases with cystic tumors does not indicate any way in which they may be anticipated prior to the institution of therapy, although their presence may be suspected in radioresistant tumors.

Discussion of Radiotherapy

The data presented here do not provide sufficient information as to the optimal mode and amount of radiotherapy. However, in combination with reports in the literature, and from the results of recent cases not included here, several tentative conclusions can be reached. The trend in therapy has been to increase the amount of total roentgen units to three or four thousand tumor doses. This is about 15 per cent more than the total dosage received by patients of Group I. X-ray treatments may be administered in single or multiple courses. Kerr[280] has stressed the effectiveness of a single course and showed that indications are if there is not improvement with this dosage extended over thirty to forty-five days, surgery should be considered. Relapses following initial radiotherapy occur in about 15 per cent in most series, including the present one.[19, 280] These cases appear to respond well to a second course of x-ray. Most observers believe that the efficacy of treatment can be prognosticated on the basis of the regression of symptoms that may result from the first course of radiotherapy.

Evans and Picciotto[153] confirm the opinion that improvement is usually noted by the fourth week of treatment. Our findings suggest that the prognosis may be surmised occasionally at an even earlier stage. If no improvement is observed, after two series of 2400 r administered in the manner described above or under more intensive conditions the tumor should not be expected to respond to further x-ray. If there is an urgent decision with regard to the management of the patient some time after the first 2400 r, the results of the first course may be considered an adequate indication of the radiosensitivity of the tumor.

It may be noted that in this series patients unresponsive to x-ray in all three groups were exposed to a dosage similar to other members of their group. In the 13 cases unresponsive to x-ray in Group I, regression of symptoms did not occur during the first course of x-ray, and of the 5 in Group II, only 1 showed transient improvement with irradiation. The statistics of others with regard to the results of radiotherapy are better than those described here but their criteria of improvement are evidently different.

Bachman[19] reports improvement in 58 per cent and Kerr[280] in 70 per cent of patients treated with x-ray. In our series 45 per cent obtained satisfactory results. Our data and conclusions drawn from them are in agreement with the current views of radiotherapists analyzing the problem with their special knowledge and judgment. There is some reluctance on the part of the English school[276] and Professor Olivecrona[20] to accept radiotherapy as a desirable primary measure; they express more confidence in surgical therapy.

The complications consequent to radiotherapy are in themselves negligible. For the systematically appraised patient x-ray treatments are without danger. Occasionally an irradiated tumor may produce a temporary increase in symptomatology because of radiation edema. During this phase, the radiotherapist is obliged to diminish the amount of roentgens administered at each exposure until this process reverses. However, a patient with hypoadrenalism may be further embarrassed during this period of stress, unless suitable measures are taken to maintain blood volume, electrolyte balance and adrenocorticoid output. We found no evidence that x-ray therapy prior to surgery increases perisellar meningeal adhesions, vascularity or friability of tissues, thereby adding to the difficulty of operation.

SURGICAL THERAPY

During the years from which this report is drawn surgery was employed as a secondary therapeutic measure. Relatively urgent cases and those in which irradiation had failed were treated surgically.

Under these conditions the present surgical results cannot give a clear picture of the efficacy of this form of therapy in the early stages of illness. Over the course of the years surgical technics were modified. However, either an intradural or extradural approach to the tumors through the transfrontal route was employed. Whether partial extirpation or intracapsular enucleation was attempted depended on the complexity of the case and the inclination of the surgeon. It is important to realize that probably in no case can a chromophobe adenoma be completely removed without doing irreversible damage to the residual pituitary body itself.

In general, patients who delayed their initial examination, those with large tumors and those with poor initial status had a less fortunate outcome. Using the criteria described in the section on radiotherapy, the results of surgery are summarized in table 23.

TABLE 23—*Results of Surgical Therapy**

Pretreatment Status	Post-treatment Status		
GROUPS	I (16)	II (6)	III (32)
I (15)	10	1	4
II (22)	5	3	14
III (17)	1	2	14

* Figures in parentheses represent total number of patients in each group.

In only one instance was surgery performed in the absence of a notable extrasellar extension. The tumor was usually large, occasionally moderate in size and involved contiguous structures. Viewed in this light the results of surgery are quite satisfactory. Operative results are comparable to those with irradiation. Forty per cent of the patients were treated successfully by surgery as compared to 45 per cent by x-ray. The complications noted in the series of 54 operated cases were: clot formations, transient edema of the retracted frontal lobe, infarction of the brain as a result of occlusion of a compressed vessel, immediate postoperative seizures, hypothalamic damage and further interference with function of the optic nerve. The mortality rate was 24 per cent, or 13 cases of the operated series. At first glance this may appear unprecedentedly high. However, all the patients who died had large tumors with extensive hypothalamic encroachment. Corresponding statistics of Jefferson[273] and Olivecrona[20] for this type of case are 33 per cent and 35 per cent respectively. In 7 of the fatal cases, post-operative symptoms of vasomotor shock, hyperpyrexia, sleepiness and diabetes insipidus were found. Aside from its typical features, terminal and fatal hypoadrenalism may manifest similar symptomatology, notably shock and hyperpyrexia. These symptoms were seen in 3 cases and could be ascribed to hypoadrenal crisis. In 1 case, accidental perforation of the internal carotid which was encircled by the tumor led to death. The remaining 2 patients died of postoperative complications related to the stress of operation.

In addition to the mortality consequent to surgery, 3 other patients died; 1 of septic meningitis subsequent to erosion of a sphenoid sinus, 1 following spread of a malignant chromophobe adenoma to involve the structures of the posterior fossa and 1 following sudden intracranial hemorrhage from a nasal extension of an adenoma. In the latter instance the patient had made an excellent postoperative recovery four years earlier.

Recurrences were found solely in patients who were classified eventually in Group III. Since a mixture of radiologic and surgical therapies was given to these patients, it was not possible to designate them as specific failures of one or another type treatment. The recurrence rate was 9 per cent. It is interesting that 2 patients had tumors which were solid adenomas at first, but, following unsuccessful radiotherapy and surgery the neoplasms appeared cystic as observed at the time of their second operation.

Of the several surgical reports,[20, 114, 239, 273] that of Cushing and Henderson remains the most complete, and some comparisons with it can be made. Of the 93 patients who had intracranial operations in their series, 5 died, 4 immediately and 1 after a recurrence of the tumor. There were 3 additional cases with intracranial extensions which terminated fatally within two weeks, a period that may be considered postoperative. Including the latter cases, the overall mortality rate rises from 4.5 per cent to 8.6 per cent in Cushing's series.

This is not to detract from the excellence of his results but rather to place his statistics on a base comparable to ours.

In our series there were, as noted, 13 postoperative deaths, an overall mortality of 11.8 per cent for the entire series. Within a five year period there were 3 additional deaths bringing the long term mortality rate to 14 per cent. It is difficult to distinguish the equivalent data in Cushing's series, since the results of intracranial operations are not always differentiated from those of transphenoidal. Recurrence rates in the Cushing-Henderson series are similar to ours. They indicate that x-ray in addition to operation decreases the incidence of symptomatic neoplastic regrowth from 35 per cent to 13 per cent, in the group operated on through the transfrontal route. Though not directly pertinent, it may be added that in cases operated on by the transphenoidal route, supplementary x-ray decreased the recurrence rate from 68 per cent to 43 per cent. There are probably accessory explanations, such as improvement of technic, size of tumor, and so forth which may influence the degree, although not the direction, of change induced by irradiation. Finally, comparison of the early results of transfrontal operations may be made. The criteria advanced by Henderson are somewhat less detailed than ours but it is probable that analogies can be made safely. If we consider his patients classified as "very good," "good" and "satisfactory," to be equivalent to Groups I and II, the results are satisfactory in 65 per cent. In our series 60 per cent of these patients responded similarly.

The purpose of this comparsion is to offer a guide to the type of treatment the patient may be advised to accept. It is obvious that the results of Cushing and Henderson depend more on the efficacy of surgical therapy than radiotherapy. This is quite the reverse of our series. A comparison of the two series indicates an overall mortality of 8.6 per cent in Cushing's series and 14.0 per cent in our own. Aside from this the final results are similar. Does this lead to the general advocacy of surgery as a first recourse in management? Following are several arguments contrary to this view.

Recent articles on radiotherapy of chromophobe adenoma indicate that with higher dosage the incidence and degree of improvement has increased. Many of our cases were treated in the early and middle periods of x-ray therapy of pituitary tumors and received what is considered now an inadequate amount. Yet this form of treatment was quite satisfactory in 45 per cent of all the cases where attempted.

Cushing's statistics indicate the effectiveness of irradiation in preventing recurrences. Moreover, the rate of recurrence in his non-irradiated cases was 35 per cent, as compared to 9 per cent in the present series in which x-ray was combined with surgery. The decline of recurrence rate in the Cushing series from 35 to 13 per cent following the utilization of irradiation is in complete harmony with the previous statement. Without proceeding further, these data establish the usefulness of x-ray in limiting regrowths and point to the radiosensitivity of many tumors upon which Dr. Cushing operated.

It is mainly the mortality rate (presented as 4.5 per cent by Henderson, said to decrease below 3 per cent for the later cases and raised for comparative reasons by ourselves to 8.6 per cent) that attracts the observer. There are some qualifications that may be made at this time. The majority of neurosurgeons do not have the range of experience and concentrated opportunity to treat the number of adenomas that Professor Cushing did. Assuming similar skill and judgment, the factors of experience and perhaps other intangibles favor Cushing over other neurosurgeons. This is borne out by the mortality and recovery statistics of other groups. It is striking to note the quantitative similarities in the results of the chief surgeons of several groups.[20, 114, 273]

Sparing 50 of 100 patients, the risks of operation may not influence the mortality rate of the remaining 50, but it will diminish the total number of patients who succumb to operation, all else being equal.

It is possible to estimate quite early in the course of radiotherapy whether or not it will be effective. Time lost in this trial period does not affect the final operative results of nonurgent cases.

There are other arguments that may be adduced but it is believed that these are sufficiently persuasive to permit the presentation of a plan of therapy which does not include routine surgery.

PLAN OF THERAPY

The type of onset, the extent of visual loss and the degree of extra-sellar involvement are guides in the choice of the initial therapy. Acutely developing visual and neurologic symptoms suggest that one of several events has occurred. Hemorrhage into the tumor, with the possibility of extravasation beyond the pituitary, or edema of the tumor may account for acute compression of optic nerves and contiguous neural structure. The sudden expression of the contents of a ruptured cyst may produce a perineural inflammatory reaction about the optic nerves and also lead to meningismus. Finally, the subacute development of a bacterial meningitis may herald the expansion of an adenoma into neighboring nasal sinuses. If, in these instances, the neurologic symptoms are marked and indicate hypothalamic compression or evident involvement of the frontal, temporal, peduncular or cavernous sinus areas, the adenoma is probably compromising the particular region fairly extensively. Moderate and slowly progressive invasion within these areas is frequently asymptomatic or just barely apparent. To avoid irreversible changes as a result of sudden pressure by the tumor, surgery is advised despite the fact that the mortality in this group is higher than average.

If, in addition, vision is affected beyond 20/50, 20/100 and the visual fields are unsatisfactory, the indications for operation are even more demanding. Surgery may afford immediate relief, whereas x-ray at best certainly requires three to four weeks for appreciable improvement and perhaps a significant fraction of this time for the actual relief of pressure on neural tissue. Acutely developing lesions do not permit adjustments to occur by means of displacement of the structures and circulatory accommodation. Usually delay is interdicted. Of the several possibilities, hemorrhage, edema, rupture of a cyst and intra-sinus extension, it is the first three that more commonly present the acutely developing picture of visual and neurologic disability. Since it is difficult to distinguish between them, the fact that radiotherapy is ineffective in the cystic cases is further support for surgical intervention. It is true that the changes due to cystic rupture may be transitory and may subside spontaneously. Moreover, the possible collapse of the wall of the cyst may afford natural decompression. In this event neurologic symptoms become less marked and following the defervescence of inflammation, visual difficulties may diminish. It is not possible to predict this state. In addition, since cystic tumors are radioresistant, operation may be anticipated at a future time. Extension of the tumor into the sinuses with consequent meningitis, usually is unaccompanied by signs of parenchymatous neural involvement. The cerebrospinal fluid findings as well as x-ray studies lead to the correct diagnosis. In the presence of infection, surgery should be withheld and antibacterial drugs and radiotherapy instituted.

It is impossible to grade formally the degree and type of involvement one may see in these acute cases. However, in those sudden forms presenting with minimum neurologic signs and moderate nonprogressive visual states (which remain better than 20/50, 20/100 with satisfactorily extensive fields), radiotherapy is a possible alternative to surgery. Repeated daily examination of the patient during the course of irradiation indicates the effectiveness of treatment. Progressive involvement or the lack of improvement within four weeks suggest that surgery is necessary.

By far the greater number of patients exhibits a history of chronic unremitting progression of symptoms. A sense of urgency need not influence the decision of the choice of treatment. All those whose initial status justifies their inclusion in Groups I and II should receive radiotherapy accompanied by the usual precaution of daily general and visual examinations. It is to be hoped that improvement will be noted in these groups during and following the first course of irradiation. The condition of these patients is, in the main, functionally satisfactory. If this state is maintained subsequent to x-ray treatment and during the immediate follow-up period, the first therapeutic goal may be considered attained. In those border-line cases of the lower fourth of Group II where the adequacy of the patients is marginal, either re-irradiation or surgery may be contemplated, if no improvement occurs after three to four thousand roentgens. Our view is that improvement with roentgen therapy is seen within four to six weeks and little is to be expected if diminution in pathologic signs is not apparent by this time. Surgery is then advised.

The cases of Group III present a problem in treatment. If the antecedent history is over six months, it is probable that the delay of one month during which radiotherapy is attempted will not affect the outcome adversely. If no progress is made during the month of radiotherapy and one additional month thereafter, surgery must be resorted to. Those cases with a shorter latency period may tentatively be tried on irradiation, but there is more substance to the argument that immediate surgical relief of pressure may prevent chronic changes from becoming established. In any event, should the patient of Group III or the lower fourth of Group II fail to respond to the first course of irradiation, it would appear that operation is preferred. In this situation, as in all others, no definitive statements as to the mode of therapy may be made.

All patients must be checked periodically within intervals of three months. Those patients whose initial response to radiotherapy is satisfactory but who relapse may receive an additional course of irradiation. This type of patient usually responds to the second course with improvement. If no improvement then occurs the patient should be treated surgically.

On the basis of the analysis of our cases and of a survey of the relevant literature, the administration of larger amounts of roentgens, up to three to four thousand (tumor dose), appears to be most effective. Whether the single or multiple course is preferable cannot be decided by us, nor have expert radiologists shown complete accord in this regard.

The surgical technics employed at present are beyond the critical scope of this review. The transfrontal route has become generally adopted and only in selective cases is the nasal approach worthy of trial.

Although both surgery and radiologic treatments have been discussed without reference to supplemental hormonal therapy the following discussion will indicate the importance attached to this form of treatment. Both irradiation and surgery are imposing loads to place upon a patient with variable pituitary insufficiency. It is necessary in the first examination to determine the extent of endocrinopathy.

MEDICAL THERAPY OF ENDOCRINE AND
METABOLIC DISTURBANCES

The individual with a chromophobe adenoma of the pituitary gland is the therapeutic paradox, par excellence. Untreated, he is one who maintains a positive nitrogen balance at the expense of regularly needed glycogen stores. When presented with a superabundance of exogenous glucose he shows a lessened rather than increased ability to draw on it in metabolic need. He tends to direct this glucose preferentially into tissue fat stores even though his liver be depleted. He stores in the face of need. In general, his untreated trend is consistently in the direction of negative overall water balance. A regime (posterior pituitary preparation) intended to correct this rarely conspicuous disturbance may also dangerously dilute serum electrolytes. Therapeutic maintenance of normal serum electrolytes, by contrast, occasionally may tend to shift the fluid balance even more toward the negative side by charging the extracellular compartment. Further, the patient with a chromophobe adenoma is one whose renal tubules may fail to reabsorb what he needs, yet conserve what he cannot use. The female patient will usually manifest hypogonadism, yet specific endocrine therapy intended to substitute for lost function may augment or aggravate tumor growth and increase local tumor symptoms. In conclusion, the patient with a chromophobe adenoma is one whose untreated physical machine is driven along at a precariously modulated subnormal metabolic pace. It is not, therefore, unfitting that therapeutic measures intended to alter that pace should claim our first attention since herein resides an important clue to successful and conservative therapy.

Observations and recommendations

Perhaps greatest hazard attends the use of thyroid products in patients with chromophobe adenomas. Most available preparations are potent in low dosage and routine studies will reveal theoretical indications for such therapy in a majority of patients. Although the precipitation of adrenal crises by thyroid substance, as reported in a few recent studies[71, 302, 343] is a complication to be anticipated, it is nonetheless uncommon.[249a] Thyroid extract, in small but increasing doses, was administered to one young woman of this series who, on a previous admission, had shown a conspicuously positive response to salt deprivation and, in the interim, had had an episode of mild adrenal insufficiency precipitated by excessive perspiration and transient gastroenteritis. A total of 0.33 Gm. of thyroid extract was administered in increasing divided doses over a ten day period. During this interval there was neither evident shift in extracellular fluids, alteration in serum electrolytes nor diuresis. However, the testimony of one case is scarcely reassuring.

Many patients with chromophobe adenomas are intolerant of thyroid preparations even in small doses and will terminate therapy on their own initiative because of disturbing subjective symptoms. The gains which might be made by urging such therapy do not justify the risk of continuing it. Certainly the use of thyroid preparations to elevate a subnormal BMR, which it will do quite effectively, is not often attended by gratifying relief of symptoms referred to such subnormal metabolism. Sluggishness, lassitude, easy fatigue, mental torpor, sensitivity to cold, dryness and scaling of the skin cannot be referred with consistency to secondary hypothyroidism alone, nor is relief of these symptoms impressive following thyroid administration. The argument that such preparations may, by enhancing intestinal absorption, combat fasting hypoglycemia with its attendant weakness and nervousness, has neither clinical nor experimental foundation. What good evidence is available would indicate that thyroid preparations may actually accentuate fasting hypoglycemia because of their stimulation of cellular metabolic processes.

Treatment of secondary hypothyroidism by thyrotrophin is theoretically attractive. Until preparations of uniform efficiency,[427] free of specific antigenic agents[18, 426, 507] are readily available and inexpensive, it will not be a practical reality. Thyroid extract or thyroxin, if used at all, should be administered under close supervision and then only to those where complete endocrine inventory is a matter of recent record. It is, of course, possible to give thyroid preparations successfully in the presence of known secondary hypoadrenalism,[517] but

symptomatic improvement may be accomplished as effectively by
other endocrine products such as testosterone derivatives.

Disturbances in gonadal function are far more conspicuous,
symptomatically, than those related to hypothyroidism since the majority of such tumors develop during the sexually active years. Potent
gonadotrophic substances of pituitary as well as extrapituitary origin
have been available for many years[142, 429] and may occasionally induce
periodic uterine bleeding in previously amenorrheic patients. The
occurrence of cyst formation in the pituitary gland after prolonged
injections of anterior pituitary preparations in animals[426] suggests the
possibility of such a complication in the tumor patient so treated.

Both natural and synthetic estrogenic substances are, in our
opinion, contraindicated in patients with chromophobe adenomas
(see section on pathogenesis). On the other hand, testosterone derivatives have a secure place in the therapeutic armamentarium. They are
more effective than any other single acceptable agent in establishing a
sense of well-being, in combating mild fatigue and lassitude and in
reapplying the veneer of active sexual life in the male. Only in high
and regular doses are they to be considered as potentially dangerous.[421]
In the human adult female patient the theoretical possibility of inhibiting gonadotrophic production from a functional pituitary remnant by gonadal preparations[295] is questioned. The tendency of testosterone preparations to induce epiphyseal closure or to accelerate that
process is matter of little importance except in the rare adolescent or
young adult patient with epiphyses still open. Overdosage with testosterone may decrease spermatogeneses and its schedule of administration
should include periods of abstention.

Selye's recent review of tumorigenic factors[423] contains the interesting observation that cistestosterone, the hormonally inactive isomer
of testosterone, is extremely effective in inhibiting the experimental
production of chromophobe adenoma-like lesions by alpha estradiol
(the acetate and propionate derivatives being even more effective).
While, as he stresses, there are many facts to warn against drawing
too close a parallel between the pituitary tumors induced by estrogens
and those occurring in man, there seems to be no clear-cut contraindica-

tion to a clinical trial of derivatives of cistestosterone under appropriately controlled conditions.

Williams and his associates,[518] among others, have noted a doca-like effect of testosterone preparations in both primary and secondary adrenal insufficiency, but this should not be overestimated. It is quite clear that none of the known sex hormones, per se, can effectively maintain the human in adrenal insufficiency. Thorn and Engel considered progesterone as a possible exception on the basis of experimental observations.[478] Clinical experience with progesterone has not, however, justified such exception.

The therapy of secondary hypoadrenalism is of maintenance and crisis types. The use of doca during crises is well established on clinical and experimental[477, 479] grounds. Cortisone has recently assumed a dominant role[366a, 531a] in the treatment of secondary adrenal insufficiency and its usefulness is particularly apparent in crisis.

The full therapeutic regime to be followed during crises is precisely that for primary Addisonian crisis, and is discussed in detail by Loeb[313, 314] and Thorn.[475a] Following subsidence of crisis, the patient with secondary hypoadrenalism usually tolerates a rapidly tapering therapeutic program. Doca can frequently be discontinued within a relatively brief period. A diet with moderate sodium supplement and reduced potassium is quite adequate in many instances. Doca itself may maintain normal or even supranormal plasma volumes[83] but serial studies in patients of our series would not justify consideration of doca as a maintenance medication except in rare instances. Because prolonged therapy with doca is so infrequently indicated, implantation of pellets is not advised even in those patients with severe episodic hypoadrenalism. The proper use of doca and of supplementary dietary salt are determined in each individual case. No set rule can be suggested.

The possibility of increasing adrenal cortical atrophy with doca[70] or, more remotely, of suppressing residual cortical function with adrenal cortical extract,[327] is of greater significance in these patients than in those with primary adrenal insufficiency. In many of the former there is sufficient functioning cortical tissue to maintain the individual in all except acutely traumatic crises. Thus, in general, doca should be used with more reservation in patients with secondary hypoadrenalism than in those with Addison's disease.

Though the scientific literature of the past several years is surfeited with reports on the actions and therapeutic applications of cortisone and ACTH, it is still premature to attempt an evaluation of these agents in the maintenance therapy of hypoadrenal states secondary to chromophobe adenoma. It is tempting to join the mass of enthusiastic students in metabolism who extoll the merits of such active and highly purified agents but rather sobering to discover that, from the patient's standpoint, life seemed quite as liveable with the help of small amounts of added salt and a regular tablet of methyltestosterone. There are, of course, a good number for whom such a simplified regime is wholly inadequate but an overenthusiastic (and frequently expensive) early resort to multi-replacement therapy may often deprive a large proportion of these patients of the simple and inexpensive aids which will carry them successfully and actively through years of productive living.

The Lahey Clinic group[531a] report gratifying results in maintaining a small group of patients with secondary hypoadrenalism on ACTH. Maintenance levels varied from 10 mg. every other day to 25 mg. daily. More recently oral cortisone has been used extensively and they report satisfactory control with daily dosage levels of approximately 25 mg. Cortisone has proved to be a highly satisfactory agent by others, as well,[366a] and undoubtedly deserves a secure place as a therapeutic tool in secondary hypoadrenalism.

Little is really known about the possible role of dietary therapy in hypopituitarism, except for salt supplements in secondary hypoadrenalism. It would be wise, however, to correct the popular misconception that a high carbohydrate diet is indicated or could be expected to correct either hypoglycemic tendencies or episodes. Studies previously reviewed indicate that hypophysectomized animals on a high carbohydrate diet have increased tolerance for carbohydrates, show increased fasting hypoglycemia and even greater insulin sensitivity. On theoretical grounds, a high fat, low carbohydrate diet would be desirable but such is neither practical nor acceptable to most patients.

It is evident that the medical management of the chronic nonemergency patient is a slowly derived, constantly evolving process based on careful clinical and laboratory evaluation and current response to instituted treatment. The patient who shows acute neurologic progression cannot be so treated. The majority of these will be operated on after a brief interval. The therapeutic regime should be designed to sustain the patient during surgical stress and should avoid the complication of cardiac failure resulting from overtreatment.

A successful preoperative program is as follows: (1) estimate plasma volume, serum electrolyte levels and cardiac status; (2) shift the equilibrium toward normal plasma volume and serum electrolytes by the use of doca and intravenous saline; (3) guard against the perilous maintenance of fluid and electrolyte balance at the expense of cardiac decompensation and pulmonary edema, by administering conservative and barely adequate medication, while estimating cardiac reserve during the process; and (4) institute cortisone therapy for its wide metabolic effects, and follow with maintenance doses of ACTH.

During operation, whole blood usually is administered under the same restrictions described in the third step above. The immediate and delayed postoperative management involves use of the same principles. Since the functional reserve of patients with secondary hypoadrenalism is greater than those with primary Addisonian deficiency, the magnitude of replacement therapy is less.

BIBLIOGRAPHY

1. ABELS, J. C., YOUNG, N. F. AND TAYLOR, H. C.: Effects of testosterone and of testosterone propionate on protein formation in man. J. Clin. Endocrinol. 1944, *4:* 198–201.
2. ABRAHAMSON, I. AND CLIMENKO, H.: A study of one hundred selected cases of pituitary disease. J.A.M.A. 1917, *69:* 281–282.
3. ADDISON, W. H. F.: The Golgi apparatus in the cells of the distal glandular portion of the hypophysis. Anat. Rec. 1916–17, *11:* 317–318.
4. ———: The cell-changes in the hypophysis of the albino rat, after castration. J. Comp. Neurol. 1917, *28:* 441–461.
5. Adrenal Cortex. Ann. New York Acad. Sc. 1949, *50:* 509–678.
6. Adrenal Cortex Conference. Josiah Macy Jr. Foundation, Caldwell, Progress Associates, 1950.
7. ADRIAN, E. D.: The Physical Background of Perception. Oxford, Clarendon Press, 1946.
8. ALLEN, E.: Physiology of the ovaries, in: Glandular Physiology and Therapy, a Symposium. Chicago, American Medical Association, 1942, pp. 143–167.
9. ALLEN, W. F.: Effects of ablating pyriform-amygdaloid areas and hippocampi on positive and negative olfactory conditioned reflexes and on conditioned olfactory differentiation. Am. J. Physiol. 1941, *132:* 81–92.
9a. ALMEIDA LIMA, P.: Cerebral Angiography. London, Oxford University Press, 1950, pp. 82–86.
10. ALPERS, B. J.: Personality and emotional disorders associated with hypothalamic lesions, in: The Hypothalamus. Research Publ. A. Nerv. & Ment. Dis. Baltimore, Williams & Wilkins, 1940, vol. 20, pp. 725–752.
11. ANDERS, J. M. AND JAMESON, H. L.: The relation of glycosuria to pituitary disease and a report of a case, with statistics. Tr. A. Am. Physicians 1914, *29:* 115–124.
12. ANDERSON, E., JOSEPH, M. AND HERRING, V.: Changes in excretion of radioactive Na and K, and in carbohydrate stores twenty-four hours following adrenalectomy. Proc. Soc. Exper. Biol. & Med. 1939, *42:* 782–785.
13. ANDERSON, E. M. AND LONG, J. A.: The hormonal influences on the secretion of insulin, in: Recent Progress in Hormone Research, New York, Academic Press, 1948, vol. 2, pp. 209–229.
14. ASCHNER, B.: Über die Funktion der Hypophyse. Pflüger's Arch. f. d. ges. Physiol. 1912, *146:* 1–146.

247

15. Astwood, E. B.: The regulation of corpus luteum function by hypophysial luteotrophin. Endocrinology 1941, *28:* 309–320.
16. ——:Mechanisms of action of various antithyroid compounds. Ann. New York Acad. Sc. 1949, *50:* 419–444.
17. Atwell, W. J.: The development of the hypophysis cerebri with special reference to the pars tuberalis. Am. J. Anat. 1926, *37:* 157–179.
18. Aub, J. C. and Karnofsky, D.: Medical progress: endocrinology: treatment of abnormalities of the anterior pituitary gland. New England J. Med. 1942, *226:* 759–768.
19. Bachman, A. L. and Harris, W.: Roentgen therapy for pituitary adenomas. Radiology 1949, *53:* 331–341.
20. Backay, L.: The results of 300 pituitary adenoma operations (Prof. Herbet Olivecrona's series). J. Neurosurg. 1950, *7:* 240–256.
21. Bailey, P.: Cytological observations on the pars buccalis of the hypophysis cerebri of man, normal and pathological. J. Med. Research 1921, *42:* 349–381.
22. ——:Tumors involving the hypothalamus and their clinical manifestations, in: The Hypothalamus. Research Publ. A. Nerv. & Ment. Dis., Baltimore, Williams & Wilkins, 1940, vol. 20, pp. 713–725.
23. —— and Bremer, F.: Experimental diabetes insipidus. Arch. Int. Med. 1921, *28:* 773–803.
24. —— and Cushing, H.: Studies in acromegaly. VII. The microscopical structures of the adenomas in acromegalic dyspituitarism (fugitive acromegaly). Am. J. Path. 1928, *4:* 545–564.
25. —— and Davidoff, L. M.: Concerning the microscopic structure of the hypophysis cerebri in acromegaly. (Based on a study of tissues removed at operation from 35 patients.) Am. J. Path. 1925, *1:* 185–208.
26. —— and Gibbs, F. A.: Surgical treatment of psychomotor epilepsy. J.A.M.A. 1951, *145:* 365–371.
27. Bailey, O. T. and Cutler, E. C.: Malignant adenomas of the chromophobe cells of the pituitary body. Arch. Path. 1940, *29:* 368–399.
28. Baird, P. C. Jr., Coloney, E. and Albright, F.: Effect of cortical hormone in preventing extreme drop in colonic temperature displayed by hypophysectomized rats upon exposure to cold with preliminary observations upon the effect of hypophyseal and other hormones. Am. J. Physiol. 1933, *104:* 489–501.
29. Baker, B. L.: A study of the parathyroid glands of the normal and hypophysectomized monkey (Macaca Mulatta). Anat. Rec. 1942, *83:* 47–73.
30. Barbour, H. G.: Hypothalamic control of water movement in response to environmental temperature, in: The Hypothalamus. Research Publ. A. Nerv. & Ment. Dis., Baltimore, Williams & Wilkins, 1940, vol. 20, pp. 449–486.
31. Bard, P.: The hypothalamus and sexual behavior, in: The Hypothalamus. Research Publ. A. Nerv. & Ment. Dis., Baltimore, Williams & Wilkins, 1940, vol. 20, pp. 551–580.
32. —— and Mountcastle, V. B.: Some forebrain mechanisms involved in expression of rage with special reference to suppression of angry behavior,

in: The Frontal Lobes. Research Publ. A. Nerv. & Ment. Dis., Baltimore, Williams & Wilkins, 1948, vol. 27, pp. 362–405.

33. BARKER, S. B.: Metabolic functions of the endocrine system. Ann. Rev. Physiol. 1949, *11:* 45–82.

34. BARNES, B. O., DIX, A. S. AND ROGOFF, J. M.: Effect of adrenalin on insulin sensitivity of partially adrenalectomized and of hypophysectomized dogs. Proc. Soc. Exper. Biol. & Med. 1934, *31:* 1145–1146.

35. BARTLETT, W., JR.: Effects upon blood amylase of variations in thyroid activity. Proc. Soc. Exper. Biol. & Med. 1937, *36:* 843–848.

36. BAUER, W. AND AUB, J. C.: Studies of calcium and phosphorus metabolism. XVI. The influence of the pituitary gland. J. Clin. Investigation 1941, *20:* 295–301.

37. BECK, H. G.: Hypophyseal disorders with special reference to Froelich's syndrome (dystrophia adiposogenitalis). Endocrinology 1920, *4:* 185–198.

38. BENDA, C.: Hypophysis cerebri, in Hirsch, M.: Handbuch der Inneren Sekretion. Leipzig, Verlag von Carl Kabitzsch, 1932, vol. 1, pp. 867–909.

39. BENNETT, H. S.: Localization of adrenal cortical hormones in the adrenal cortex of the cat. Proc. Soc. Exper. Biol. & Med. 1939, 42: 786–788.

40. BENNETT, L. L.: The interrelation of the pituitary and adrenal glands in the control of carbohydrate levels in the rat. Endocrinology 1938, *22:* 193–196.

41. —— AND EVANS, H. M.: The hypophysis and diabetes mellitus, in: The Hormones. New York, Academic Press, 1950, vol. 2, pp. 405–427.

42. —— AND LI, C. H.: The effects of the pituitary growth and adrenocorticotrophic hormones on the urinary glucose and nitrogen of diabetic rats. Am. J. Physiol. 1947, *150:* 400–404.

43. BERLINGER, W.: Pathologie und Pathologische Morphologie der Hypophyse des Menschen, in Hirsch, M.: Handbuch der Inneren Sekretion. Leipzig, Verlag von Carl Kabitzsch, 1932, vol. 1, pp. 910–1097.

44. BERGMAN, A. G. AND TURNER, C. W.: Gonadotropic hormone in the anterior pituitary of male and female rabbits during growth. Endocrinology 1942, *30:* 11–15.

45. BIEDL, A.: Die Wechselbeziehungen der Organe mit Innerer Sekretion. Tr. 17th International Cong. of Med., London, 1913, Section VI, 109–115.

46. ——: Die Hypophyse, in: Innere Sekretion. Ihre Physiologischen Grundlagen und ihre Bedeutung für die Pathologie, ed. 3. Urban & Schwarzenberg, Berlin and Vienna, 1916, vol. 11, pp. 82–187.

47. BIELSCHOWSKY, A.: Lectures on Motor Anomalies. Hanover, Dartmouth College Publications, 1945, vol. 122.

48. BLOOMFIELD, A. L.: The coincidence of diabetes mellitus and Addison's disease. Bull. Johns Hopkins Hosp. 1939, *65:* 456–465.

49. VON BONIN, G.: Classification of tumors of the pituitary body. Brit. M. J. 1913, *1:* 934.

50. BOON, A. A.: Comparative anatomy and physiopathology of the autonomic hypothalamic centres. Acta psychiat. & neurol. 1938, supp. 18: 1–129.

51. BORELL, U.: On the transport route of the thyrotropic hormone, the occur-

rence of the latter in different parts of the brain and its effect on the thyroidea. Acta Med. Scandinav. 1945, Suppl. 161, pp. 1–220.

52. BRITTON, S. W.: Adrenal insufficiency and related considerations. Physiol. Rev. 1930, *10:* 617–682.

53. —— AND COREY, E. L.: Antagonistic adrenal and pituitary effects on body salts and water. Science 1941, *93:* 405–406.

54. ——, SILVETTE, H. AND KLINE, R.: Carbohydrate and electrolyte changes in adrenal insufficiency in the dog. Am. J. Physiol. 1938, *122:* 446–454.

55. BROBECK, J. R.: Mechanism of the development of obesity in animals with hypothalamic lesions. Physiol. Rev. 1946, *26:* 541–560.

56. ——, MAGOUN, H. W. AND RANSON, S. W.: Insulin sensitivity of monkeys after section of the hypophyseal stalk. Proc. Soc. Exper. Biol. & Med. 1939, *42:* 622–624.

57. ——, TEPPERMAN, J. AND LONG, C. N. H.: Experimental hypothalamic hyperphagia in the albino rat. Yale J. Biol. & Med. 1943, *15:* 831–855.

58. ——, ——, AND —: The effect of experimental obesity upon carbohydrate metabolism. Yale J. Biol. & Med. 1943, *15:* 893–905.

59. BRONK, D. W., PITTS, R. F. AND LARRABEE, M. G.: Role of hypothalamus in cardiovascular regulation, in: The Hypothalamus. Research Publ. A. Nerv. & Ment. Dis., Baltimore, Williams & Wilkins, 1940, vol. 20, pp. 323–341.

60. BRONSTEIN, I. P., LUHAN, J. A. AND MAVRELIS, W. B.: Sexual precocity associated with hyperplastic abnormality of the tuber cinereum. Am. J. Dis. Child. 1942, *64:* 211–220.

61. BROOKHART, J. M. AND DEY, F. L.: Reduction of sexual behavior in male guinea pigs by hypothalamic lesions. Am. J. Physiol. 1941, *133:* 551–554.

62. BROOKS, C. Mc C.: A study of the mechanism whereby coitus excites the ovulation producing activity of the rabbit's pituitary. Am. J. Physiol. 1938, *121:* 157–177.

63. —— AND GERSH, I.: Innervation of the hypophysis of the rabbit and rat. Endocrinology 1941, *28:* 1–5.

64. BUCY, P. C.: The pars nervosa of the bovine hypophysis. J. Comp. Neurol. 1930, *50:* 505–511.

65. ——: Comments on presentation, in Bard, P. and Mountcastle, V. B., p. 397.[82]

66. CAJAL, S. R.: cited in Harris.[219]

67. ——: cited in Friedgood.[179]

68. CAMUS, J., AND ROUSSY, G.: Experimental researches on the pituitary body. Diabetes insipidus, glycosuria and those dystrophies considered as hypophyseal in origin. Endocrinology 1920, *4:* 507–522.

69. —— AND —: Les syndromes hypophysaires. Rev. neurol. 1922, *38:* 622–639.

70. CARNES, W. H., RAGAN, C., FERREBEE, J. W. AND O'NEILL, J.: Effects of desoxycorticosterone acetate in the albino rat. Endocrinology 1941, *29:* 144–149.

71. CASTLEMAN, J. AND HERTZ, S.: Pituitary fibrosis with myxedema. Arch. Path. 1939, *27:* 69–79.

72. CATCHPOLE, H. R., HAMILTON, J. B. AND HUBERT, G. R.: Effect of male hormone therapy on urinary gonadotropins in man. J. Clin. Endocrinol. 1942, 2: 181–186.

73. CHAIKOFF, I. L., ENTENMAN, C., CHANGUS, G. W. AND REICHERT, E. L.: Influence of thyroidectomy on blood lipids of the dog. Endocrinology 1941, 28: 797–805.

74. ——, ——, RINEHART, J. F. AND REICHERT, F. L.: Development of cirrhosis in the livers of dogs deprived of both pituitary and thyroid glands. Proc. Soc. Exper. Biol. & Med. 1943, 54: 170–171.

75. ——, GIBBS, G. E., HOLTON, G. F. AND REICHERT, F. L.: The lipid metabolism of the hypophysectomized dog and the lipid and carbohydrate metabolism of the hypophysectomized-depancreatized dog. Am. J. Physiol. 1936, 116: 543–550.

76. —— AND TAUROG, A.: Studies on the formation of organically bound iodine compounds in the thyroid gland and their appearance by the use of radioactive iodine. Ann. New York Acad. Sc. 1949, 50: 377–403.

77. CHAPMAN, A.: The relation of the thyroid and the pituitary glands to iodine metabolism. Endocrinology 1941, 29: 680–685.

78. CHOW, B. F., VAN DYKE, H. B., GREEP, R. O., ROTHEN, A. AND SHEDLOVSKY, T.: Gonadotrophins of swine pituitary. II. Endocrinology 1942, 30: 650–656.

79. CHOROBSKI, J. AND PENFIELD, W.: Cerebral vasodilatator nerves and their pathway from the medulla oblongata. Arch. Neurol. & Psychiat. 1932, 28: 1257–1289.

80. CLARK, E. R.: cited in Friedgood.[179]

81. CLAUDE, H. AND GOUGEROT: L'insuffisance pluriglandulaire totale tardive et les syndromes pluriglandulaires. Tr. 17th International Cong. of Med., London 1913, Section VI: 173–183.

82. CLEGHORN, R. A., ARMSTRONG, C. W. J. AND AUSTEN, D. C.: Clinical and chemical observations on adrenalectomized dogs maintained by a diet high in sodium salts and low in potassium. Endocrinology 1939, 25: 888–898.

83. CLINTON, M., JR., THORN, G. W., EISENBERG, H. AND STEIN, K. E.: Effect of synthetic desoxycorticosterone acetate therapy on plasma volume and electrolyte balance in normal dogs. Endocrinology 1942, 31: 578–581.

84. COBB, W. A.: Rhythmic slow discharges in the electroencephalogram. J. Neurosurg. & Psychiat. 1945, 8: 65–78.

85. COLLINS, V.: Effects of destruction of hypothalamus by tumor. Arch. Neurol. & Psychiat. 1942, 48: 774–788.

86. COLLIP, J. B.: Corticotropic (adrenotropic), thyrotropic, and parathyrotropic factors, in: Glandular Physiology and Therapy, a Symposium. Chicago, American Medical Association, 1942, pp. 33–50.

87. ——, SELYE, H. AND WILLIAMSON, J. E.: Changes in the hypophysis and the ovaries of rats chronically treated with an anterior pituitary extract. Endocrinology 1938, 23: 279–284.

88. COLOWICK, S. P., CORI, G. T. AND STEIN, M. W.: The effect of adrenal cortex and anterior pituitary extracts and insulin on the hexokinase reaction. J. Biol. Chem. 1947, 168: 583–596.

89. Cope, O., Hagströmer, A. and Blatt, H.: The activity of the blood serum amylase in the hypophysectomized dog. Am. J. Physiol. 1938, *122*: 428–434.

90. ——, Kapnick, I., Lambert, A., Pratt, T. D. and Verlot, M. G.: Endocrine function and amylase activity. II. Changes in activity of blood serum amylase in response to changes in adrenal cortical function in dog and rabbit. Endocrinology 1939, *25*: 236–247.

91. ——, ——, ——, ——, and —: Endocrine function and amylase activity. III. Further observations of blood serum amylase activity in relation to pituitary, pancreas, and thyroid function in the dog and rabbit. Endocrinology 1939, *25*: 248–276.

92. Corey, E. L. and Britton, S. W.: Blood cellular changes in adrenal insufficiency and the effects of corticoadrenal extracts. Am. J. Physiol. 1932, *102*: 699–706.

93. —— and —: Hypophyseal and adrenal interrelationships and carbohydrate metabolism. Am. J. Physiol. 1939, *126*: 148–154.

94. —— and —: The antagonistic action of desoxycorticosterone and post-pituitary extract on chloride and water balance. Am. J. Physiol. 1941, *133*: 511–519.

95. ——, Silvette, H., and Britton, S. W.: Hypophyseal and adrenal influences on renal function in the rat. Am. J. Physiol. 1939, *125*: 644–651.

96. Crafts, R. C.: The effects of iron, copper, and thyroxine on the anemia induced by hypophysectomy in the adult female rat. Am. J. Anat. 1946, *79*: 267–284.

97. Crandall, L. A., Jr. and Cherry, I. S.: The effect of insulin and glycine on hepatic glucose output in normal, hypophysectomized, adrenal denervated, and adrenalectomized dogs. Am. J. Physiol. 1939, *125*: 658–673 .

98. Crooke, A. C. and Russell, D. S.: The pituitary gland in Addison's disease. J. Path. & Bact. 1935, *40*: 255–283.

99. Crowe, S. J., Cushing, H. and Homans, J.: Experimental hypophysectomy. Bull. Johns Hopkins Hosp. 1910, *21*: 127–169.

100. Cushing, Harvey: The Pituitary Body and Its Disorders. Clinical States Produced by Disorders of the Hypophysis Cerebri. Philadelphia and London, Lippincott, 1912.

101. ——: The pituitary gland as now known. Lancet 1925, *2*: 899–906.

102. ——: Neurohypophyseal mechanisms from a clinical standpoint. (Lister Memorial Lecture.) Lancet 1930, *2*: 119–127, 175–184.

103. ——: "Dyspituitarism": Twenty years later, with special consideration of the pituitary adenomas. Arch. Int. Med. 1933, *51*: 487–557.

104. —— and Bordley, J. Jr.: Observations on experimentally induced choked discs. Bull. Johns Hopkins Hosp. 1909, *20*: 95–101.

105. —— and Davidoff, L. M.: Studies in acromegaly. IV. The basal metabolism. Arch. Int. Med. 1927, *39*: 673–697.

106. —— and Walker, C. B.: Distortion of the visual fields in cases of brain tumor. Chiasmal lesions with special reference to bitemporal hemianopsia. Brain 1915, *37*: 341–400.

107. CYON, E. V.: Zur Physiologie der Hypophyse. Arch. f. d. ges. Physiol. 1901, 87: 565–593.
108. DAGGS, R. G. AND EATON, A. G.: Metabolic studies in partially hypophysectomized dogs. Am. J. Physiol. 1933, 106: 299–308.
109. DALE, H. H.: The action of extracts of the pituitary body. Biochem. J. 1909, 4: 427–448.
110. DANDY, W. E.: The nerve supply to the pituitary body. Am. J. Anat. 1913, 15: 333–343.
111. ——: Section of the human hypophyseal stalk. J. A. M. A. 1940, 114: 312–314.
112. —— AND GOETSCH, E.: The blood supply of the pituitary body. Am. J. Anat. 1911, II: 137–150.
113. DAVIDOFF, L. M. AND CUSHING, H.: Studies in acromegaly. VI. The disturbances of carbohydrate metabolism. Arch. Int. Med. 1927, 39: 751–779.
114. —— AND FEIRING, E. H.: Surgical treatment of tumors of the pituitary body. Am. J. Surg. 1948, 75: 99–136.
115. DAVISON, C.: Disturbances of temperature regulation in man, in: The Hypothalamus. Research Publ. A. Nerv. & Ment. Dis., Baltimore, Williams & Wilkins, 1940, pp. 774–824.
116. —— AND DEMUTH, E. L.: Disturbances in the sleep mechanism. A clinicopathologic study. Arch. Neurol. & Psychiat. 1946, 55: 111–134, 365–382.
117. DAWSON, A. B.: Mitosis in the anterior pituitary of the monkey. Endocrinology 1942, 30: 516–518.
118. DEANE, H. W. AND GREEP, R. O.: A morphological and histochemical study of the rat's adrenal cortex after hypophysectomy with comments on the liver. Am. J. Anat. 1946, 79: 117–146.
118a. DEGROOT, J. AND HARRIS, G. W.: Hypothalamic control of the anterior pituitary and blood lymphocytes. J. Physiol. 1950, 3: 335–375.
119. DE LA BALZE, F. A., REIFENSTEIN, E. C. JR. AND ALBRIGHT, F.: Differential blood counts in certain adrenal cortical disorders (Cushing's syndrome, Addison's disease and panhypopituitarism). J. Clin. Endocrinol. 1946, 6: 315–319.
120. DELAY, J., BERTRAND, I. AND GUILLAIN, J.: L'electroencephalogramme dans le myoxedème. Compt. rend. Soc. de biol. 1938, 129: 395–398.
121. DEMPSEY, E. W.: The relationship between the central nervous system and the reproductive cycle in the female guinea pig. Am. J. Physiol. 1939, 126: 758–765.
122. ——: Some recent advances in experimental endocrinology. J. Clin. Endocrinol. 1944, 4: 211–216.
123. DENNY BROWN D. AND BRENNEN, C.: Paralysis of nerve induced by direct pressure and by tourniquet. Arch. Neurol. & Psychiat. 1944, 51: 1–27.
124. DERCUM, F. X. AND MCCARTHY, D. J.: Autopsy in a case of adiposis dolorosa. Am. J. M. Sc. (N. S.) 1902, 124: 994–1006.
125. DE ROBERTIS, E.: Cytological and cytochemical bases of thyroid function. Ann. N. Y. Acad. Sc. 1949, 50: 317–336.

126. DEY, F. L.: Genital changes in female guinea pigs resulting from destruction of the median eminence. Anat. Rec. 1943, *87:* 85–90.

127. ——, FISHER, C. AND RANSON, S. W.: Disturbances in pregnancy and labor in guinea pigs with hypothalamic lesions. Am. J. Obstet. & Gynecol. 1941, *42:* 459–466.

128. DOHAN, F. C., CHAMBERS, A. H. AND FISH, C. A.: The metabolism of dogs with permanent diabetes produced by anterior pituitary extract. Endocrinology 1941, *28:* 566–579.

129. DORFMAN, R. I.: Biochemistry of androgens, in: The Hormones. New York, Academic Press, 1950, vol. 1, pp. 467–549.

130. DOTT, N. M.: An investigation into the functions of the pituitary and thyroid glands. Quart. J. Exper. Physiol. 1923, *13:* 241–282.

131. —— AND BAILEY, P.: A consideration of the hypophyseal adenomata. Brit. J. Surg. 1925–26, *13:* 314–366.

132. DOUGHERTY, THOMAS F. AND WHITE, A.: The influence of hormones on lymphoid tissue structure and function. The role of the pituitary adrenotrophic hormone in the regulation of lymphocytes and other cellular elements of the blood. Endocrinology 1944, *35:* 1–14.

132a. DRUCKMAN, R.: A critique of "suppression" with additional observations in the cat. Brain 1952, *75:* 226–243.

133. DUKE ELDER, W. S.: Diseases of the inner eye, in: Textbook of Opthalmology. St. Louis, C. V. Mosby, 1949, vol. 3, p. 2944.

134. DVOSKIN, S.: Local maintenance of spermatogenesis in hypophysectomized rats with low dosages of testosterone from intratesticular pellets. Proc. Soc. Exper. Biol. & Med. 1943, *54:* 111–113.

135. DYKE, C. G.: Roentgen ray diagnosis of diseases of the skull and intracranial contents, in: Diagnostic Radiology. New York, Thomas Nelson & Sons, 1948, vol. 1, pp. 1–35.

136. —— AND HARE, C. C.: Roentgen therapy of pituitary tumors, in: The Pituitary Gland. Research Publ. A. Nerv. & Ment. Dis., Baltimore, Williams & Wilkins, 1938, vol. 17, p. 654.

137. EAGLE, E., BRITTON, S. W. AND KLINE, R.: The influence of corticoadrenal extract on energy output. Am. J. Physiol. 1932, *102:* 707–713.

138. EIDELBERG, J.: The pituitary and the sugar tolerance curve. Ann. Int. Med. 1932, *6:* 201–206.

139. ELMER, A. W.: Iodine metabolism and thyroid function. London, Oxford University Press, 1938.

140. ENGEL, G. L. AND MARGOLIN, S. G.: Neuropsychiatric disturbances in Addison's disease and role of impaired carbohydrate metabolism in production of abnormal cerebral function. Arch. Neurol. & Psychiat. 1941, *45:* 881–883.

141. ENGELBACH, W.: Classification of disorders of the hypophysis. Endocrinology 1920, *20:* 347–365.

142. ENGLE, E. T. AND LEVIN, L.: Gonadotrophins of the anterior lobe of the pituitary and of chorionic tissue. J. A. M. A. 1941, *116:* 47–52.

143. ENTENMAN, C., CHAIKOFF, I. L. AND REICHERT, F. L.: The role of nutrition in response of blood lipids to thyroidectomy. Endocrinology 1942, *30:* 794–801.

144. ——, ——, AND —: Blood lipids of the hypophysectomized-thyroidectomized dog. Endocrinology 1942, *30:* 802–815.

145. ERDHEIM J. AND STUMME E.: Über die Schwangerschaftsveränderung der Hypophyse. Beitr. z. path. Anat. u. z. allg. Path. 1909, *46:* 1–132.

146. ESCAMILLA, R. F. AND LISSER, H.: Simmonds' disease: A clinical study with review of the literature; differentiation from anorexia nervosa by statistical analysis of 595 cases, 101 of which were proved pathologically. J. Clin. Endocrinol. 1942 *2:* 65–96.

147. EVANS, H. M. AND GORBMAN, A.: Urinary gonadotrophins in normal men. Proc. Soc. Exper. Biol. & Med. 1942, *49:* 674–678.

148. ——, MEYER, K., PENCHARZ, R. AND SIMPSON, M. E.: Cure of the cachexia following hypophysectomy by administration of the growth hormone and its relation to the resulting adreno-cortical repair. Science 1932, *75:* 442–443.

149. —— AND SIMPSON, M. E.: Hormones of the anterior hypophysis. Am. J. Physiol. 1931, *98:* 511–546.

150. —— AND —: Physiology of the gonadotrophins, in: The Hormones. New York, Academic Press, 1950, vol. 2, pp. 351–405.

151. ——, — AND TURPEINEM, K.: Stimulation of deciduomata around threads on administration of lactogenic and adrenocorticotropic hormones. Anat. Rec. 1938, *70:* supp. 3, 26.

152. EVANS, J. N. AND BROWDER, J.: A problem of split macula. Study of visual fields. Arch. Ophthalmol. 1944, *31:* 43–54.

153. EVANS, W. G. AND PICIOTTO, G.: Chromophobe adenoma of the pituitary. Brit. J. Radiol. 1948, *21:* 330–336.

154. FALTA, WILHELM: Die Erkrankungen der Blutdrüsen, ed. 2. Vienna and Berlin, Julius Springer, 1928.

155. FARKAS, K.: Untersuchung des Zusammenhanges zwischen Zelltätigkeit und Golgi-Apparat in der Hypophyse; Zugleich eine Bemerkung zur Kritik von Prof. Romeis über meine in Virchows Archiv, bd. 305, erschienene Arbeit. Virchows arch. f. Path. Anat. 1941, *307:* 314–326.

156. FEE, A. R. AND PARKES, A. S.: Studies on ovulation. 1. The relation of the anterior pituitary body to ovulation in the rabbit. J. Physiol. 1929, *67:* 383–388.

157. FELDMAN, F., ROBERTS, J. B., SUSSELMAN, S. AND LIPETZ, B.: Coincidence of diabetes mellitus and hypopituitarism. Arch. Int. Med. 1947, *79:* 322–332.

158. FERGUSON, J. K. W.: A study of the motility of the intact uterus at term. Surg., Gynec. & Obst. 1941, *73:* 359–366.

159. FEVOLD, H. L.: Synergism of the follicle stimulating and luteinizing hormones in producing estrogen secretion. Endocrinology 1941, *28:* 33–36.

160. FICHERA, G.: Sur l'hypertrophie de la glande pituitaire consècutive á la castration. Arch. Ital. de Biol. 1905, *43:* 405–426.

161. FISCHEL, E. E., LE MAY, M. AND KABAT, E. A.: The effect of ACTH and x-ray on the amount of circulating antibodies. J. Immunol. 1949, *61:* 89–93.

162. FISHER, C., INGRAM, W. R. AND RANSON, S. W.: Diabetes Insipidus and the Neurohumoral Control of Water Balance. Ann. Arbor, Edward Bros., 1938.

163. ——, MAGOUN, H. W. AND RANSON, S. W.: Dystocia in diabetes insipidus. The relation of pituitary oxytocin to parturition. Am. J. Obst. & Gynec. 1938, *36:* 1–9.

164. FISHER, R. A.: Statistical Methods for Research Workers, ed. 10. Edinburgh and London, Oliver & Boyd, 1948.

165. FISHER, R. E., RUSSELL, J. A. AND CORI, C. F.: Glycogen disappearance and carbohydrate oxidation in hypophysectomized rats. J. Biol. Chem. 1936, *15:* 627–634.

166. FLAUM, G.: Insulin insensitivity: Its possible relation to the pituitary gland. Endocrinology 1938, *24:* 630–636.

167. FOLEY, M.P., SNELL, A. M. AND CRAIG, W. McK.: Anterior pituitary tumor associated with cachexia, hypoglycemia, and duodenal ulcer. Am. J. M. Sc. 1939, *118:* 1–8.

168. FOSTER, M. A., FOSTER, R. C. AND HISAW, F. L.: The interrelationships of the pituitary sex hormones on ovulation, corpus luteum formation and corpus luteum secretion in the hypophysectomized rabbit. Endocrinology 1937, *21:* 249–259.

169. —— AND HISAW, F. L.: Experimental ovulation and the resulting pseudopregnancy in anoestrous cats. Anat. Rec. 1935, *62:* 75–95.

170. —— AND McCARTER, J. C.: Hypopituitarism; Simmonds' disease associated with pernicious anemia, with bioassay of large chromophobe adenoma. J. Clin. Endocrinol. 1941, *1:* 436–441.

171. FRAENKEL-CONRAT, H. L., HERRING, V. V., SIMPSON, M. E. AND EVANS, H. M.: Effects of purified pituitary preparations on the insulin content of the rat's pancreas. Am. J. Physiol. 1942, *135:* 404–410.

172. ——, SIMPSON, M. E. AND EVANS, H. M.: Purification of follicle stimulating hormone of anterior pituitary. An. Fac. de med. de Montevideo 1940, *25:* 617–626.

173. ——, —, AND —: Effect of hypophysectomy and of purified pituitary hormones on liver arginase activity of rats. Am. J. Physiol. 1943, *138:* 439–449.

174. FRASER, R., ALBRIGHT, F. AND SMITH, P. H.: Carbohydrate metabolism: the value of the glucose tolerance test, the insulin tolerance test, and the glucose-insulin tolerance test in the diagnosis of endocrinologic disorders of glucose metabolism. J. Clin. Endocrinol. 1941, *1:* 297–306.

175. —— AND SMITH, P. H.: Simmonds' disease or panhypopituitarism (anterior). Its clinical diagnosis by the combined use of two objective tests (insulin tolerance test and urinary 17-keto-steroid assay). Quart. J. Med. 1941, *10:* 297–330.

176. FRAZIER, C. H.: Interrelationship of the pituitary to the endocrine system with remarks on treatment of pituitary disorders; observations of 334 cases. Surg., Gynec. & Obst. 1931, *52:* 1069–1074.

177. —— AND GRANT, F. C.: Pituitary disorder. A digest of one hundred cases with remarks on the surgical treatment. J. A. M. A. 1925, *85:* 1103–1106.

178. FREEMAN, H., LOONEY, J. M. AND HOSKINS, R. G.: Spontaneous variability of oral glucose tolerance. J. Clin. Endocrinol. 1942, 2: 431.
179. FRIEDGOOD, H. B.: Endocrine Function of the Hypophysis. New York, Oxford University Press, 1946.
180. —— AND DAWSON, A. B.: Inhibition of the carmine-cell reaction in the pituitaries of cats which mate but do not ovulate. Endocrinology 1942, 30: 252–257.
181. FRÖHLICH, A.: Ein Fall von Tumor Hypophysis cerebri ohne Akromegalie. Wien klin. Rundschau 1901, 15: 883–906.
182. FROMENT, M. J.: Les syndromes hypophysaires. Clinique et therapeutique. Rev. neurol. 1922, 38: 649–670.
183. FRYKMAN, H. M.: A quantitative study of the paraventricular nucleus and its alterations in hypophysectomy. Endocrinology 1942, 31: 23–29.
184. FULTON, J. F.: Physiology of the Nervous System. New York, Oxford University Press, 1949, pp. 243, 245–255.
185. FULTON, M. N. AND CUSHING, H.: The specific dynamic action of protein in patients with pituitary diseases. Arch. Int. Med. 1932, 50: 649–667.
186. GARDNER, W. U.: The persistence and growth of spontaneous mammary tumors and hyperplastic nodules in hypophysectomized mice. Cancer Research 1942, 2: 476–488.
187. —— AND ALLEN, E.: Effects of hypophysectomy at mid-pregnancy in the mouse. Anat. Rec. 1942, 83: 75–98.
188. GAUNT, R., POTTS, H. E. AND LOOMIS, E.: Postadrenalectomy diuresis: Effects of cortical extracts, salts, and estrone. Endocrinology 1938, 23: 216–222.
189. GEILING, E. M. K.: The pituitary body. Physiol. Rev. 1926, 6: 62–123.
190. GEISS, M. A.: Differential cell counts of anterior lobe of pituitary glands of rats showing diabetic traits. Proc. Soc. Exper. Biol. & Med. 1941, 47: 121–123.
191. GERGELY, J.: Einfluss der Hypophysenexstirpation auf den Kalkhaushalt. Pflüger's Arch. f. d. ges. Physiol. 1941, 245: 342–352.
192. GERHARDT: Fälle von Hypophysentumor. München med. Wchnschr. 1918, 65: 950.
193. GERMAN, W. J.: The endocrine effects of pituitary tumors. A clinical review. Surgery 1944, 16: 47–81.
194. GERSH, I. AND GROLLMAN, A.: Kidney function in adrenal cortical insufficiency. Am. J. Physiol. 1939, 125: 66–73.
195. GIBBS, E. L., FUSTIN, B. AND GIBBS, F. A.: Psychomotor Epilepsy. Private publication, 1948.
196. GILBERT, M. S.: Some factors influencing the early development of the mammalian hypophysis. Anat. Rec. 1935, 62: 337–360.
197. GILFORD, H.: The Hunterian lectures on infantilism. Lancet 1914, 1: 587–595, 644–673.
198. GILMAN, H.: Experimental sodium loss analogous to adrenal insufficiency: The resulting water shift and sensitivity to hemorrhage. Am. J. Physiol. 1934, 108: 662–669.

199. Giroud, A. and Desclaux, P.: Bases histologiques des localisations fonc-tionelles dans le lobe anterieur de l'hypophyse. Ann. d'endocrinol. 1947, *8:* 276–280.

200. Globus, J. H., Goldfarb, A. I. and Silver, S.: Hypophysio-hypothalamic interfunctions and dysfunctions. J. Mt. Sinai Hosp. 1947, *14:* 308–346.

201. Glusman, M.: Personal communication.

202. Goetsch, E.: A critical review, the pituitary body. Quart. J. Med. 1914, *7:* 173–208.

203. Goldzieher, M. A.: The relation of the anterior lobe to the specific dynamic action of protein. A. Research Nerv. & Ment. Dis., Proc. 1938, *17:* 536–546.

204. —— and Kaldor, J.: Studies of the relation of the pituitary to water metabolism. Proc. Soc. Exper. Biol. & Med. 1930, *27:* 799–801.

205. Gorbman, A.: The comparative anatomy and physiology of the anterior pituitary. Quart. Rev. Biol. 1941, *16:* 294–310.

206. Green, J. D.: The histology of the hypophyseal stalk and median eminence in man with special reference to blood vessels, nerve fibers and a peculiar neurovascular zone in this region. Anat. Rec. 1948, *100:* 273–288.

207. Greep, R. O., Van Dyke, H. B. and Chow, B. F.: Separation in nearly pure form of luteinizing (interstitial cell-stimulating) and follicle stimulating (gametogenic) hormones of the pituitary gland. J. Biol. Chem. 1940, *133:* 289–290.

208. ——, — and —: 1. Gonadotrophins of swine pituitary. Endocrinology 1942, *30:* 635–649.

208a. Greer, M. A.: The role of the hypothalamus in the control of thyroid function. J. Clin. Endocrinol. & Metab. 1952, *12:* 1259–1268.

209. Gregersen, M. I.: A practical method for the determination of blood volume with the dye T–1824. J. Lab. & Clin. Med. 1944, *29:* 1266–1286.

210. —— and Stewart, J. D.: Simultaneous determinations of the plasma volume with T–1824 and the "available fluid" volume with sodium thiocyanate. Am. J. Physiol. 1939, *125:* 142–152.

211. Griffiths, M. and Young, F. G.: Does the hypophysis secrete a pancreatropic hormone. Nature, London 1940, *146:* 266–267.

212. Grollman, A.: The relation of the adrenal cortex to carbohydrate metabolism. Am. J. Physiol. 1938, *122:* 460–471.

213. —— and Firor, W. M.: The role of the hypophysis in experimental chronic adrenal insufficiency. Am. J. Physiol. 1935, *112:* 310–319.

214. Gross, R. E.: Neoplasms producing endocrine disturbances in childhood. Am. J. Dis. Child. 1940, *59:* 579–628.

215. Grunbrecht, P., Keller, F. and Loeser, A.: Die Wirkung von Röntgenstrahlen auf Struktur und Funktion des Hypophysenvorderlappens. Klin. Wchnschr. 1938, *17:* 801–805.

216. Grüter: Hypophysentumor mit Dystrophia adiposogenitalis. München. med. Wchnschr. 1915, *62:* 199.

216a. Halstead, W. C.: Brain and Intelligence. Chicago, University of Chicago Press, 1947.

217. HAMMAN, L. AND HIRSCHMAN, I. I.: Studies on blood sugar. I. Alimentary hyperglycemia and glycosuria as a test of sugar tolerance. Arch. Int. Med. 1917, 20: 761–808.
218. HANN, V. F.: Über die Bedeutung der Hypophysenveränderungen bei Diabetes Insipidus. Frankfurt Ztschr. Path. 1918, 21: 337–366.
219. HARRIS, G. W.: Neural control of pituitary gland. Physiol. Rev. 1948, 28: 139–180.
220. HARRISON, H. C. AND HARRISON, H. E.: The effect of injection of a saline extract of anterior pituitary on the glucose tolerance of rats. Endocrinology 1942, 30: 121–128.
221. —— AND LONG, C. N. H.: Effects of anterior pituitary extracts in the fasted animal. Endocrinology 1940, 26: 971–978.
222. —— AND DARROW, D. C.: Renal function in experimental adrenal insufficiency. Am. J. Physiol. 1939, 125: 631–644.
223. HARROP, G. A., WEINSTEIN, A., SOFFER, L. J. AND TRESCHER, J. H.: The diagnosis and treatment of Addison's disease. J. A. M. A. 1933, 100: 1850–1855.
224. ——, NICHOLSON, W. M., SOFFER, L. J. AND STRAUSS, M.: Extracellular and intracellular water loss during suprarenal insufficiency in the dog. Proc. Soc. Exper. Biol. & Med. 1935, 32: 1312–1315.
225. ——, SOFFER, L. J., ELLSWORTH, R. AND TRESCHER, J. H.: Studies on the suprarenal cortex. III. Plasma electrolytes and electrolyte excretion during suprarenal insufficiency in the dog. J. Exper. Med. 1933, 58: 17–38.
226. ——, WEINSTEIN, A., SOFFER, L. J. AND TRESCHER, J. H.: Studies on the suprarenal cortex. II. Metabolism, circulation, and blood concentration during suprarenal insufficiency in the dog. J. Exper. Med. 1933, 58: 1–16.
227. HARTMAN, F. A. AND WINTER, C. A.: Irreversibility in adrenal insufficiency. Endocrinology 1933, 17: 180–186.
228. HARTOCH, W.: Die Merkmale der sogenannten Dystrophia adiposogenitalis. Eine Kritik des endokrinologischen Schriftum. Virchows Arch. f. path. Anat. 1928, 270: 561–604.
229. HATERIUS, H. O.: The genital-pituitary pathway. Non-effect of stimulation of superior cervical ganglia. Proc. Soc. Exper. Biol. & Med. 1934, 31: 1112–1113.
230. HAYNE, R. A., BELINSON, L. AND GIBBS, F. A.: Electrical activity of subcortical areas in epilepsy. E. E. G. Clin. Neurophysiol. 1949, 1: 437–445.
230a. HAYNES, R., SAVARD, K. AND DORFMAN, R. I.: The action of ACTH on adrenal slices. Science 1952, 116: 690.
231. HEINBECKER, P., SOMOGYI, M. AND WEICHSELBAUM, T. E.: The effect of diet on insulin response in normal and hypophysectomized dogs. Proc. Soc. Exper. Biol. & Med. 1937, 36: 804–805.
232. —— AND WHITE, H. L.: The hypothalamico-hypophysial system and its relation to water balance in the dog. Am. J. Physiol. 1941, 133: 582–593.
233. ——, — AND ROLF, D.: The relation of the adeno- and the neuro-hypophysis to insulin sensitivity and sugar tolerance in the dog. Am. J. Physiol. 1942, 136: 592–594.

234. ——, — AND —: The essential lesion in experimental diabetes insipidus. Endocrinology 1947, *40:* 104–113.
235. HELLER, H.: The action of the antidiuretic principle of posterior pituitary extracts in the urine excretion of anesthetized animals. J. Physiol. 1940, *98:* 405–419.
236. HELLER, C. G., FARNEY, J. P., MORGAN, D. N. AND MYERS, G. B.: A correlation of the ovarian and endometrial histology, vaginal epithelium, gonadotrophic hormonal excretion and the day of the menstrual cycle in 28 women. J. Clin. Endocrinol. 1944, *4:* 95–100.
237. ——, HELLER, E. J. AND SEVRINGHAUS, E. L.: Does estrogen substitution materially inhibit pituitary gonadotrophic potency? Endocrinology 1942, *30:* 309–316.
238. HENDERSON, W. R.: Sexual dysfunction in adenomas of the pituitary body. Endocrinology 1931, *15:* 111–127.
239. ——: The pituitary adenomata—a follow-up study of the surgical results in 338 cases. (Dr. Harvey Cushing's Series.) Brit. J. Surg. 1939, *26:* 811–921.
240. HERRING, V. V. AND EVANS, H. M.: Effects of purified antero-pituitary hormones on the carbohydrate stores of hypophysectomized rats. Am. J. Physiol. 1943, *140:* 452–459.
241. ——, FRAENKEL-CONRAT, H. AND EVANS, H. M.: The lack of effect of thyroxin on blood sugar and glycogen stores of fasted, hypophysectomized rats. Endocrinology 1942, *30:* 483–484.
242. HETHERINGTON, A. W.: Nonproduction of hypothalamic obesity in the rat by lesions rostral or dorsal to the ventro-medial hypothalamic nuclei. J. Comp. Neurol. 1944, *80:* 33–47.
243. —— AND RANSON, S. W.: Hypothalamic lesions and adiposity in the rat. Anat. Rec. 1940, *78:* 149–173.
244. —— AND —: The effect of early hypophysectomy on hypothalamic obesity. Endocrinology 1942, *31:* 30–34.
245. HILLARP, N. A.: Studies on the localization of hypothalamic centres controlling the gonadotrophic function of the hypophysis. Acta Endocrinologica 1949, *2:* 11–24.
246. HIMWICH, H. E., FAZEKAS, J. F. AND SPIERS, M. A.: Studies on sodium loss. Proc. Soc. Exper. Biol. & Med. 1936, *34:* 450–451.
247. HIRSCH, O.: Contribution a la clinique des tumeurs hypophysaires, baseé sur 100 cas opérés par l'auteur d'après sa propre méthode endonasale. Presse méd. 1926, *34:* 578–580.
248. HOBERMAN, H.: Endocrines in amino acid and protein metabolism. Yale J. Biol. & Med. 1950, *22:* 341–367.
249. HOFFMAN, W. C., LEWIS, R. A. AND THORN, G. W.: Electroencephalogram in Addison's disease. Bull. John Hopkins Hosp. 1942, *70:* 335–361.
249a. HORRAX, G., HARE, H. F., POPPEN, J. L., HURXTHAL, L. M. AND YOUNG-HUSBAND, O. Z.: Chromophobe pituitary tumors. II Treatment. J. Clin. Endocrinol. & Metab. 1952, *12:* 631–641.
250. HORVATH, S. M.: The response to cold following double adrenalectomy. Endocrinology 1938, *23:* 223–227.

251. HOUSSAY, B. A.: What we have learned from the toad concerning hypophyseal functions. New England J. Med. 1936, *214:* 913–926.

252. ——: The hypophysis and metabolism. New England J. Med. 1936, *214:* 961–971.

253. ——: Carbohydrate metabolism. New England J. Med. 1936, *214:* 971–986.

254. ——: Advancement of knowledge of the role of the hypophysis in carbohydrate metabolism during the last 25 years. Endocrinology 1942, *30:* 884–897.

255. ——: Thyroid and metathyroid diabetes. Endocrinology 1944, *35:* 158–172.

256. ——: The role of the hypophysis in carbohydrate metabolism and in diabetes, in: Les Prix Nobel en 1947. Stockholm, Norstedt and Soner, 1949, pp. 129–136.

257. —— AND BIASOTTI, A.: The hypophysis, carbohydrate metabolism, and diabetes. Endocrinology 1931, *15:* 511–523.

258. ——, FOGLIA, V. G. AND FUSTINONI, O.: The intestinal absorption of sugar in the toad with hypophyseal or adrenal insufficiency. Endocrinology 1941, *28:* 915–922.

259. HOWE, H. S.: Normal and abnormal variations in the pituitary fossa. Neurol. Bull. 1919, *2:* 233–238.

260. HUBBLE, D.: The influence of the endocrine system in blood disorders. Lancet 1933, *2:* 113–120.

261. HUME, D. M. AND WITTENSTEIN, G. J.: The relationship of the hypothalamus to pituitary adrenocortical function, in: Proceedings of the First Clinical ACTH Conference. Philadelphia, Blakiston, 1950, pp. 134–148.

262. HUNT, T. E.: Mitotic activity in the anterior hypophysis of female rats of different age groups and at different periods of the day. Endocrinology 1943, *32:* 334–339.

263. HURXTHAL, L. M.: Blood cholesterol and hypometabolism. Suprarenal and pituitary deficiency, obesity, and miscellaneous conditions. Arch. Int. Med. 1934, *53:* 825–831.

264. —— AND HUNT, H. M.: Clinical relationships of blood cholesterol with a summary of our present knowledge of cholesterol metabolism. Ann. Int. Med. 1935, *9:* 717–727.

265. Hypothalamus, The. Research Publ. A. Nerv. & Ment. Dis., Baltimore, Williams & Wilkins, 1940, vol. 20, p. 943.

266. ILLIG, W.: Geschwülste der Hypophyse bzw. der Hypophysengegend und Zwischenhirn. Virchows Arch. f. path. Anat. 1928, *270:* 549–560.

267. INGELBRECHT, P.: Influence du système nerveux central sur la mamelle lactante chez le rat blanc. Compt. rend. Soc. de biol. 1935, *120:* 1369–1371.

268. INGRAM, W. R. AND WINTER, C. A.: The effects of adrenalectomy upon the water exchange of cats with diabetes insipidus. Am. J. Physiol. 1938, *122:* 143–150.

269. IRVING, G. W., JR. AND DU VIGNEAUD, V.: Hormones of the posterior lobe of the pituitary gland. Ann. New York. Acad. Sc. 1943, *43:* 273–309.

270. VON ISSEKUTZ, B., JR. AND VERZÀR, F.: Die Rolle des Hypophysenvorderlappens und des Nebenniere bei der Fettwanderung. Arch. f. d. ges Physiol. 1938, *240:* 624.

271. JAILER, J. W., SPERRY, W. M., ENGLE, E. T. AND SMELSER, G.: Experimental hypothyroidism in the monkey. Endocrinology 1944, *35:* 27–37.

272. JASPER, H. H.: Diffuse projection systems. The integrative action of the thalamic reticular system. E. E. G. Clin. Neurophysiol. 1949, *1:* 405–420.

273. JEFFERSON, G.: Extrasellar extensions of pituitary adenomas. Proc. Roy. Soc. Med. 1940, *33:* 433–458.

274. JENSEN, D.: The effect of androgen on spermatogenesis in the rat. Anat. Rec. 1948, *100:* 680.

275. JOHN, H. J.: Hypopituitarism and diabetes. Endocrinology 1925, *9:* 397–402.

276. KAHN, E. A. AND CROOKE, A. C.: Indications for and effects of irradiation of the pituitary gland. Brit. J. Surg. 1944, *17:* 133–139.

277. KELLER, A. D.: Protection by peripheral nerve section of the gastrointestinal tract from ulceration following hypothalamic lesions. Arch. Path. 1936, *21:* 165–184.

278. —— AND D'AMOUR, M. C.: Ulceration in the digestive tract of the dog following hypophysectomy. Arch. Path. 1936, *21:* 185–201.

279. —— AND HAMILTON, J. W., JR.: Normal sex functions following section of the hypophyseal stalk in the dog. Am. J. Physiol. 1937, *119:* 349–350.

280. KERR, H. D.: Irradiation of pituitary tumors: results in fifty cases. Am. J. Roentgenol. 1948, *60:* 348–358.

281. KESTENBAUM, A.: Clinical Methods of Neuro-ophthalmologic Examination. New York, Grune & Stratton, 1947, p. 373.

282. KIMELDORF, D. J.: The excretion of 17-ketosteroids by male rabbits during altered gonadal function. Endocrinology 1948, *43:* 83–88.

283. KLISIECKY, A., PICKFORD, M., ROTHSCHILD, P. AND VERNEY, E. B.: The absorption and excretion of water by the mammal. I. The relation between absorption of water and its excretion by the innervated and denervated kidney. Proc. Roy. Soc., London, s. B. 1933, *112:* 496–521.

284. ——, —, — AND —: The absorption and excretion of water by the mammal. II. Factors influencing the response of the kidney to water ingestion. Proc. Roy. Soc., London, s. B. 1933, *112:* 521–547.

285. KNOWLTON, A. I., JAILER, J. W., HAMILTON, H. AND WEST, R.: Effects of pituitary adrenotropic hormone in panhypopituitarism of long standing and in myxedema. Am. J. Med. 1950, *8:* 269–284.

286. KOFFKA, K.: Principles of Gestalt Psychology. New York, Harcourt, Brace, 1935, p. 716.

287. KONEFF, A. A.: Effect of adrenocorticotropic hormone on the anterior pituitary of the normal young male rat. Endocrinology 1944, *34:* 77–82.

288. KORNBLUM, K. AND OSMOND, L. H.: Deformation of the sella turcica by tumors in the pituitary fossa. Ann. Surg. 1935, *101:* 201–211.

289. KRAUS, E. J.: Die Hypophyse, in: v. Hanke, F. and Lubarsch, O.: Drüsen mit Inneren Sekretion, Handbuch d. Spez. Path. Anat. u. Histologie. Berlin, J. Springer, 1926, vol. 8, pp. 810–950.

290. ——: Bemerkungen zu Kiyono's Nachtrag zu der Arbeit "Die Histo-pathologie der Hypophyse" in Virchows Archiv., Band 262, Heft. 1. Virchows Arch. f. path. Anat. 1927, *264:* 214–216.

291. KRAUS, F.: Correlation of organs of internal secretion and their disturbances. Tr. 17th International Cong. of Med., London, 1913, Sect. VI, 117–135.

292. KRAUS, J. E.: Hyperplastic disease of the adenohypophysis. J. Clin. Endocrinol. 1945, *5:* 42–51.

293. KRISTIANSEN, K. AND COURTOIS, G.: Rhythmic electrical activity from isolated cerebral cortex. E. E. G. Clin. Neurophysiol. 1949, *1:* 265–271.

294. LANGWORTHY, O.: The influence of suprasegmental levels on nervous activity, in: The Hypothalamus. Research Publ. A. Nerv. & Ment. Dis., Baltimore, Williams & Wilkins, 1940, vol. 20, pp. 617–623.

295. LAQUEUR, G. L. AND FLUHMANN, C. F.: The action of testosterone on the female rat hypophysis. Endocrinology 1942, *31:* 300–302.

296. LAUNOIS, P. E. AND CLÉRET, M.: Le syndrome hypophysaire adiposogénital. Gaz. des hôp. 1910, *83:* 57–64, 79–86.

297. LAWSON, H. D., GOLDIN, J. B. AND SEVRINGHAUS, E. L.: The gonado-trophin content of the hypophysis throughout the life cycle of the normal female rat. Am. J. Physiol. 1939, *125:* 396–404.

298. LEATHEM, J. H. AND DRILL, V. A.: The role of the hypophysis and adrenals in the control of systolic blood pressure in the rat. Endocrinology 1944, *35:* 112–120.

299. LENNON, G. G.: Chromophobe adenomata of the hypophysis cerebri. J. Obst. & Gynaec. Brit. Emp. 1943, *50:* 369–371.

300. LENNOX, M. A. AND BRODY, B. S.: Paroxysmal slow waves in the ence-phalograms of patients with epilepsy and with subcortical lesions. J. Nerv. & Ment. Dis. 1946, *104:* 237–248.

301. LEQUIME, J.: Le debit cardiaque dans les états pathologiques a métabolisme abaissé. Compt. rend. Soc. de Biol. 1939, *130:* 807–809.

302. LERMAN, J. AND STEBBINS, H. D.: The pituitary type of myxedema. Further observations. J. A. M. A. 1942, *119:* 391–395.

303. LEVIN, L., LEATHEM, J. H. AND CRAFTS, R. C.: The effects of adrenal-ectomy and replacement therapy on the serum protein levels of the cat. Am. J. Physiol. 1942, *136:* 776–782.

304. LEWIS, D. D.: Tumors of the hypophysis; their relation to acromegaly and Fröhlichs' syndrome. Tr. Am. Acad. Ophth. 1911, *16:* 255–266.

305. LEYENDECKER, R.: Cited in Stevenson.[460]

305a. LI, C. H.: The chemistry of gonadotrophic hormones, in: Vitamins and Hormones. New York, Academic Press, 1949, vol. 7, pp. 224–254.

306. ——: Growth and adrenocorticotrophic hormones of the anterior pituitary, in: The Harvey Lectures. Springfield, Charles C Thomas, 1950–1951, pp. 180–217.

307. —— AND EVANS, H. M.: The isolation of pituitary growth hormone. Science 1944, *99:* 183–184.

308. LILIENFELD, A.: The use of the low salt diet in the diagnosis of Addison's disease. J. A. M. A. 1938, *110:* 804–805.

309. LINDSLEY, D. B., BROWDER, J. AND MAGOÙN, H. W.: Effect of hypothalamic lesions on the E. E. G. E. E. G. Clin. Neurophysiol, 1949, *1:* 519.

310. LISSER, H. AND ESCAMILLA, R. F.: The clinical diagnosis of Simmonds' disease (hypophyseal cachexia). A critical statistical comparison of 69 verified, 134 unverified cases. Tr. A. Am. Physicians 1938, *53:* 210–220.

311. LIVINGSTON, R, B., FULTON, J. F., DELGADO, J. M. R., SACHS, E., JR., BRENDLER, S. J. AND DAVIS, G. D.: Stimulation and regional ablation of orbital surface of frontal lobe, in: The Frontal Lobes. Research Publ. A. Nerv. & Ment. Dis., Baltimore, Williams & Wilkins, 1948, vol. 27, pp. 405–420.

312. LOEB, R. F.: Adrenal insufficiency. Bull. New York Acad. Med. 1940, *16:* 347–367.

313. ——: The adrenal cortex and electrolyte behavior, in: The Harvey Lectures. Lancaster, Science Press Printing Co., 1941–1942, pp. 100–129.

314. ——: Adrenal cortex insufficiency, in: Glandular Physiology and Therapy, a Symposium. Chicago, American Medical Association, 1942, pp. 287–306.

315. —— AND ATCHLEY, D. W.: The significance of certain chemical abnormalities found in the blood in Addison's disease. Tr. A. Am. Physicians 1937, *52:* 228–235.

316. ——, —, BENEDICT, E. M. AND LELAND, J.: Electrolyte balance studies in adrenalectomized dogs with particular reference to the excretion of sodium. J. Exper. Med. 1933, *57:* 775–792.

317. LOESER, A. AND THOMPSON, K. W.: Hypophysenvorderlappen, Jod und Schilddrüse. Der Mechanismus der Schilddrüsenwirkung des Jods. Endokrinologie 1934, *14:* 144–150.

318. LONG, C. N. H.: The influence of the pituitary and adrenal glands upon pancreatic diabetes. Medicine 1937, *16:* 214–247.

319. ——: Evidence for and against control of carbohydrate metabolism by the hypothalamus, in: The Hypothalamus. Research Publ. A. Nerv. & Ment. Dis., Baltimore, Williams & Wilkins, 1940, vol. 20, pp. 486–501.

320. ——: Adrenal Cortex Conference. Josiah Macy, Jr. Foundation, Caldwell, Progress Associates, 1950, p. 81.

321. LÖWENSTEIN, C.: Die Entwicklung der Hypophysisadenome. Ein Beitrag zur Lehre von den Geschwülsten. Virchows Arch. f. path. Anat. 1907, *188:* 44–65.

322. LOZNER, E. L., WINKLER, A. W., TAYLOR, F. H. L. AND PETERS, J. P.: The intravenous glucose tolerance test. J. Clin. Investigation 1941, *20:* 507–515.

323. LUKENS, F. D. W.: Pituitary diabetes. Am. J. M. Sc. 1946, *212:* 229–240.

324. —— AND DOHAN, F. C.: Further observations on the relation of the adrenal cortex to experimental diabetes. Endocrinology 1938, *22:* 51–58.

325. —— AND —: Pituitary diabetes in the cat; recovery following insulin or dietary treatment. Endocrinology 1942, *30:* 175–202.

326. MACKAY, E. M. AND BARNES, R. H.: Fasting ketosis in the pregnant rat as influenced by adrenalectomy. Proc. Soc. Exper. Biol. & Med. 1936, *34:* 682–683.

327. —— AND MacKAY, L. L.: The influence of adrenal cortex extract upon compensatory hypertrophy of the adrenal cortex. Endocrinology 1938, *23:* 237–240.

328. —— AND WICK, A. N.: The influence of adrenalectomy on the blood and urine ketones during fasting and anterior pituitary extract administration. Am. J. Physiol. 1939, *126:* 753–757.

329. McCULLAGH, E. P. AND LEWIS, L. A.: Tiselius electrophoresis studies of plasma proteins in Addison's disease. Am. J. M. Sc. 1945, *210:* 81–86.

330. McCULLOCH, W.: Mechanisms for the spread of epileptic activation of the brain. E. E. G. Clin. Neurophysiol. 1949, *1:* 19–24.

331. MAGOUN, H. W., RANSON, S. W., HARRISON, F. AND BROBECK, J. R.: Activation of heat loss mechanisms by local heating of the brain. J. Neurophysiol. 1938, *1:* 101–114.

332. —— AND RHINES, R.: Spasticity, the Stretch Reflex, and Extrapyramidal Systems. Springfield, Charles C Thomas, 1948, p. 59.

333. MAHONEY, W. AND SHEEHAN, D.: Pituitary-hypothalamic mechanisms: Experimental occlusion of the pituitary stalk. Brain 1936, *59:* 61–75.

334. MAJOR, S. G. AND MANN, F. G.: The formation of glycogen following pancreatectomy. Am. J. Physiol. 1932, *102:* 409–421.

335. MARINESCO, M. G.: De la destruction de la glande pituitaire chez le chat. Compt. rend. Soc. de biol. 1892, *44:* 509–510.

336. MARKEE, J. E., SAWYER, C. H. AND HOLLINSHEAD, W. H.: Activation of the anterior hypophysis by electrical stimulation in the rabbit. Endocrinology 1946, *38:* 345–357.

337. MARKS, H. P. AND YOUNG, F. G.: Observations on the metabolism of dogs made permanently diabetic by treatment with anterior pituitary extract. J. Endocrinol. 1939, *1:* 470–507.

338. MARTIN, S. J., HERRLICH, H. C. AND FAZEKAS, J. F.: The relation between electrolyte imbalance and excretion of an anti-diuretic substance in adrenalectomized cats. Am. J. Physiol. 1939, *127:* 51–57.

339. MARTIUS, K.: Hypophysistumor ohne Akromegalie. Frankfurt. Ztschr. f. Path., vol. 11, no. 1., abstracted, Berl. klin. Wchnschr. 1912, *49:* 2041.

340. MARX, W. AND EVANS, H. M.: The Chemistry and Physiology of Hormones. Washington, Am. Assoc. Adv. Sc., 1944, pp. 47–57.

341. MASSERMAN, J.: The hypothalamus in psychiatry. Am. J. Psychiat. 1942, *98:* 633–637.

342. MAYER. L. L., STROUSE, C. D. AND SOSKIN, S.: Lack of perimetric evidence for pituitary hypertrophy in diabetes. J. Clin. Endocrinol. 1941, *1:* 604–606.

343. MEANS, J. H., HERTZ, S. AND LERMAN, J.: The pituitary type of myxedema or Simmonds' disease masquerading as myxedema. Tr. A. Am. Physicians 1940, *55:* 32–53.

344. MEYER, O. O., THEIVELIS, E. W. AND RUSCH, H. P.: The hypophysis and hematopoiesis. Endocrinology 1940, *27:* 932–944.

345. MIRSKY, I. A.: The site and mechanism of the antiketogenic action of insulin. Am. J. Physiol. 1936, *116*: 322–326.

346. ——: The influence of adrenalectomy on anterior pituitary ketogenesis in rats. Science 1938, *88*: 332–333.

347. ——: The influence of the anterior pituitary gland on protein metabolism. Endocrinology 1939, *25*: 52–56.

348. VON MONAKOW, P.: Zur Pathologie der Hypophyse. Schweiz. Arch f. Neurol. u. Psychiat. 1921, *8*: 200–207.

349. MORTON, M. E., PERLMAN, I. AND CHAIKOFF, I. L.: Radioactive iodine as an indicator of the metabolism of iodine. III. The effect of thyrotropic hormone on the turnover of thyroxine and diiodotyrosine in the thyroid gland and plasma. J. Biol. Chem. 1941, *140*: 603–611.

350. MOSONYI J.: Über die allmähliche Rückbildung der Ausfallerscheinungen bei hypophysektomierten Hunden. Klin. Wchnschr. 1941, *20*: 818.

351. MOSSBERGER, J. I.: Perforated duodenal ulcer and neoplasm of the tuber cinereum. J. Neuropath. & Exper. Neurol. 1947, *6*: 391–400.

352. MÜNZER, A.: Die Hypophysis. Berl. klin. Wchnschr. 1910, 47: 341–344.

353. MURPHY, J. P. AND GELLHORN, E.: Influence on hypothalamic stimulation on cortically induced movements and on action potentials of the cortex. J. Neurophysiol. 1945, *8*: 341–365.

354. NETTROUR, W. S. AND RYNEARSON, E. H.: A salt-poor diet as a provocative test for Addison's disease. Proc. Staff Meet., Mayo Clin. 1934, *9*: 550–556.

355. NICHOLSON, W. M.: Observations on the pathological changes in suprarenalectomized dogs with particular reference to the anterior lobe of the hypophysis. Bull. Johns Hopkins Hosp. 1936, *58*: 405–417.

356. NONNE: Symptomatik von Hypophysiserkrankungen, unter Ausschluss der Akromegalie. Deutsche med. Wchnschr. 1916, *42*: 1338–1339.

357. NORTHFIELD, D. W. C.: Some observations on headache. Brain 1938, *61*: 133–162.

358. ONODI, A.: The Optic Nerves and Accessory Sinuses of the Nose. New York, Williams & Wood, 1910, p. 101.

359. PANCOAST, H. K.: The interpretation of roentgenograms of pituitary tumors. Explanations of some of the sources of error confusing the clinical and roentgenological diagnoses. Am. J. Roentgenol. 1932, *27*: 697–712.

360. ——, PENDERGRASS, E. P. AND SCHAEFFER, J. P.: Head and Neck in Roentgen Diagnosis. Springfield, Charles C Thomas, 1942, p. 905.

361. PARDEE, I. H.: Some neurological and therapeutic aspects of hypophyseal tumors. New York Med. J. 1923, *117*: 415–419.

362. PARKER, R. L.: The use of a salt-poor diet in the diagnosis of Addison's disease. Proc. Staff Meet., Mayo Clin. 1935, *10*: 344–348.

362a. PASCHKIS, K. E. AND CANTAROW, A.: Hypopituitarism: studies in pituitary tumors and Simmonds' disease. Ann. Int. Med. 1951, *43*: 669.

363. PENCHARZ, R. I. AND LONG, J. A.: Hypophysectomy in the pregnant cat. Am. J. Anat. 1933, *53*: 117–140.

364. PENFIELD, W.: Epileptic manifestations of cortical and supracortical discharge. E. E. G. Clin. Neurophysiol. 1949, *1:* 3–10.
365. —— AND ERICKSON, T. C.: Epilepsy and Cerebral Localization. Baltimore, Charles C Thomas, 1941.
366. PERERA, GEORGE A.: Acetyl-beta-methylcholine in Addison's disease. J. A. M. A. 1945, *128:* 1018–1020.
366a. PERKINS, R. F. AND RYNEARSON, E. H.: Practical aspects of insufficiency of the anterior pituitary gland in the adult. J. Clin. Endocrinol. & Metab. 1952, *12:* 574–603.
367. PERLA, D.: Hemorrhagic changes in the suprarenal cortex of adult rats following pituitarectomy. Proc. Soc. Exper. Biol. & Med. 1935, *32:* 655–658.
368. —— AND ROSEN, S. H.: The effect of hypophysectomy on natural resistance of adult albino rats to histamine poisoning. Arch. Path. 1935, *20:* 222–232.
369. PETERS, J. P. AND MAN, E. B.: The interrelations of serum lipids in normal persons. J. Clin. Investigation 1943, *22:* 707.
370. —— AND VAN SLYKE, D. D.: Interpretation. Quantitative Clinical Chemistry. Baltimore, Williams & Wilkins, 1946, vol. 1, p. 165.
371. PICKERING, G. W.: Experimental observations on headache. Brit. M. J. 1939, *1:* 907–912.
372. PICKFORD, M.: Control of the secretion of antidiuretic hormone from the pars nervosa of the pituitary gland. Physiol. Rev. 1945, *25:* 573–596.
373. Pituitary Gland, The. Research Publ. A. Nerv. & Ment. Dis., Baltimore, Williams & Wilkins, 1938, vol. 17, p. 725.
374. POMERAT, G. R.: Mitotic activity in the pituitary of the white rat following castration. Am. J. Anat. 1941, *69:* 89–122.
375. POPA, G. AND FIELDING, U.: Portal circulation from pituitary to the hypothalamic region. J. Anat. 1930, *65:* 88–91.
376. Proceedings of the First Clinical ACTH Conference. New York, Blakiston, 1950.
377. Proceedings of the Second Clinical ACTH Conference. Research; Therapeutics. New York, Blakiston, 1951, vols. 1 and 2.
378. PRICE, W. H., CORI, C. F. AND COLOWICK, S. P.: The effect of anterior pituitary extract and of insulin on the hexokinase reaction. J. Biol. Chem. 1945, *160:* 633.
379. PRUITT, B. S.: On the dimensions of the hypophyseal fossa in man. Am. J. Phys. Anthropol. 1927, *11:* 205–222.
380. RANDOLPH, T. G. AND ROLLINS, J. P.: Eosinophil observations in adrenocorticotrophic hormone, in: Proc. of the First Clinical ACTH Conference. New York, Blakiston, 1950, pp. 1–14.
381. RANSON, S. W.: Somnolence caused by hypothalamic lesions in the monkey. Arch. Neurol. & Psychiat. 1939, *41:* 1–23.
382. ——: The hypothalamus as a thermostat regulating body temperature. Psychosom. Med. 1939, *1:* 486–495.
383. ——, KABAT, H. AND MAGOUN, H. W.: Autonomic responses to electrical

stimulation of hypothalamus, preoptic region, and septum. Arch. Neurol. & Psychiat. 1935, *33:* 467–477.

384. —— AND MAGOUN, H. W.: The hypothalamus. Ergebn. Physiol. 1939, *41:* 56–163.

385. RANSTRÖM, S.: The hypothalamus and sleep regulation, an experimental and morphological study. Acta. Path. & Microbiol. Scandinav., Supp. 70, 1947, 1–90.

386. RASMUSSEN, A. T.: The percentage of the different types of cells in the male adult human hypophysis. Am. J. Path. 1929, *5:* 263–274.

387. ——: Innervation of the hypophysis. Endocrinology 1938, *23:* 263–278.

388. ——: The growth of the hypophysis cerebri (pituitary gland) and its major subdivisions during childhood. Am. J. Anat. 1947, *80:* 95–116.

389. RAWSON, R. W.: Physiological reactions of thyroid stimulating hormone. Ann. New York Acad. Sc. 1949, *50:* 491–507.

390. REDLICH, E.: Zur Symptomatologie der Hypophysentumoren mit Hinweisen auf die Simmondsche hypophysäre Kachexie. Jahrb. f. Psychiat. u. Neurol. 1927, *45:* 276–291.

391. REESE, J. D., KONEFF, A. A. AND AKIMOTO, M. B.: Anterior pituitary changes following adrenalectomy. Anat. Rec. 1939, *75:* 373–404.

391a. RENOLD, A. E., JENKINS, D., FORSHAM, P. H. AND THORN, G. W.: Intravenous ACTH: A study in quantitative adrenocortical stimulation. J. Clin. Endocrinol. & Metab. 1952, *12:* 763–798.

392. RICHARDSON, C. H.: An Introduction to Statistical Analysis. War Dept. E. M. 327. U. S. Armed Forces Inst., New York, Harcourt, Brace, 1944.

392a. RICHTER, R. B.: True hamartoma of the hypothalamus associated with pubertas praecox. J. Neuropathol. & Exper. Neurol. 1951, *10:* 368–383.

393. RIOCH, D. McK.: Paths of secretion from the hypophysis, in: The Pituitary. Research Publ. A. Nerv. & Ment. Dis., Baltimore, Williams & Wilkins, 1938, vol. 17, pp. 151–175.

394. ROMANO, J. AND ENGEL, G. L.: Delirium 1. Electroencephalographic data. Arch. Neurol. & Psychiat. 1944, *51:* 356–377.

395. ROSE, B.: The effect of cortin and desoxycorticosterone acetate on the ability of the adrenalectomized rat to inactivate histamine. Am. J. Physiol. 1939, *127:* 780–784.

396. ROSE, J. AND WOOLSEY, C. N.: Organization of the mammalian thalamus and its relationships to the cerebral cortex. E. E. G. Clin. Neurophysiol. 1949, *1:* 391–404.

397. ROWE, A. W. AND LAWRENCE, C. H.: Studies of the endocrine glands. II. The pituitary. Endocrinology 1928, *12:* 245–322.

398. ROUSSY, G. AND CLUNET, J.: Les tumeurs du lobe anterieur de l'hypophyse. Essai de classification histologique. Rev. neurol. 1911, *22:* 313–320.

399. —— AND MOSINGER, M.: L'innervation de l'hypophyse: Son importance dans l'interpretation des syndromes dits hypophysaires. Rev. neurol., 1940, *72:* 437–447.

400. RUBINSTEIN, H. S. AND SOLOMON, M. L.: The growth-depressing effect of

large doses of testosterone propionate in the castrate albino rat. Endocrinology 1941, *28:* 112–114.

401. RUSSELL, JANE A.: The relation of the anterior pituitary to carbohydrate metabolism. Physiol. Rev. 1938, *18:* 1–28.

402. ——: The effect of thyroxin on the carbohydrate metabolism of hypophysectomized rats. Am. J. Physiol. 1938, *122:* 547–550.

403. SALTER, W. T.: 1. The chemistry and physiology of thyroid hormone. 2. The control of thyroid activity, in: The Hormones. New York, Academic Press, 1950, vol. 1, pp. 181–351.

404. ——, CORTELL, R. E. AND McKAY, E. A.: Goitrogenic agents and thyroidal iodine: their pharmacodynamic interplay upon thyroid function. J. Pharmacol. & Exper. Therap. 1945, *85:* 310–323.

405. SAMUELS, L. T., REINECKE, R. M. AND BALL, H. A.: Balance studies in hypophysectomized and normal rats fed on equicaloric high carbohydrate and high fat diets. Endocrinology 1942, *31:* 35–41.

406. ——, ——, AND ——: Effect of diet on glucose tolerance and liver and muscle glycogen of hypophysectomized and normal rats. Endocrinology 1942, *31:* 42–45.

407. ——, — AND BAUMAN, K. L.: Growth and metabolism of young hypophysectomized rats fed by stomach tube. Endocrinology 1943, *33:* 87–95.

408. SATTLER, D. G., AND INGRAM, W. R.: Experimental hypertension and the neurohypophysis. Endocrinology 1941, *29:* 952–957.

409. SAXTON, J. A., JR.: The relation of age to the occurrence of adenoma-like lesions in the rat hypophysis and to their growth after transplantation. Cancer Research 1941, *1:* 277–282.

410. SAYERS, G. AND SAYERS, M. A.: The pituitary-adrenal system. Ann. New York Acad. Sc. 1949, *50:* 522–540.

411. SCHÄFER, E. A.: Croonian lecture: The functions of the pituitary body. Proc. Roy. Soc., London, s. B. 1909, *81:* 442–468.

412. ——: An Introduction to the Study of the Endocrine Glands and Internal Secretions. Stanford, Stanford University Press, 1914.

413. SCHAEFFER, J. P.: Some points in the regional anatomy of the optic pathway, with special reference to tumors of the hypophysis cerebri and resulting ocular changes. Anat. Rec. 1924, *28:* 243–280.

414. SCHARRER, E. AND SCHARRER, B.: Secretory cells within the hypothalamus, in: The Hypothalamus. Res. Publ. A. Nerv. & Ment. Dis., Baltimore, Williams & Wilkins, 1940, vol. 20, pp. 170–195.

415. SCHAUR, I. AND ROGOFF, J. M.: The influence of the adrenal glands on calcium metabolism. Science 1936, *83:* 267–268.

416. SCHNITKER, M. T., CUTLER, E. C., BAILER, O. T. AND VAUGHAN, W. W.: The chromophobe adenomas of the pituitary: Pathologic features and response to irradiation based on a study of 81 verified cases. Am. J. Roentgenol. 1938, *40:* 645–659.

417. SCHOCKAERT, J. A. AND FOSTER, G. J.: Influence of the anterior pituitary substances on the total iodine of the thyroid gland in the young duck. J. Biol. Chem. 1932, *95:* 82–94.

418. SEIBERT, W. J. AND SMITH, R. S.: Cited by Albert, A.: The biochemistry of the thyrotropic hormone. Ann. New York Acad. Sc. 1949, *50:* 466–488.

419. SEIDLIN, S. M.: The metabolism of the thyrotrophic and gonadotrophic hormones. Endocrinology 1940, *26:* 696–702.

420. SELYE, H.: On the nervous control of lactation. Am. J. Physiol. 1934, *107:* 535–538.

421. ——: Morphological changes in female mice receiving large doses of testosterone. J. Endocrinol. 1939, *1:* 208–215.

422. ——: Atypical cell proliferation in anterior lobe adenomas of estradiol-(estrogen)-treated rats. Cancer Research 1944, *4:* 349–351.

423. ——: Experimental investigations concerning the role of the pituitary in tumorigenesis. Surgery 1944, *16:* 33–46.

424. ——: Interaction between the adrenocorticotropic hormone (ACTH) and the somatotrophic hormone (STH) in respect to their effects upon the kidney and the cardiovascular apparatus, in: Proceedings of the Second Clinical ACTH Conference. Philadelphia, Blakiston, 1951, vol. 1, pp. 95–108.

425. SEVERINGHAUS, A. E.: Cellular changes in the anterior hypophysis with special reference to its secretory activities. Physiol. Rev. 1937, *17:* 556–588.

426. —— AND THOMPSON, K. W.: Cytological changes induced in the hypophysis by the prolonged administration of pituitary extract. Am. J. Path. 1939, *15:* 391–412.

427. SEVRINGHAUS, E. L.: Dysfunctions of the anterior lobe of the pituitary and their treatment (including use of pituitary preparations). J. A. M. A. 1941, *116:* 221–225.

428. SHANNON, J. A.: Control of renal excretion of water. 1. The effect of variations in the state of hydration on water excretion in dogs with diabetes insipidus. J. Exper. Med. 1942, *76:* 371–387.

429. ——: Control of renal excretion of water. 2. The rate of liberation of the posterior pituitary antidiuretic hormone in the dog. J. Exper. Med. 1942, *76:* 387–401.

430. SHEDLOVSKY, T., ROTHEN, A., GREEP, R. O., VAN DYKE, H. B. AND CHOW, B. F.: The isolation in pure form of the interstitial stimulating (luteinizing) hormone of the anterior lobe of the pituitary gland. Science 1940, *92:* 178–180.

431. SHEEHAN, D.: The hypothalamus and gastrointestinal regulation, in: The Hypothalamus. Research Publ. A. Nerv. & Ment. Dis., Baltimore, Williams & Wilkins, 1940, vol. 20, pp. 589–616.

432. SHEEHAN, H. L.: Simmonds' disease due to postpartum necrosis of the anterior pituitary. Quart. J. Med. 1939, *8:* 277–309.

433. SILBERBERG, M.: Effects of combined administration of extracts of anterior lobe of pituitary and potassium iodide on thyroid gland. Proc. Soc. Exper. Biol. & Med. 1929, *27:* 166–170.

434. SILVERS, S.: Simmonds' disease (cachexia hypophyseopriva): Report of a case with postmortem observations and a review of the literature. Arch Int. Med. 1933, *51:* 175–199.

435. SILVETTE, H.: Chloride, carbohydrate, and water metabolism in adrenal insufficiency and other conditions. Am. J. Physiol. 1934, *108:* 535–544.

436. ——, BRITTON, S. W. AND KLINE, R.: Carbohydrate changes in various animals following potassium administration. Am. J. Physiol. 1938, *122:* 524–529.

437. SIMMONDS, M.: Zur Pathologie der Hypophysis. Verhandl. d. deutsch. path. Gesellsch. 1914, *17:* 208–212.

438. ——: Ueber Hypophysisschwund mit tödlichem Ausgang. Deutsch. med. Wchnschr. 1914, *40:* 322–323.

439. ——: Atrophie des Hypophysisvorderlappens und hypophysäre Kachexie. Deutsche. med. Wchnschr. 1918, *44:* 852–854.

440. SIMPSON, M. E., EVANS, H. M., FRAENKEL-CONRAT, H. L. AND LI, C. H.: Synergism of estrogens with pituitary gonadotropins in hypophysectomized rats. Endocrinology 1941, *28:* 37–41.

441. SIMPSON, S. L.: The Pituitary. Major Endocrine Disorders, ed. 2. London, New York, Toronto, Oxford University Press, 1948, vol. 1.

442. SMITH, P. E.: The effect of hypophysectomy in the early embryo upon the growth and development of the frog. A preliminary report. Anat. Rec. 1916, *11:* 57–64.

443. ——: Hypophysectomy and a replacement therapy in the rat. Am. J. Anat. 1930, *45:* 205–273.

444. ——: The relations of the activity of the pituitary and thyroid glands, in: Harvey Lectures. Baltimore, Williams & Wilkins, 1931, Series 25, pp. 129–143.

445. ——: The non-essentiality of the posterior hypophysis in parturition. Am. J. Physiol. 1932, *99:* 345–348.

446. ——: Effect of equine gonadotropin on testes of hypophysectomized monkeys. Endocrinology 1942, *31:* 1–12.

447. ——, TYNDALE, H. H., DOTTI, L., AND ENGLE, E. T.: Response of normal and hypophysectomized Rhesus monkeys to insulin. Proc. Soc. Exper. Biol. & Med. 1936, *34:* 250–251.

448. SNYDER, F. H. AND TWEEDY, W. R.: Effect of anterior hypophyseal extract upon serum calcium and phosphorus. Proc. Soc. Exper. Biol. & Med. 1941, *47:* 234–236.

449. SOSKIN, S.: Role of the endocrines in the regulation of blood sugar. J. Clin. Endocrinol. 1944, *4:* 75–88.

450. ——, LEVINE, R. AND HELLER, R. E.: The role of the thyroid in carbohydrate disturbances which follow hypophysectomy. Am. J. Physiol 1939, *125:* 220–226.

451. SOULAIRAC, A.: La regulation neuro-endocrinienne de l'absorption intestinale des glucides. Ann. d'Endocrinol. 1947, *8:* 377–393.

452. —— AND DESCLAUX, P.: Modifications hypophysaires après lesions hypothalamiques. Action de la phloridzine. Ann. d'Endocrinol. 1947, *8:* 343–346.

453. SPERRY, W. M., JAILER, J. W. AND ENGLE, E. T.: The influence of diet on the cholesterol concentration of the blood serum in normal, spayed, and hypothyroid monkeys. Endocrinology 1944, *35:* 38–48.

454. SPIEGEL, E. A. AND SOMMER, I.: Neurology of the Eye, Ear, Nose, and Throat. New York, Grune & Stratton, 1944, pp. 3–363.

455. STADIE, W. C. AND HAUGGARD, N.: The hexokinase reaction in tissue extracts from normal and diabetic rats. J. Biol. Chem. 1949, *177:* 311–324.

456. STARR, P. AND DAVIS, L.: Endocrine studies of patients after subtotal hypophysectomy. Ann. Surg. 1941, *113:* 778–790.

456a. STEHLE, R. L.: The physiological action of the hormones of the posterior lobe of the pituitary gland, in: Vitamins and Hormones. New York, The Academic Press, 1950, vol. 8, pp. 215–254.

457. STEIN, K. F. AND LISLE, M.: The gonad-stimulating potency of the pituitary of hypothyroid young male rats. Endocrinology 1942, *30:* 16–24.

458. STEPHENS, D. J.: Hypopituitarism. Internat. Clin. 1939, *1:* 97–109.

459. ———: Chloride excretion in hypopituitarism with reference to adrenocortical function. Am. J. M. Sc. 1940, *199:* 67-75.

460. STEVENSON, J. A. F.: Effects of hypothalamic lesions in water and energy metabolism in the rat, in: Recent Progress in Hormone Research. New York, Academic Press, 1949, vol. 4, pp. 363–394.

461. SUNDERLAND, S. E.: The meningeal relations of the human hypophysis cerebri. J. Anat. 1945, *79:* 33–38.

462. SWANN, H. G.: Sodium chloride and diabetes insipidus. Am. J. Physiol. 1939, *126:* 341–346.

463. ———: The pituitary—adrenocortical relationship. Physiol. Rev. 1940, *20:* 493–521.

464. SWINGLE, W. W., PARKINS, W. M. AND TAYLOR, A. R.: Revival from insufficiency and maintenance of adrenalectomized dogs with low serum sodium and chloride levels. Proc. Soc. Exper. Biol. & Med. 1936, *34:* 75–77.

465. ———, — AND —: Experiments on intact and adrenalectomized dogs subjected to sodium and chloride depletion by intraperitoneal injections of glucose. Am. J. Physiol. 1936, *116:* 430–437.

466. ———, —, — AND HAYS, H. W.: The relation of serum sodium and chloride levels to alterations of body water in the intact and adrenalectomized dog, and the influence of adrenal cortical hormone on fluid distribution. Am. J. Physiol. 1936, *116:* 438–445.

467. ———, —, — AND —: A study of the circulatory failure of adrenal insufficiency and analogous shock-like conditions. Am. J. Physiol. 1938, *123:* 659.

468. ———, PFIFFNER, J. J., VARS, H. M., BOTT, P. A. AND PARKINS, W. M.: The function of the adrenal cortical hormone and the cause of death from adrenal insufficiency. Science 1933, *77:* 58–64.

469. ———, —, — AND PARKINS, W. M.: The effect of hemorrhage on the normal and adrenalectomized dog. Am. J. Physiol. 1934, *107:* 259–274.

470. SZÁNTÓ, J.: Pluriglanduläre Veränderungen bei Hypophysentumoren. Deutsch. med. Wchnschr. 1926, *52:* 103–105.

471. TALBOT, W. B. AND BUTLER, A. M.: Urinary 17-ketosteroid assays in clinical medicine. J. Clin. Endocrinol. 1942, *2:* 724–727.

472. TALBOTT, J. H., PECORA, L. J., MELVILLE, R. S. AND CONSOLAZIO, W. V.:

Renal function in patients with Addison's disease and in patients with adrenal insufficiency secondary to pituitary pan-hypofunction. J. Clin. Investigation 1942, *21:* 107–119.

473. TEPPERMAN, J., BROBECK, J. R. AND LONG, C. N. H.: The effect of hypothalamic hyperphagia and of alterations in feeding habits on the metabolism of the albino rat. Yale J. Biol. & Med. 1943, *15:* 855–875.

474. THOMPSON, K. W. AND LONG, C. N. H.: The effect of hypophysectomy upon hypercholesteremia of dogs. Endocrinology 1941, *28:* 715–722.

475. THOREK, P.: Vagus section in the treatment of peptic ulcers. J. A. M. A. 1947, *135:* 1141–1145.

475a. THORN, G. W.: The diagnosis and treatment of adrenal insufficiency, in: American Lectures in Endocrinology, Thompson, W. O., editor. Springfield, Charles C Thomas, 1949.

476. —— AND CLINTON, M., JR.: Metabolic changes in a patient with Addison's disease following the onset of diabetes mellitus. J. Clin. Endocrinol. 1943, *3:* 335–345.

477. —— AND EISENBERG, H.: Studies on desoxycorticosterone, a synthetic adrenal cortical hormone. Endocrinology 1939, *25:* 39–46.

478. —— AND ENGEL, L. L.: The effect of sex hormones on the renal excretion of electrolytes. J. Exper. Med. 1938, *68:* 299–312.

479. ——, — AND EISENBERG, H.: The effects of corticosterone and related compounds on the renal excretion of electrolytes. J. Exper. Med. 1938, *68:* 161–171.

480. TILNEY, F.: Contribution to the study of the hypophysis cerebri with especial reference to its comparative histology, in: Memoirs of Wistar Institute of Anatomy and Biology. Baltimore, Williams & Wilkins, 1911, vol. 2, p. 92.

481. ——: The morphology of the diencephalic floor—a contribution to the study of craniate homology. J. Comp. Neurol. 1915, *25:* 213–282.

482. ——: The development and constituents of the human hypophysis. Bull. Neurol. Inst. New York 1936, *5:* 387–437.

483. TÖRNBLOM, N.: On the functional relationship between the pituitary gland and the parathyroids. Acta Endocrinologica supp. 4, 1949, 5–76.

484. TRAQUAIR, H. M.: The field of vision and the anatomy of the visual neural path. Edinburgh M. J. 1939, *46:* 83–94.

485. TROLAND, C. E. AND BROWN, C. A.: Precocious puberty of intracranial origin. J. Neurosurg. 1948, *5:* 541–556.

486. TRUETA, J. R.: Studies of the Renal Circulation. Oxford, Blackwell, 1947, p. 187.

487. UOTILA, U. U.: Role of the pituitary stalk in regulation of thyrotropic and thyroid activity. Proc. Soc. Exper. Biol. & Med. 1939, *41:* 106–108.

488. ——: Hypothalamic control of anterior pituitary function, in: The Hypothalamus. Research Publ. A. Nerv. & Ment Dis., 1940, vol. 20, pp. 580–589.

489. VAN DYKE, H. B., CHOW, B. F., GREEP, R. O. AND ROTHEN, A.: The isolation of a protein from the pars neuralis of the ox pituitary with constant oxytocic, pressor, and diuresis inhibiting activities. J. Pharmacol. & Exper. Therap. 1942, *74:* 190–207.

490. VARNEY, R. F., KENYON, A. T. AND KOCH, F. C.: Association of short stature, retarded sexual development and high urinary gonadotropin titers in women; ovarian dwarfism. J. Clin. Endocrinol. 1942, *2:* 137–145.

491. VENNING, E. H. AND BROWNE, J. S. L.: Studies on corpus luteum func· tion. 1. The urinary excretion of sodium pregnanediol glucuronidate in the human menstrual cycle. Endocrinology 1937, *21:* 711–721.

492. VERNEY, E. B.: The antidiuretic hormone and the factors which determine its release. Proc. Roy. Soc., London, s. B. 1947, *135:* 25–106.

493. VOLLMER, E. P. AND GORDON, A. S.: Effect of sex and gonadotrophic hormones on the blood picture of the rat. Endocrinology 1941, *29:* 828–837.

494. WADDINGTON, C. H.: Organisers and Genes. Cambridge Biol. Studies. Cambridge, Cambridge University Press, 1940, p. 159.

495. WAGENER, H. P., WOLTMAN, H. W. AND LOVE, J. G.: Pituitary tumor associated with choked disks and normal peripheral fields of vision. Report of a case. Proc. Staff Meet. Mayo Clin. 1939, *14:* 417–419.

496. WAGNER, H. P.: Visual hallucinations. Am. J. M. Sc. 1948, *215:* 226–232.

497. WALTER, W. G. AND DOVEY, V. J.: Electroencephalography in cases of subcortical tumors. J. Neurol., Neurosurg., & Psychiat. 1944, *7:* 57–65.

498. WARING, H. AND LANDGREBE, F. W.: Hormones of the posterior pituitary, in: The Hormones. New York, Academic Press, 1950, vol. 2, p. 431.

498a. WATERHOUSE, C., KEUTMANN, E. H. AND FENNINGER, L. D.: Studies of electrolyte metabolism in 2 patients with pituitary insufficiency. J. Clin. Endocrinol. & Metab. 1952, *12:* 798–820.

499. WATSON, B. A.: An analysis of 583 glucose tolerance tests. Endocrinology 1939, *25:* 845–852.

500. WATTS, J. W. AND FULTON, J. F.: Intussusception. The relation of the cerebral cortex to intestinal motility in the monkey. New England J. Med. 1934, *210:* 883–896.

501. WEAVER, T. A., AND BUCY, P. C.: The anatomical relationships of the hypophyseal stem and the median eminence. Endocrinology 1940, *27:* 227–235.

502. WEIL, A. AND HETHERINGTON, A. W.: Experimental tumor of the hypophysis of the white rat. J. Mt. Sinai Hosp. 1942, *9:* 842–849.

503. —— AND ZONDEK, B.: The histopathology of the pituitary of the white rat injected with follicular hormone. Endocrinology 1939, *25:* 114–122.

504. WEINBERGER, L. M., ADLER, F. H. AND GRANT, F. C.: Primary pituitary adenoma and the syndrome of the cavernous sinus: a clinical anatomic study. Arch. Ophthalmol. 1940, *24:* 1197–1237.

505. —— AND GRANT, F. C.: Visual hallucinations and their neuroptical correlates. Arch. Ophthalmol. 1940, *23:* 166–199.

506. —— AND —: Precocious puberty and tumors of the hypothalamus. Arch. Int. Med. 1941, *67:* 762–793.

507. WERNER, S. C.: The thyrotropic hormone and the antihormone problem. Endocrinology 1938, *22:* 291–300.

508. ——: A quantitative study of urinary excretion of hypophyseal gonadotropin, estrogen, and androgen of normal women. J. Clin. Investigation 1941, *20:* 21–30.

509. ——,QUIMBY, E. H. AND SCHMIDT, C.: The clinical use of radioactive iodine. Bull. New York Acad. Med. 1948, *24:* 549–560.

510. WESTMAN, A. AND JACOBSOHN, D.: Endokrinologische Untersuchungen an Ratten mit durchtrenntem Hypophysenstiel. Acta path. et microbiol. Scandinav. 1938, *15:* 301–306.

511. WHEATLEY, M. D.: The hypothalamus and affective behavior in cats. Arch. Neurol & Psychiat. 1944, *52:* 296–317.

511a. WHITE, A.: Chemistry and physiology of adenohypophyseal luteotropin, in: Vitamins and Hormones. New York, Academic Press, 1949, vol. 7, pp. 254–288.

512. —— AND DOUGHERTY, T. F.: The role of the lymphocytes in normal and immune globulin production and the mode of release of globulin from lymphocytes. Ann. New York Acad. Sc. 1946, *46:* 859–882.

513. WHITE, J. C. AND WARREN, S.: Unusual size and extension of a pituitary adenoma. J. Neurosurg. 1935, *2:* 126–139.

514. WHITE, H. L., HEINBECKER, P. AND ROLF, D.: Effects of hypophysectomy on some renal functions. Proc. Soc. Exper. Biol. & Med. 1941, *46:* 44–47.

515. ——, — AND —: Effects of the removal of the anterior lobe of the hypophysis on some renal functions. Am. J. Physiol. 1942, *136:* 584–591.

516. WILBRAND AND SAENGER: Cited in Traquair, H. M.: An Introduction to Clinical Perimetry, St. Louis, C. V. Mosby, 1944, p. 274.

517. WILLIAMS, R. H. AND WHITTENBERGER, J. L.: Treatment of Simmonds' disease. J. Clin. Endocrinol. 1942, *2:* 539–550.

518. ——, —, BISSELL, G. W. AND WEINGLASS, A. R.: Treatment (with special reference to androgens) of adrenal insufficiency (in Simmonds' disease). J. Clin. Endocrinol. 1945, *5:* 163–180.

519. WIMMER, A.: Chronic Epidemic Encephalitis. London, W. Heinemann, 1924, p. 335.

520. WINTER, C. A., INGRAM, W. R. AND GROSS, E. G.: Effects of pitressin injections on serum electrolytes and water exchange of cats with diabetes insipidus and adrenal insufficiency. Am. J. Physiol. 1939, *127:* 64–70.

521. WISLOCKI, G. B.: The meningeal relations of the hypophysis cerebri. 1. Relations in adult mammals. Anat. Rec. 1937, *67:* 273–295.

522. ——: The vascular supply of the hypophysis cerebri of the cat. Anat. Rec. 1937, *69:* 361–387.

523. ——: The vascular supply of the hypophysis cerebri of the Rhesus monkey and man, in: The Pituitary Gland. Research Publ. A. Nerv. & Ment. Dis., Baltimore, Williams & Wilkins 1938, vol. 17, pp. 48–69.

524. WOLFE, J. M.: Effects of testosterone propionate on the structure of the anterior pituitaries of old male rats. Endocrinology 1941, *29:* 969–974.

525. ——: The effects of advancing age on the structure of the anterior hypophysis and ovaries of female rats. Am. J. Anat. 1943, *72:* 361–383.

526. ——, BRYAN, W. R. AND WRIGHT, A. W.: Histologic observations on the anterior pituitaries of old rats with particular reference to the spontaneous appearance of pituitary adenomata. Am. J. Cancer 1938, *34:* 352–372.

527. WOLFF, H. G.: Headache and Other Head Pain. New York, Oxford University Press, 1948, p. 642.

528. WORTIS, H. AND MAURER, W. S.: Sham rage in man. Am. J. Psychiat. 1942, *98:* 638–644.
529. WYMAN, L. C. AND TUM SUDEN, C.: Studies on suprarenal insufficiency: VIII: The blood volume of the rat in suprarenal insufficiency, anaphylactic shock, and histamine shock. Am. J. Physiol. 1930, *94:* 579–585.
530. —— AND —: Studies on suprarenal insufficiency: IX: Vascular responses to histamine in normal and in suprarenalectomized rats. Am. J. Physiol. 1932, *99:* 285–297.
531. YOUNG, F. G.: Permanent experimental diabetes produced by pituitary (anterior lobe) injections. Lancet 1937, *2:* 372–374.
531a. YOUNGHUSBAND, O. Z., HORRAX, G., HURXTHAL, L. M., HARE, H. F. AND POPPEN, J. L.: Chromophobe pituitary tumors. II. Treatment. J. Clin. Endocrinol. & Metab. 1952, *12:* 611–630.
532. ZACHARIAS, L. R.: Further studies of the vidian ganglion as a source of innervation of the anterior lobe of the hypophysis. Endocrinology 1942, *31:* 638–643.
533. ZONDEK, H.: Die Krankheiten der Endokrinen Drüsen. Berlin, J. Springer, 1923.

INDEX

Numbers appearing in italics refer to illustration pages.